Veterinary Toxicology

Veterinary Toxicology

Radhey Mohan Tiwari
Malini Sinha

Oxford Book Company
Jaipur ▪ New Delhi

Published By

Oxford Book Company

Regd. Off. "Bony Residency", Gate No. 2
Opp. Tilak Public School, Vishweswariya Nagar,
Gopalpura Road, Jaipur - 302018, India
Ph: 0141 - 2761280, Telefax: 2761381
email - oxfordbookjpr@gmail.com
website - oxfordbookcompany.com

Delhi Office: 102, 1st Floor, Satyam House,
4327/3, Ansari Road, Darya Ganj,
New Delhi - 110002, India
Ph: 011-45652440

Distributed by
KEYA INTERNATIONAL PRESS LLP
E-mail: keyainternationalpressllp@gmail.com

Published in India, 2025

ISBN : 9789380179285

Typeset by Shivangi Computers, Jaipur

Printed and bound in India by Replika Press Pvt. Ltd.

Preface

A vast number of substances potentially toxic to animals exist, including pesticides, household cleaning products, agricultural chemicals, automotive products, human prescription and non-prescription drugs, herbal remedies, and poisonous plants and animals. With such huge numbers of potential toxins, it is impossible for veterinarians to be knowledgeable about all of them. But because some poisonings can cause illness or even death within only minutes to hours after exposure, immediate access to reliable information on diagnosis and treatment is essential. Often intoxications involve new drugs or chemical products for which very little or no published veterinary toxicity data is available.

The present book is a unique single reference that teaches the basic principles of veterinary toxicology to any student at the graduate and postgraduage level and will continue to serve as a clinical reference for practising veterinary toxicologists, poison control centres, marine biologists, environmentalists, and animal scientists. While most comparable texts are primarily directed toward the field of human toxicology, this is the one text needed to thoroughly prepare future veterinarians on the newest approaches for diagnosing poisoning cases in all animals from chemicals and plants of a diverse nature as a result of inadvertent, accidental, or malicious intents. Many chapters are provided on topics not covered in any previous books such as target organ toxicity, radiation and radioactive materials, and ethics in veterinary toxicology.

The strengths of this book comprise the inclusion of large and small animal species; the broad range of topics encompassing regulatory, diagnostic, pathologic, and clinical toxicology; and the affordable cost. It will be a useful source of information for the veterinary clinician, student, toxicologist, and a nice addition to any veterinarian's library. This book can be considered a cornerstone upon which a deeper understanding of the issues and individual toxicants in veterinary toxicology can be based. The topics covered are of interest to not only toxicologists and researchers, but also to clinicians who do not have an extensive background in toxicology.

Radhey Mohan Tiwari
Malini Sinha

Contents

1

Introduction to Toxicology

Toxicology is a science of poisons. Fogleman refers to toxicology as a "many splendored thing." Although its spendour may not be obvious to the physician dealing with a hopeless case of heroin addiction or to the veterinarian faced with an outbreak of malicious poisoning in domestic pets, the many facets of toxicology are beyond dispute. It has frontiers with pharmacology, physiology and pathology; with chemistry, biochemistry and biology; with agriculture, industry and economics; with forensic science and clinical medicine; with ecology, with pollution, and hence with the whole future of life on this planet. To understand it properly calls for a knowledge of all these subjects, a breadth of learning impossible of achievement. Hence the discipline is usually divided into several branches such as clinical toxicology, chemical toxicology, forensic toxicology, industrial toxicology and veterinary toxicology.

Mathieu Orfila is considered to be the modern father of toxicology, having given the subject its first formal treatment in 1813 in his *Traité des poisons*, also called *Toxicologie générale*. Theophrastus Phillipus Auroleus Bombastus von Hohenheim (1493–1541) (also referred to as Paracelsus, from his belief that his studies were above or beyond the work of Celsus—a Roman physician from the first century) is also considered "the father" of toxicology. He is credited with the classic toxicology maxim, "Alle Dinge sind Gift und nichts ist ohne Gift; allein die Dosis macht, dass ein Ding kein Gift ist." which translates as, "All things are poison and nothing is without poison; only the dose makes a thing not a poison." This is often condensed to: "The dose makes the poison".

In the last century, our society has become chemically oriented. Along with benefits, problems related to health hazards have arisen. Toxicology, a science that deals with the harmful effects of chemical substances on biological mechanisms, is attempting to study these problems scientifically and to find practical solutions. The research techniques of toxicology are those of classical medical sciences: biochemistry, pharmacology, pathology, etc. Modern toxicology is a multidisciplinary field and borrows freely, in addition to the aforementioned areas, from veterinary sciences, environmental sciences and several others. No matter which has provided his major basic training, a toxicologist should always be interested in the dynamic aspects of chemico-biological interactions. On the occasion, he will also have some interest in their forensic implications.

Veterinary toxicology faces problems related to the general increase in the use of chemicals and especially to their increased use in livestock husbandry and agriculture. Since these two industries supply mankind with much of what he eats, careful considerations must be given to the possible effects on the human population of the use of chemicals on animals and crops. Toxicologists must bear in mind possible public health hazards when evaluating the toxicity of chemical agents. Veterinary toxicologists are also involved in the evaluation of the toxic effects of chemicals, which are primarily intended for use in or on humans, since these compounds must be evaluated in animal system prior to their limited or widespread use in man.

The principles of the preclinical evaluation of the safety of new compounds for their proposed use in veterinary medicine and in human medicine remain the same. Thus, it is quite evident that veterinary toxicology and human toxicology are so closely interrelated that they are indeed inseparable.

DEFINITION OF A POISON

It is difficult to arrive at a completely satisfactory definition of a poison. A poison may be defined as any substance or matter (solid, liquid, or gaseous) which, when applied to the body outwardly, or in any way introduced into it in a very small dose, can destroy life by its own inherent qualities, without acting mechanically, and irrespective of temperature.

It is doubtful if anymore modern definition describes it better, because a poison is almost impossible to define, and any attempt to do so is a exercise in semantics rather than in toxicology. Whether or not a substance is poisonous depends on the quantity taken, the species to which it is given, and the route by which it enters the body.

A small intake of vitamin A is essential to prevent night blindness, but excess may lead to serious gastrointestinal disorders, as arctic explorers who have eaten polar bear liver have found to their cost. To the layman, sugar and salt are the epitome of the non-toxic, but cattle have been poisoned by sugar, and salt poisoning in pigs is well known. Cobra venom may be drunk with impurity, but isl ethal if administered parenterally. It would be difficult to find a definition adequately to cover retinal, sucrose, sodium chloride and cobra toxin.

TOXICITY

There are different types of toxicity:

1. *Acute toxicity*: Effect or response that chemical produces when given to an animal in a single dose. It is measured by the median lethal dose, or LD50. This is the dose that will kill 50% of a group of animals under stated conditions.
2. *LC50*: It is another way of exposing a species to a series of concentrations and recording mortality at those concentrations. Here, we measure the concentration at which 50% of the entire population is killed.
3. *LT50*: Here the animals are exposed to one dose and the time at which 50% of the population is killed is recorded.
4. *Chronic toxicity*: Type of toxicity that produces functional and/or anatomical changes in animals with repeated exposure or dosing. The response is measured for a smaller dose over a prolonged period of time, usually lasting 2 years for rodents such as rats.
5. *Subacute or subchronic toxicity*: Similar to chronic toxicity, but the duration lasts for 3 months or less.

Dose-response Relationships

Frequency response: There are two of the more common methods of predicting responses to dosages by observation of large number of animals. If an adequate dose is given to a very large number of animals and fixed single effect (e.g., convulsions seizures) is measured, a variety of differences will be observed.

The data obtained from such an experiment may be plotted in the form of a distribution or frequency-response curve that includes percent responding on its ordinate and dosage levels on its abscissa. Such a curve follows the laws represented by the normal Gaussian distribution pattern and permits the use of statistical procedure applicable to such curves. But, these curves are not particularly useful or determining LD50 values.

Cumulative response: It is generally more useful to plot cumulative response (such as death) against dosage. These curves are commonly known as dose-response curves. Such plot can be developed for only a single response, for example, death. From this plot, one can draw a horizontal line across from the 50% death mark to an intersection with the curve, then a vertical line to the dosage scale. The dosage indicated will be the LD50.

One of the criteria that maybe used to determine relative toxicities of the two compounds is LD50, or equal effect. It is common practice to use the term "potent" for a chemical if the lethal dose is small i.e.a few milligrams.

Several guidelines have been developed as aids in classifying the relative toxicities of compounds. The following table shows one such classification.

Table 1. Toxicity Ratings

Rating Class	Oral LD50 in rats mg/kg	Probable lethal dose in man	Example
6 Super toxic	less than 5	5 drops	Strychnine
5 Extremely toxic	5-50	1 teaspoon	Parathion
4 Very toxic	50-500	1 ounce	Phenobarbital
3 Moderately toxic	500-5000	1 lb (or 1 pt)	Ethanol
2 Slightly toxic	50000-15000	1 quart	Ethanol
1 Practically Nontoxic	over 15000	over 1 quart	Linseed oil

Margin of Safety

The LD50 value is usually based on the effects of a single oral exposure with the rats observed for several days after the chemical administered. The slope of a dose-response curve is an indicator of the range of dosage levels that will elicit a desired effect. If the range is wider the slope will be flatter; if the dosage range is smaller the curve will be steep. The slope of the dose-response curve is therefore an index of the margin of safety of a compound. Thus, the margin of safety is the magnitude of the range of doses involved in progressing from a non-effective dose to a lethal dose.

Any LD50 is a calculated value which represents the best estimation of the dose required to produce death in 50% of the animals and the error of the value can be estimated statistically since the curves follow the laws of normal Gaussian distribution. LD50 is obtained graphically. Other values such as LD95 or LD5 may be obtained in the same manner. If LD84 (lethal dose for 84% of the animals) represents + 1 S.D. from the LD50, then the LD16 represents -1 S.D. from the LD50. The percent mortality may be converted to probits, which are numbers assigned to percentage so that 50% mortality equals a probit of 5, 50% mortality +2 S.D.equals a probit of 7 or, 3 etc. If we plot cumulative % response vs log dose, we get a sigmoid curve. If the cumulative % response units are converted to probits and plotted against log dose we get a straight line. Thus probits are useful to convert a sigmoid to a straight line plot.

Safety Testing

It involves assessment of the safety and toxicity of new drugs for human and veterinary use, new agricultural chemicals, new feed additives, and a wide variety of industrial chemicals. It is done prior to release of a new product. Testing costs millions of dollars per chemical.

Toxicologic tests conducted to determine safety of a new product include:

1. *General Tests*—Acute, subacute and chronic toxicity
2. *Special Tests*—Specific effects on reproduction; fertility; potentiation; teratogenicity; carcinogenicity; mutagenicity; skin, eye, muscle, subcutaneous or intramammary irritation; hemolysis; and behavior.

In general, rats and dogs are the most commonly used animal species. Other animals used include mice, rabbits, guinea pigs, hamsters, and gerbils. Primates are frequently used. The compound should be chemically as pure as possible. If vehicle is used, it should be inert. The most common route of exposure for general testing is oral.

CLASSIFICATION OF POISONS

The graduate veterinarian's ability to serve his clientele is no better than his ability to accurately differentiate between the various possible causes of the illnesses presented to him. It should be noted that mere memorization of clinical signs is not the only way to recall a certain toxicological problem. Perhaps, a better method of recognition is to classify the common toxicoses according to their specific lesions. Since there are many plants, feed additives, insecticides, herbicides, fungicides, and heavy metals that may fall under a specific lesion, each lesion could be subdivided and indexed to help with differential diagnosis. The following classification based on toxic effects of poisons is far from complete, but it may act as a starting point for future indices of diagnostic classifications.

Gastrointestinal Syndrome

This is seen in poisoning from oak, acute copper, E.coli, Salmonella, carbamate fungicides, ANTU, acute crotalaria, paraquat herbicides, thallium, bracken fern, warfarin, etc. The important clinical signs include: bloody diarrhea, hematuria, enteritis, sometimes GI irritation. Death may occur within one to a few days. In case of wild indigo, staphylococcus, peptides and amides, and borates deaths seldom occur. Severe gastrointestinal syndrome is caused by pokeweed, sneezweed, inorganic arsenic herbicides. Death may occur within 1-2 days with bloody diarrhea, hemolytic crisis (pokeweed), and excess salivation (sneezweed).

Neuromuscular (paresis) Effects

Some poisons causing these effects act rapidly, some act slowly. Oleander, buttercup, buckeye, lead (in poultry)act rapidly causing death in 1-2 days. Others include: death comas, poison hemlock, organophosphates. All the above cause in coordination plus GI syndrome where as jimsonweed, 2, 4-D, organic tin, ticks cause only in coordination. Other examples of toxicants causing CNS effects include botulism, horse tail, bracken fern (in horses), pigweed, etc.

Bone-Teeth-Hoof-Hair Deformities

Ergot—sloughing of tips of tail, ears, teats, etc.

Fluoride—bone and teeth lesions

Selenium (chronic), poisonvetch, copper deficiency, chronic thallium, lead nitrate, chlorinated naphthalene, are all associated with hair problem.

Kidney Lesions

Depending on the types of renal damage caused by toxicants kidney lesions are categorized as follows:

a. *Hematuria*: This may be accompanied by fever as in the case of bracken fern or there may be no fever as seen in poisoning from oak, cassia, inorganic mercury or cadmium.

b. *Hemoglobinuria*: This is caused by crucifers (mustard) with photosensitization. Similar condition is seen in chronic copper toxicity.

c. *Oxalates*: These are formed in poisoning from amaranthus (which also causes perirenal edema), halogeton, black greasewood, rhubarb, and ethylene glycol.

d. *Perirenal Edema*: Amaranthus and oak (with as cites); nightshade (no as cites).

e. *Degenerative Changes in Kidneys*: These can be caused by chronic organic mercury compounds, chronic thallium, sulfonamides and so forth.

Liver Lesions

These are caused by several toxicants such as selenium (acute,) aflatoxins, crotalaria, tannic acid, carbon tetrachloride, phenothiazines, gossypol, tarweed, etc.

Photosensitization

Phenolic fungicides (necrosis of contact tissue); vehicles for insecticides; blue-green algae (death within 1-2 days); crucifers (with hemoglobinuria), snow-on-the-mountain (without hemoglobinuria); phenothiazines, alfalfa; St. Johnswort, horse brush.

Hemorrhagic Syndrome

Bracken fern (with fever); those that do not have fevers include: sweet clover, warfarin, pindone, radiation, mycotoxins, crotalaria.

Fevers

Castorbean, oleander, have rapidly acting toxic materials and death may occur within 1-2 days. On the other hand, milkweed, bracken fern, buckeye, locust, etc. are known to be slow-acting.

Abortions and/or Anomalies

Fusarium fungal metabolities, poisonvetch, lupine, broomweed, ergot, 2, 4, 5-T, nitrates. The following cause birth defects: chronic selenium, veratrum, oak, locoweed, jimsonweed, hem-lock, lead, and mercury.

The classification of poisons made in the previous section is based on the organ or system that is the 'target' site for the effect of the toxic chemical. Such classification that is based on the toxic effects of poisons on the body may be unsatisfactory because the same substance can have different effects on different organs of the body. It can also vary in its action between one species and another. Therefore a relatively simple classification can be made on the basis of the structural features of the toxic chemicals that are responsible for their toxic properties and their affinity for 'target' sites in the animal body. Various diverse chemical compounds can be thus divided into two groups, namely, inorganic and organic compounds.

Inorganic compounds include metals, metalloids, their salts and acids and alkalis. Organic compounds on the other hand include all carbon compounds other than carbonates, and the metallic carbides and cyanides. Furthermore, an analytical toxicologist endeavours to separate poisons into characteristic groups and several classifications can be made according to the analytical procedures involved. A typical subdivision is: (1) volatile poisons, (2) metallic poisons, (3) toxic anions, (4) non-volatile organic poisons isolated by solvent extractions, (5) miscellaneous poisons. Finally, poisons may often be classified conveniently by their origin (plant poisons) or use (pesticides).

TYPES OF POISONING

It has been customary to subdivide poisoning into acute, a sudden violent syndrome caused by a single large dose of poison and chronic, a persistent, lingering condition brought on by small repeated doses, with subacute poisoning somewhere in between. This subdivision, however, is not really tenable, as there are types of poisoning which would be difficult to fit into any of these categories. 'Chronic'copper poisoning in sheep only becomes manifesting an acute hemolytic crisis. Symptoms of bracken poisoning may not appear until months after the plant has been ingested. In addition to these types of poisoning, there are other unto-ward effects due to 'poisonous' substances.

(1) Allergy, an immunological response due to sensitization of the subject by a previous dose, although less common in animals than in man, is still quite well known.

(2) Carcinogenicity, in which the agent is responsible for the formation of neoplasia, bracken and the cycads are examples;

(3) Teratogenicity, in which material ingested by the mother at some definite stage in pregnancy produces abnormalities in the off-spring. The classical example in veterinary toxicology is the cyclopean malformation in lambs due to Veratrum californicum.

METABOLISM OF TOXICANTS

Absorption

In order to exert their toxic effects most poisons must be absorbed into the blood stream. Under natural conditions toxicants may enter the body through the lungs, gut and skin. Substances may be injected into the body subcutaneously, intramuscularly, intravenously and intraperitoneally.

1. *Respiratory tract*: The very extensive highly vascular pulmonary mucous membrane affords an excellent channel of absorption for gases and for solids and liquids, particularly when in a fine state of dispersal (as aerosols or dusts).
2. *Alimentary tract*: It is the most usual route of entry of a poison. In all species, much absorption occurs in the small intestine; in the dog it can also take place from the stomach, in the ruminant from the rumen and reticulum, and in all species, especially in non-ruminant herbivora, from the large gut. The contents of the alimentary tract can modify the action of poison. The hydrochloric acid present in gastric juice may aid the solution of originally insoluble materials. A full stomach or rumen may delay symptoms of poisoning or may dilute the poison to such an extent that it is relatively harmless.
3. *Dermal exposure*: The unbroken skin does not offer a favorable channel of absorption to most compounds. Nicotine is one of the exceptions which in aqueous solutions,

is very efficiently absorbed through intact skin. Absorption takes place more readily from oily solutions or emulsions.

Absorption through damaged or abraded skin or a wound occurs as through moist mucous membranes. Subcutaneous or intramuscular injection is equally effective, while intravenous administration is the fastest way of introducing a poison into the blood stream.

Distribution and Accumulation

Hepatic storage: All foreign compounds entering the body pass to the liver which is the major detoxifying organ in the body and by virtue of this fact many poisons accumulate in this organ. It is therefore not unexpected to find hepatic lesions as a consequence of exposure to many toxicants.

Extra hepatic storage: Some poisons are selectively deposited in certain organs or tissues. Iodine is largely taken up by the thyroid glands; strontium, fluorine and lead are deposited in the bones. A knowledge of the distribution of a particular poison is of great help in the selection of organs for chemical analysis.

Biotransformation and Detoxication

Many foreign compounds that are introduced into the body undergo chemical transformation, and this process is generally referred to as metabolic transformation or biotransformation.Very frequently this process is referred to as the detoxication mechanism. However, this term is misleading because the metabolic transformation of a foreign compound may result into increased or decreased toxicity of the product. Two categories of enzyme systems are known to exist in mammals that cause chemical transformation of foreign compounds.

One category consists of enzymes that normally occur in the tissues and are responsible for transformation of normal endogenous substances in tissues as well as foreign chemical e.g., alcohol dehydrogenase. Second category consists of an enzymes system that is very important in toxicology. These are known as drug metabolizing enzymes, which are present in many tissues but are particularly in liver cells. These enzymes are located in small particles called microsomes which in turn are located in the smooth surface of endoplasmic reticulum. These microsomal enzymes are capable of catalyzing a variety of biotransformation reactions, the major ones being oxidation, reduction, and hydrolysis.

The drug metabolizing enzymes system is also called as mixed function oxidase (MFO) enzyme system for the obvious reason that is capable of catalyzing various types of reactions. The oxidase system requires the presence of a cofactor NADPH, and molecular oxygen for its activity. NADPH reduces a component of the microsomes which reacts with molecular oxygen to form an active oxygen intermediate which oxidizes the drug or the foreign chemical. The components of microsomes which is reduced by NADPH is a heme protein called cytochrome P-450.

R.T. Williams divided the biotransformation mechanism of foreign chemicals into two major types:

(1) the non synthetic reactions involving oxidation, reduction and hydrolysis, and

(2) the synthetic or conjugations involving production of a product that is biosynthesized from the chemical (or its metabolite) plus an endogenous metabolite such as glycine.

If we call the non synthetic reactions as phase 1 of biotransformation mechanism, then conjugation reactions will be phase II, which are described below.

- *Conjugation Reactions*: These are reactions in which a poisoner ametabolite is combined with some compound provided by the animal body. Following is the list of some of these processes.
- *Glycine Conjugations*: Benzoic acid combines with glycine to form hippuric acid.
- *Glucuronic Acid*: Conjugation with this occurs in may cases. e.g., dinitrophenol, chloral hydrate.
- *Sulfate Conjugation*: Some phenols conjugate with $=SO_4$ to form ethereal sulfates.
- *Cysteine Conjugation*: Arsenic trioxide and mainly benzene, polycyclic hydrocarbons, and certain halogenated hydrocarbons conjugate with cysteine to form mercapturic acids.
- *Acetylation Reactions*: This takes place between CoASH and amino groups of aromatic compounds, e.g., sulfanilamide derivatives. Dog is deficient to acetylate aromatic amine groups.
- *Methylation Reactions*: It is relatively uncommon form of detoxication and is confined to the heterocyclic nitrogen atoms in compound of the pyridine and quinoline type.
- *Thiocyanate Formations*: Inorganic cyanides are converted by the enzymerhodanese to thiocyanate. It is a true detoxication, for sodium thiocyanate is nearly 200 times less toxic than sodium cyanide and is slowly excreted in the urine.
- *Glutamine and Ornithine Conjugation*: Conjugation processes with glutamine and ornithine occur in man and bird, respectively.

Inhibition of Biotransformation Mechanisms

The microsomal enzyme systems can be inhibited by several compounds in concentrations which by themselves have little pharmacologic activity. The most common example of such inhibitor is SKF 525A (diethyl aminoethanol ester of diphenyl propyl acetic acid). Thus, the inhibition of the microsomal enzyme system would result into the inhibition of the metabolism of toxic foreign compound, the presence of which may cause increased toxicity. On the other hand, when the product of metabolic transformation is of greater toxicity than that of the parent compound, the inhibition of the microsomal enzymes by SKF525A would be expected to protect the animal from toxicity resulting from metabolism of the parent compound.

Induction of Biotransformation Mechanisms

The total quantity of microsomal drug metabolizing enzymes can be increased in humans and in animals by prior administration of large variety of chemical substances. Such substances include the anesthetics, such as nitrous oxide; the sedatives, such as barbiturates; the analgesics, such as phenylbutazone; and the insecticides, such as chlordane.

Induction of increased enzyme activity usually involves repeated exposure to the inducing agent. It is usually temporary and lasts for two to four weeks following the administration of the inducing chemical. Since metabolic transformation has been shown to result in the formation of more or less toxic products as compared to the parent compound, enzyme induction may be protective to the animal (when detoxication is involved) or detrimental to the animal (when toxication is involved).

Elimination

Following are the major ways through which poisons and their metabolites are excreted.

1. *Fecal excretion*. Ingestation of a relatively insoluble poison (e.g., lead arsenate) is followed by excretion of the major part in the feces. Substances may also find their way into faeces via bile; metals stored in the liver are slowly excreted in this way.

2. *Pulmonary excretion*. Volatile poisons may be mainly excreted in the expired air, e.g., CS_2, cyanide. In phosphorus poisoning the breath may smell of garlic odor and glow in the dark. Diagnosis of hemlock poisoning may be made from the characteristic "mouse-like" odor of coniine in the exhaled air (and also in urine). The lesions found in the lungs in paraffin poisoning are probably due to irritant effect caused by pulmonary excretion.

3. *Urinary excretion*. This is the most important pathway of the excretion of a poison. Irritant poisons cause damage to kidney. Urine is often a convenient material for

diagnostic analysis. In veterinary field it is of great importance in detecting the pasture contamination with fluorides.

4. *Milk and dermal excretion.* Excretion can also take place through skin, e.g., arsenic, and in lactating animals in milk. Many of the insecticides are fat soluble and it has been shown that DDT, aldrin, and several other chlorinated hydrocarbons can be detected in minute amounts in cow's milk.

TOXICOKINETICS

Toxicokinetics involves the relationship between tissue concentration of a toxicant and time. There are two types of kinetics:

1. Zero-order kinetics and
2. First order kinetics.

In zero-order kinetics, a toxicant is eliminated from the body at a fixed amount per unit time. This occurs when the toxicant elimination process is saturated and a fixed amount of toxicant (e.g., mg or g) is excreted per unit time.

Many toxicants are eliminated from animal tissues in a fixed-order manner. Thus, in first-order kinetics a constant fraction of a toxicant/drug is eliminated per unit time. For example, if the initial level were 500 mg and it took ten days to reach 250 mg, then it will take additional 10 days to reach 125 mg. During the first 10 days a total of 250 mg toxicant was excreted and during the next 10 days only 125 mg. In each case, the amount excreted was a constant fraction (i.e., 50%)of the original amount. The ten-day period is called half-life of the toxicant. Various species handle excretion of a toxicant in different manner and therefore a given toxicant will have different half-lives in different species.

MODE OF ACTION OF TOXICANTS

In a broader sense, mode of action of poisons may be divided as physical and chemical disruption of the living process.

Physical Action: Because of their physical properties such as lipid solubility, some substances exert a non-specific inhibitory effect on enzyme systems by virtue of the fact that their physical nature is such as to bring about their accumulation in vital parts of cells where they depress cellular functions. Many compounds, including hypnotics and anesthetics such as hydrocarbons, chlorinated hydrocarbons, alcohols, ethers, ketones exert their inhibitory effects in this way.

Chemical Action: Majority of poisons produce their effect as a result of their chemical interactions with cell components. It is the enzymes concerned in cell oxidation and oxidative phosphorylation which seem to be most vulnerable to the action of poisons. Enzymes have active sites and the toxic compounds may occupy those active sites thus preventing normal substrates to combine.

The enzyme inhibition caused by a toxicant may be irreversible (asin the case of certain organophosphates) or reversible (as in the case of carbamates). Some of the factors that may affect the enzyme inhibition are: chemical structure of the inhibitor, cell permeability, enzyme inhibitor concentrations, the presence of an antagonist of the inhibitor, lethal synthesis, presence of an antidote.

FACTORS AFFECTING ACTIONS OF TOXICANTS

Numerous factors influence the action of poisonous substances. In addition to those already described (e.g., route of absorption, biotransformation), they include (1) dosage, (2) the physical and chemical nature of the poison (3) the source of the poison (4) repeated exposure to the poison (5) species (6)size, age and sex (7) general state of health of the animal.

Dosage

Harmful effect of a toxic compound is largely dependent on the amount of that compound absorbed into the body.

Physical and Chemical Nature

The physical state, e.g., whether solid, powder, orin solution will affect the dose of a poison. Coarsely crystalline arsenic trioxideis slowly absorbed and so has relatively low toxicity; finely powdered arsenic is highly toxic. Many substances are readily absorbed from oily than from aqueous solution, e.g., insecticides.

Chemical nature is important in regard to toxicity, yellow phosphorus is a most poisonous substance, its allotrope red phosphorus is inert when taken in body, it is in soluble and is excreted unchanged. Compounds containing trivalent arsenic are much more toxic than those containing the pentavalent form. Barium carbonate is intensely toxic than barium sulfate.

Sources of Poisons.

Under certain circumstances poisoning from a particular compound may be enhanced or reduced. Some plant poisons are destroyed by drying or storage and hay contaminated by them is harmless (e.g., buttercups). Presence of oils in the diet will enhance the absorption and so toxicity of poison e.g., phosphorus. Accumulation of copper in the liver may be mobilized by administering molybdenum and vice versa.

Repeated Exposure

It is logical that several doses of a poison will be effective than a single dose. The degree of harmfulness of repeated small doses also depends on whether the poison accumulates in body and whether its effects are cumulative (e.g., carcinogen). Carcinogens are the example of such chronic toxicity.

Species

There are extraordinary wide variations in response to a particular poison between species.

Size, Age and Sex

In general, the amount of a poison required to produce toxic symptoms is related to the weight of the animals.This relationship between weight and dose may vary between species.

Very young and very old animals are usually more susceptible to poisons. There are few instances of sex difference in response to poisons in animals. For example, red squill has about twice the toxicity for female rats than for males.

General State of Heath

Debilitated animals are more susceptible to poisons and drugs because their general resistance and detoxication mechanisms are defective. For example, hepatic or renal disease may enormously increase the susceptibility to poisons.

COMMON CAUSES OF TOXICOSES

Accidental poisoning occurs in animals and maybe divided roughly into:

(1) poisoning by naturally-occurring toxicants and

(2) poisoning by man-made chemicals.

But there is no clear cut dividing line between these categories. Naturally occurring toxicological hazards include poisonous minerals and poisonous plants; man-made hazards include industrial contaminants, pesticides, domestic materials, unsuitable food and water, use of drugs, etc.

COMMON TOXICOLOGICAL PROBLEM IN DOMESTIC AND FARM ANIMALS

Dogs and Cats

Pesticides, garbage, ethylene glycol, heavy metals, biotoxins (toads, snakes, ticks), phyto toxins, mycotoxins, drug reactions.

Poultry

Pesticides (very sensitive to insecticides), feed and water additives, fungi, bacterial toxins, gases and fumigants, heavy metals.

Zoo Animals

Largely malacious and quite variable situations, drug reactions, poisonous plants, accidental-organophosphates and warfarin baits.

Exotic Animals

Largely due to feed additives.

Mink—Botulism, chronic lead, phenolic wood preservatives, stilbesterol, etc.

Rabbits—milkweed, toxic plants, neck paralysis and in coordination common.

Turtles—paint on shell produces lump-back deformities.

Cattle

Heavy metals, pesticides, dietary and environmental contaminants (e.g., urea, nitrate, cyanide, mycotoxins), poisonous plants; snake and insect bites, drug adverse reactions.

Sheep and Goats

Poisonous plants—photo sensitizers, cyanogenetic, selenium, oxalate, lupine, sneezeweed, laurels, white snake root, larkspur, etc; pesticides, anthelmintics, others—lead, nitrate, sulfur, fluoride.

Horses

Poisonous plants—oleander, bracken fern, castor bean, locoweed, lupine, selenium-containing, groundsel, crotalaria, cyanide; pesticides, drug adverse reactions, snake and insect bites, other aflatoxins, heavy metals, toxic gases.

Swine

Salt, coal-tar (pitch)and petroleum products, nitrates, wood preservatives, heavy metals, organic arsenicals, fungal toxins, poisonous plants, gossypol, insecticides, botulism, edema disease (endotoxins), rodenticides.

REFERENCES

Barkan, B.A. and F.W. Oehme. 1975. "A Classification of Common Midwestern Animal Toxicosis". *Vet. Tox*. 17:37-49.

Buck, et. al., *Clinical and Diagnostic Veterinary Toxicology*. 2nd ed. 1976. pp. 25-37.

Clarke, E.G.C. and M.L. Clarke, (eds.) *Veterinary Toxicology*. 1975. The Williams and Wilkins Company, Baltimore.

Casarett, L.J. and J. Doull. (eds.) *Toxicology: The Basic Science of Poisons*. 2nd Ed. Ch. 3-5, 9-12, 14-15.

Doull, J., C.D. Klaassen and M.O. Amdur, (eds.). 1980. *Casarett and Doull's Toxicology: The Basic Science of Poisons*. 2nd. ed., pp. 3-27. Macmillan Publishing Company, New York.

Loomis, T.A. (ed). 1976, *Essentials of Toxicology*. 2nd Ed., pp. 1-23. Lea and Febiger, Philadelphia.

Osweiler, G.D., T.L. Carson, W.B. Buck and G.A. Van Gelder (eds.). 1985. *Clinical and Diagnostic Veterinary Toxicology*. Kendall-Hunt Publishing Company, Iowa.

2

Toxicology of Insecticides

The greatly increased use of pesticides of all kinds which has taken place. The greatly increased use of pesticides of all kinds which has taken place since the end of the second world war has introduced a new hazard to livestock. Some of the compounds at present in use, particularly the organophosphorus insecticides, can be dangerous when mishandled or wrongly used, and there have been numerous accidents, in both human beings and animals, arising from negligence or forgetfulness, from the taking of calculated risks, or from failure to give or heed information and advice. It is imperative that every livestock owner should be aware of the potential danger to himself, his family and his animals, from misuse of the more poisonous compounds.

The striving for higher agricultural production as one of the main prerequisites for improving the population's standard of living involves the use of various pesticides to prevent losses of cultivated plants, foods and feeds from pests. Pesticides are divided according to their biological effects into insecticides, herbicides, fungicides, rodenticides and others. The use of pesticides not only reduces the losses caused by various pests but also facilitates large scale use of modern and progressive methods agriculture and improvement of the quality of farm products.

However, large scale use of pesticides, often very toxic or with other undesirable properties, has brought about many problems. In the last decade, researchers have been increasingly interested in the study of the acute toxicity of pesticides, their accumulation in the animal body, occurrence of residues in foodstuffs and their effect on the human body. In particular, many questions have been raised about increasing levels of residues in foodstuffs, implying great danger to the public health.

In agricultural practice, the insecticides are usually employed as sprays applied to soil or to the vegetation. Some of them are highly persistent, e. g., chlorinated hydrocarbons. The organophosphate compounds are potentially dangerous. They are known to be cholinesterase inhibitors. Carbamate insecticides acting similar way. These are synthetic insecticides. The older insecticides of vegetable origin, including pyrethrins, rotenones, nicotinoids have been replaced by the synthetic organic insecticides.

Pesticide labels must carry warnings against use on unapproved species or under untested circumstances. These warnings may pertain to acute or chronic toxicity, or to residues in meat, milk, or other animal products. Because labels change to meet current government regulations, it is important that label directions accompanying the product *always* be read and followed.

Each exposure, no matter how brief or small, results in some of the compound being absorbed and perhaps stored. Repeated short exposures may eventually result in intoxication. Every precaution should be taken to minimise human exposure. This may include frequent changes of clothing with bathing at each change, or if necessary, the use of respirators, rain gear, and gloves impervious to pesticides. Respirators must have filters approved for the type of insecticide being used (eg, ordinary dust filters will not protect the operator from phosphorous fumes). Such measures are generally sufficient to guard against intoxication. Overexposure to chlorinated hydrocarbon insecticides is difficult to measure except by the occurrence of signs of poisoning.

The cholinesterase-inhibiting property of organophosphates may be used to indicate degree of exposure if the activity of the blood enzyme is determined frequently. In humans, serum esterase is usually inhibited first and, in the absence of declining RBC activity, indicates a recent exposure of only moderate degree. Depression of the RBC-enzyme activity indicates a more severe acute exposure or chronic exposure. (Normal cholinesterase activity values vary a great deal in unexposed individuals, and a determination of activity has significance only when compared with the normal value for that individual.)

In addition to their effects on humans, organic pesticides may have deleterious effects on fish and wildlife as well as on domestic species. In no event should amounts greater than those specifically recommended be used, and maximum precautions should be taken to prevent drift or drainage to adjoining fields, pastures, ponds, streams, or other premises outside the treatment area.

The safety and exposure level of these compounds in target species has been carefully established, and application recommendations and regulations must be followed. Individuals, including veterinarians, have been prosecuted for failure to follow label directions or to heed label warnings and for failure to warn animal owners of the necessary precautions.

An ideal insecticide or acaricide should be efficacious without risk to livestock or persons making the application and without leaving residues in tissues, eggs, or milk. Few compounds satisfy all these requirements.

Poisoning by organic insecticides and acaricides may be caused by direct application, by ingestion of contaminated feed or forage treated for controlling of plant parasites, or by accidental exposure. This discussion is limited to only those insecticides or acaricides most frequently hazardous to livestock or likely to leave residues in animal products.

Chemical synthesis rarely yields 100% of the product of interest, and normally there are, in variable proportions, structurally related compounds that have biologic effects different from the compound sought. A prime example is tetrachlorodiphenylethane (TDE or "Rhothane, " also called DDD): the p, p¢-isomer is an effective insecticide of low toxicity for most mammals; the isomers causes necrosis of the adrenal glands of humans and dogs and is used to treat certain adrenal malfunctions.

Products stored under temperature extremes or held in partially emptied containers for long periods may deteriorate. Storing a chemical in anything but the original container is hazardous as in time its identity may be forgotten. Accidental contact with animals or humans may then have disastrous consequences. Consumer-mixed and unapproved combinations can be very dangerous and should never be used.

A number of carbamate and organophosphate insecticides that bind serine esterases (eg, carbaryl, dichlorvos, methiocarb, carbofuran, paraoxon, mevinophos, aldicarb, and monocrotophos) are also immunotoxic. Impaired macrophage signalling through interleukin I and II appears to be involved, and the insecticide levels that cause this effect are very low. This can lead to subtle but damaging influences on the health of exposed animals.

ORGANOPHOSPHATE INSECTICIDES

Organophosphates resulted from studies of nerve gases in World War II. Chemically, they are esters of phosphoric acid and poorly soluble in water. They have good knock-down ability with little residue problem. Organophosphate are noncumulative and not stored in body fat as do the chlorinated hydrocarbons. Commonly used as deforming agents—alone or in combination with other agents. May be used on livestock or on buildings and premises as sprays, dips and fogs or as pour-ons on the back of animals for absorption and circulation throughout the body. Are also given orally to dogs to control fleas.

Organophosphates (OP) have replaced the banned organochlorine compounds and are a major cause of animal poisoning. They vary greatly in toxicity, residue levels, and excretion. Many OP have been developed for plant and animal protection, and in general, they offer a distinct advantage by producing little tissue and environmental residue.

Many of the OP now used as pesticides are not potent inhibitors of esterases until activated in the liver by microsomal oxidation enzymes; they are generally less toxic, and intoxication occurs more slowly. Certain OP preparations are microencapsulated, and the active compound is released slowly; this increases the duration of activity and reduces their toxicity, but the toxic properties are still present.

Mechanism of Toxicity

Some organophosphates are extremely toxic—some much more than others. Mechanism of toxicity is the same for insects and mammals. Organophosphates complex with and tie-up cholinesterases (inhibit cholinesterase), causing a build-up of acetylcholine at the myoneural junction. Enzyme is phosporylated and as such is inactive. Organophosphates have the ability to fit and phosphorylate a specific amino acid (serine)on the cholinesterase. Reversal of complex depends on the substituent groups of the specific organophosphate. Some are less easily reversible, thus are more toxic to mammals than others.

The longer the complex ages, the tighter and more toxic it becomes. Inactive cholinesterases allow acetylcholine to build up and become excessive. Toxicity is caused by excess acetylcholine and an uncontrolled parasympathetic predominance resulting in following signs of toxicity.

Signs of Poisoning

Muscarinic type

a. Profuse salivation

b. Hypermotility of g. i. tract

c. Abdominal cramps

d. Vomiting, diarrhea, lacrimation, sweating

e. Dyspnea, miosis, pallor, cyanosis, urination

Nicotinic type

Excessive stimulation of skeletal muscle resulting in twitching of muscles of face, eyelids and tongue. Generalized tetany causing the animal to walk in a sea-horse, stiff-legged fashion followed by weakness and paralysis of skeletal and respiratory muscle.

CNS type

Vary with species; domestic food-producing animals may exhibit excessive stimulation of CNS but rarely convulsive seizures (but seen in dogs and cats). This is followed by CNS depression, and death.

Clinical Findings

In general, OP pesticides have a narrow margin of safety, and the dose-response curve is quite steep. Signs of OP poisoning are those of cholinergic overstimulation, which can be grouped under 3 categories: muscarinic, nicotinic, and central. Muscarinic signs, which are usually first to appear, include hypersalivation, miosis, frequent urination, diarrhea, vomiting, colic, and dyspnea due to increased bronchial secretions and bronchoconstriction. Nicotinic effects include muscle fasciculations and weakness. The central effects include nervousness, ataxia, apprehension, and seizures. Cattle and sheep commonly show severe depression. CNS stimulation in dogs and cats usually progresses to convulsions. Some OP (eg, amidothioates) do not enter the brain easily, so that CNS signs are mild. Onset of signs after exposure is usually within hours but may be delayed for >2 days. Severity and course of intoxication is influenced principally by the dosage and route of exposure. In acute poisoning, the primary clinical signs may be respiratory distress and collapse followed by death due to respiratory muscle paralysis.

Diagnosis

An important diagnostic aid is the cholinesterase activity in blood and brain. Unfortunately, the depression of blood cholinesterase does not necessarily correlate with the severity of poisoning; signs are seen when nerve cholinesterase is inhibited, and the enzyme in blood reflects, only in a general way, the levels in nervous tissue. The key factor appears to be the rate at which the enzyme activity is reduced. Analyses performed after exposure may be negative because OP do not remain long in tissues as the parent compound. Chlorinated OP compounds have greater potential for tissue residue. Frozen stomach and rumen samples should be analysed for the pesticide because OP are generally more stable in acids.

Lesions

Animals with acute OP poisoning have nonspecific or no lesions. Pulmonary edema and congestion, hemorrhages, and edema of the bowel and other organs may be found. Animals surviving >1 day may become emaciated and dehydrated.

Treatment

Three categories of drugs are used to treat OP poisoning: 1) muscarinic blocking agents, 2) cholinesterase reactivators, and 3) emetics, cathartics, and adsorbants to decrease further absorption. Atropine sulfate blocks the central and peripheral muscarinic effects of OP; it is administered to effect in dogs and cats, usually at a dosage of 0. 2-2 mg/kg body wt (cats are dosed at the lower end of the range), every 3-6 hr or as often as clinical signs indicate. For horses and pigs, the dosage is 0. 1-0. 2 mg/kg, IV, repeated every 10 min as needed; for cattle and sheep, the dosage is 0. 6-1 mg/kg, one-third given IV, the remainder IM or SC, and repeated as needed. Atropinisation is adequate when the pupils are dilated, salivation ceases, and the animal appears more alert. Animals initially respond well to atropine sulfate; however, the response diminishes after repeated treatments. Overtreatment with atropine should be avoided. Atropine does not alleviate the nicotinic cholinergic effects, such as muscle fasciculations and muscle paralysis, so that death from massive overdoses of OP can still occur. Including diazepam in the treatment reduced the incidence of seizures and increased survival of nonhuman primates experimentally. Using barbiturates to treat the convulsions must be done very carefully, as they seem to be potentiated by anticholinesterases.

An improved treatment combines atropine with the cholinesterase-reactivating oxime, 2-pyridine aldoxime methchloride (2-PAM, pralidoxime chloride). The dosage of 2-PAM is 20-50 mg/kg body wt, given as a 5% solution IM or by slow IV (over 5-10 min), repeated as needed. IV 2-PAM must be given very slowly to avoid musculoskeletal paralysis and respiratory arrest. Response to cholinesterase reactivators decreases with time after exposure; therefore, treatment with oximes must be instituted as soon as possible (within 24-48 hr). The rate at which the enzyme/organophosphate complex becomes unresponsive to activators varies with the particular pesticide.

Removal of the poison from the animal also should be attempted. If exposure was dermal, the animal should be washed with detergent and water (about room temperature) but without scrubbing and irritating the skin. Emesis should be induced if oral exposure occurred <2 hr previously; emesis is contraindicated if the animal is depressed. Oral administration of mineral oil decreases absorption of pesticide from the GI tract. Activated charcoal (3-6 g/kg as a water slurry) adsorbs OP and helps elimination in the feces. This is particularly recommended in cattle. Continued absorption of OP from the large amount of ingesta in the rumen has caused prolonged toxicosis in cattle. Artificial respiration or administration of oxygen may be required. Phenothiazine tranquilizers should be avoided, as well as the xanthine stimulants theophylline and aminophylline. Succinylcholine should not be used for at least 10 days after OP exposure.

Various Organophosphate Insecticides

Details of some major organophosphate insecticides are listed below:

Azinphos-methyl (or -ethyl): The maximum nontoxic oral dose is 0. 44 mg/kg body wt for calves, 2. 2 mg/kg for cattle and goats, and 4. 8 mg/kg for sheep.

Chlorpyrifos: The oral LD50 is 500 mg/kg body wt in goats and 97 mg/kg in rats. In comparison with calves, steers, and cows, bulls (particularly of the exotic breeds) are highly susceptible to a single dose of chlorpyrifos.

Coumaphos: Coumaphos is used against cattle grubs and a number of other ectoparasites and for treatment of premises. The maximum concentration that may be safely used on adult cattle, horses, and pigs is 0.5%. Young calves and all ages of sheep and goats must not be sprayed with concentrations >0.25%; 0.5% concentrations may be lethal. Adult cattle may show mild toxicity at 1% concentrations.

Diazinon: Young calves appear to tolerate 0.05% spray but are poisoned by 0.1% concentrations. Adult cattle may be sprayed at weekly intervals with 0.1% concentrations without inducing poisoning. Young calves tolerate 0.44 mg/kg body wt, PO, but are poisoned by 0.88 mg/kg. Cattle tolerate 8.8 mg/kg, PO, but are poisoned by 22 mg/kg. Sheep tolerate 17.6 mg/kg but are poisoned by 26 mg/kg.

Dichlorvos: Dichlorvos has many uses on both plants and animals. It is rapidly metabolised and excreted, and residues in meat and milk are not a problem if label directions are followed. It is of moderate toxicity, with a minimum toxic dose of 10 mg/kg body wt in young calves and 25 mg/kg in horses and sheep. The LD50 in rats is 25-80 mg/kg, PO. A 1% dust was not toxic to cattle. Flea collars containing dichlorvos may cause skin reactions in some pets.

Dimethoate: When administered PO, the minimum toxic dose for young dairy calves was ~48 mg/kg body wt, while 22 mg/kg was lethal for cattle 1 yr old. Daily doses of 10 mg/kg for 5 days in adult cattle lowered blood cholinesterase activity to 20% of normal but did not produce poisoning. Horses have been poisoned by doses of 60-80 mg/kg, PO. When applied topically, 1% sprays have been tolerated by calves, cattle, and adult sheep.

Disulfoton: The maximum nontoxic oral dose is 0.88 mg/kg body wt for young calves, 2.2 mg/kg for cattle and goats, and 4.8 mg/kg for sheep. Poisoning has occurred in cattle after consuming harvested forages previously sprayed with this insecticide.

Fenthion: Minimum toxic dose, PO, is 25 mg/kg body wt for cattle; 50 mg/kg is lethal to sheep.

Malathion: Malathion is one of the safest organophosphates. Young calves tolerate 0.5% but not 1% sprays; adult cattle tolerate 2% sprays. Given PO, it is toxic at 100 mg/kg but not 55 mg/kg body wt; young calves tolerate 11 mg/kg but are poisoned by 22 mg/kg. Malathion is excreted in cow's milk.

Methyl Parathion: The LD50 in rats from a single oral dose is 9-25 mg/kg body wt compared with 3-13 mg/kg for ethyl parathion. Microencapsulation of this compound decreases its toxicity, and the lethal dose in cattle has been increased from a 0.5% to a 2% spray.

Oxydemeton-methyl: The maximum nontoxic oral dose is 0.88 mg/kg body wt for young calves, 2.2 mg/kg for cattle, and 4.8 mg/kg for sheep and goats.

Parathion: Parathion (diethyl parathion) is widely used for control of plant pests and is approximately one-half as toxic as TEPP. It is used as a dip and spray for cattle in some countries (not in the USA). Most cases of occupational insecticide poisonings in humans have been attributed to parathion or its degradation products. As a 0.02% spray, it produces signs of poisoning in young calves and occasional transitory signs at 0.01%. Parathion is lethal to sheep at 22 mg/kg body wt, PO, but not at 11 mg/kg. Young dairy calves are poisoned by 0.44 mg/kg, while 44 mg/kg is required to poison older cattle. Parathion is used extensively to control mosquitos and insects in orchards and on market garden crops. Normally, because so little is used per acre, it presents no hazard to livestock. However, because of its potency, care should be taken to prevent accidental exposure. Parathion does not produce significant residues in animal tissues.

Phorate: The minimum toxic dose PO is 0.25 mg/kg body wt in calves, 0.75 mg/kg in sheep, and 1 mg/kg in cattle.

Phosmet: The minimum oral toxic dose PO is 25 mg/kg body wt in cattle and calves and 50 mg/kg in sheep.

Temephos: The oral LD50 for rats is 1 g (or more)/kg body wt, while the dermal LD50 is >4 g/kg.

Tetrachlorvinphos: Tetrachlorvinphos has low toxicity in dogs; chronic feeding studies indicate the lowest effect level (LEL) was 50 mg/kg/day and the no observed effect level (NOEL) 3.13 mg/kg/day. The minimum toxic dose in pigs is 100 mg/kg.

Trichlorfon: As a spray, trichlorfon at a 1% concentration is tolerated by adult cattle; given PO, it is tolerated by young dairy calves at 4.4 mg/kg body wt but produces poisoning at 8.8 mg/kg. Adult cattle, sheep, and horses appear to tolerate 44 mg/kg, while 88 mg/kg produces poisoning. Dogs were unaffected when fed 1,000 ppm of trichlorfon for 4 mo. Trichlorfon is metabolised rapidly.

Carbophenothion: Dairy calves <2 wk of age sprayed with water-based formulations showed poisoning at 0.05% or higher concentrations, and adult cattle were poisoned by spraying with 1%. Sheep and goats have been poisoned by 22 mg/kg body wt, PO, but not by 8 mg/kg. The LD50 for rats is ~31 mg/kg; a daily dosage of 2.2 mg/kg for 90 days produced poisoning. Dogs tolerated a diet containing 32 ppm for 90 days.

Chlorfenvinphos: Adult cattle were poisoned by 5% or higher sprays, while young calves were poisoned only when the concentration was raised to 2%. The minimum oral toxic dose appears to be ~22 mg/kg for cattle of all ages. The acute oral LD50 for rats is 10-39 mg/kg.

Crotoxyphos: Crotoxyphos is of rather low toxicity; however, Brahman cattle are markedly more susceptible than European breeds. Cattle (except as above), sheep, goats, and pigs all tolerate sprays containing crotoxyphos at 0.5% levels or higher. Toxic doses appears to be in the 2% range, except for in Brahman cattle, in which 0.144%-0.3% may be toxic.

Demeton: The oral LD50 is 8 mg/kg body wt in goats and 2 mg/kg in rats; the dermal LD50 in rats is 8 mg/kg.

Dioxathion: Dioxathion is a mixture of cis- and trans-isomers (70%) and reaction products (30%). Used on both plants and animals, it is rapidly metabolised and not likely to produce residues in meat greater than the 1 ppm official tolerance. Concentrations of 0.15% or greater are generally used on animals. The minimum toxic dose in calves is 5 mg/kg body wt. Sprays of 0.5% in cattle and sheep or 0.25% in goats and pigs are nontoxic. Dioxathion at 8.8 mg/kg, PO, has killed young calves, and it produced intoxication at 4.4 mg/kg.

EPN: EPN is related to parathion and is about one-half as toxic when applied externally; when given PO, it is about equally toxic. Dogs were not poisoned at doses >100 mg/kg.

Famphur: The maximum nontoxic dose is 10 mg/kg body wt in calves and 50 mg/kg in cattle, sheep, and horses. This compound is effective against warbles in cattle, but (as for all grubicides) directions must be followed as to time of application; larvae killed while migrating and the resultant local reaction can cause serious problems.

Mevinphos: The LD50 in rats is 3 mg/kg body wt, PO or topically.

Ronnel (Fenchlorphos): Ronnel produces mild signs of poisoning in cattle at 132 mg/kg body wt, but severe signs do not appear until the dosage is >400 mg/kg. The minimum toxic dose in sheep is 400 mg/kg. Concentrations as high as 2.5% in sprays have failed to produce poisoning of cattle, young dairy calves, or sheep. Poisoning usually occurs in 2 stages. The animal first becomes weak and, although able to move about normally, may be placid. Diarrhea, often flecked with blood, may also be seen. Salivation and dyspnea then appear if the dose was high enough. Blood cholinesterase activity declines slowly over 5-7 days. Ronnel produces residues in meat and milk; strict adherence to label restrictions is essential. The residues may be removed by giving the animal activated charcoal for several days.

Ruelene: Ruelene is active both as a systemic and contact insecticide in livestock, has some anthelmintic activity, and has rather low toxicity. Dairy calves have been poisoned by 44 mg/kg body wt, PO, while adult cattle require 88 mg/kg for the same effect. Sheep are moderately intoxicated by 176 mg/kg; Angora goats are about twice as sensitive. Pigs have been poisoned by 11 mg/kg and horses by 44 mg/kg. Most livestock tolerate a 2% topical spray.

Terbufos: This soil insecticide is used to control corn rootworms. The minimum oral toxic dose is ~1.5 mg/kg body wt for sheep and cattle. Cases of intoxication in cattle have occurred. Ingestion of 7.5 mg/kg was lethal to heifers.

Tetraethyl Pyrophosphate (TEPP): TEPP is one of the most acutely toxic insecticides. Although not used on animals, accidental exposure occurs occasionally. One herd of 29 cattle (including calves and adults) was accidentally sprayed with 0.33% TEPP emulsion; all died within 40 min.

Delayed Neurotoxicity from Triaryl Phosphates

For some time, compounds known as triaryl phosphates (e.g., triosthocresyl phosphate) have been used as flame retardants, plasticizers, lubricating oils, and hydraulic fluids. They are weak cholinesterase inhibitors, but do inhibit "neurotoxic esterase," located in the brain and spinal cord. A form of delayed neurotoxicity results from the inhibition of neurotoxic esterase. Triaryl phosphates have caused accidental poisonings in humans and other species (mostly cattle). Some OP insecticides (e.g., PEN, leptophos) can also cause delayed neurotoxicity; however, field cases have been rare. The lesions associated with delayed neurotoxicity include demyelination of peripheral and spinal motor tracts due to loss of neurotoxic esterase function. Clinical signs associated with delayed neurotoxicity include muscle weakness and ataxia that progresses to flaccid paralysis of the hindlimbs. Signs are usually not manifest until 8-21 days after exposure to a neurotoxic triaryl phosphate. There are no specific antidotes.

Pesticide Potentiating Agents

Piperonyl butoxide is used as a potentiator in many pesticide formulations including pyrethrins, pyrethroids, and d-limonene. It decreases breakdown of the chemical in the animal or insect's body by inhibiting mixed function oxidase enzymes and makes the pesticide more toxic to the insect—and the host. Animals that are debilitated or have decreased drug metabolising capability become more susceptible to the pesticide. However, toxins that must be activated in the body to a toxic form are frequently less toxic when piperonyl butoxide exposure occurs at the same time. This effect has been seen in many species, including cats, dogs, rats, humans, etc. Cimetidine, a drug that reduces stomach acid secretion by blocking gastric H_2 receptors, and the antibiotic chloramphenicol have the same effect.

Solvents and Emulsifiers: Solvents and emulsifiers are required in most liquid insecticide preparations. Usually they have low toxicity, but like the petroleum products (which many are), they must be considered as possible causes of poisoning. In direct treatment with pesticides, emulsification must be thorough with an average droplet size of 5 microns (preferably smaller), or excessive amounts may stick to treated animals. Treatment should be as for petroleum product poisoning.

Acetone: GI irritation, narcosis, and kidney and liver damage are the main signs. Treatment consists of gastric lavage, oxygen, and a low-fat diet. Additional supportive treatment to alleviate clinical signs may be given.

Isopropyl Alcohol: The signs are GI pain, cramps, vomiting, diarrhea, and CNS depression (dizziness, stupor, coma, death from respiratory paralysis). The liver and kidneys are reversibly affected. Dehydration and pneumonia may occur. Treatment consists of emetics, gastric lavage, milk PO, oxygen, and artificial respiration.

Methanol: Nausea, vomiting, gastric pain, reflex hyperexcitability, opisthotonos, convulsions, fixed pupils, and acute peripheral neuritis are typical. Large overdoses can lead to blindness. Toxic effects are due in part to the alcohol itself, and in part to formic acid produced by its oxidation. Treatment should include emetics (apomorphine) followed by gastric lavage with 4% sodium bicarbonate, saline laxative, oxygen therapy, sodium bicarbonate solution IV, and analgesics; however, the prognosis is poor. Intensive and prolonged alkalinisation is the mainstay of treatment. Ethanol retards the oxidation of methanol and may be given as an adjunct therapy.

Sulfur and Lime-sulfur: Sulfur and lime-sulfur are 2 of the oldest insecticides. Elemental sulfur is practically devoid of toxicity, although poisoning has occurred occasionally when large amounts were mixed in cattle feed. Specific toxic dosages are not known but probably exceed 4 g/kg body wt. Lime-sulfur, which is a complex of sulfides, may cause irritation, discomfort, or blistering but rarely causes death. Treatment consists of removing residual material and applying bland protective ointments plus any supportive measures that may be indicated

CARBAMATE INSECTICIDES

The carbamate insecticides are the derivatives of the basic compound, carbamic acid NH_2-COOH. This acid is very unstable so it is the derivative that is used as insecticide.

Dimethyl derivatives were the first substituted compounds, e. g., Isolan. Among the N-methyl derivatives, carbaryl, 1-naphthyl N-methylcarbamate, (Sevin) is most widely used insecticide of this group. In poisoning by carbamates, acetylcholinesterase is reversibly inhibited by carbamylation. Onset of symptoms is much more rapid than in the case of organophospahtes. Cholinesterase reactivation is spontaneous and rapid. Carbamates react with cholin- esterase in a way precisely analogous to the reactions of organophosphates and acetyl choline but the binding is weaker and less stable. In all cases there is an enzyme-complex formation with cholinesterase, which is spontaneously hydrolyzed.

CHLORINATED HYDROCARBON INSECTICIDES

These compounds are poisonous to insects on contact, have good knock-down capacity, and kill quickly. They are absorbed through the chitinous cuticle of the insect, their residual effect is long lasting everywhere, including in the environment. Many chlorinated hydrocarbons are known or suspected to be carcinogenic.

Due to tissue residues and chronic toxicity, use of these agents is drastically curtailed. Only lindane and methoxychlor are approved for use on or around livestock. Nevertheless, in a recent surveillance study, 51% of the cattle (mainly originating from Colorado) had detectable residues of chlorinated hydrocarbon insecticides including heptachlor, heptachlor epoxide, lindane, and oxychlordane.

Aldrin is a potent insecticide similar to dieldrin with the same order of toxicity. It is no longer registered in the USA but was used for termite control.

Benzene hexachloride (BHC, hexachlorocyclohexane) was a useful insecticide for large animals and dogs but is highly toxic to cats in the concentrations necessary for parasite control.

Cattle in good condition have tolerated 0.2% lindane applications, but stressed, emaciated cattle have been poisoned from spraying or dipping in 0.075% lindane. Horses and pigs appear to tolerate 0.2-0.5%, and sheep and goats ordinarily tolerate 0.5% applications. Emaciation and lactation increase the susceptibility of animals to poisoning by lindane; such animals should be treated with extreme caution. Young calves are very susceptible to lindane and are poisoned by a single oral dose of 4.4 mg/kg body wt. Mild signs appear in sheep given 22 mg/kg, and death occurs at 100 mg/kg. Adult cattle have tolerated 13 mg/kg without signs. BHC is stored in body fat and excreted in milk.

Chlordane is no longer registered as an insecticide in the USA. Exposure occurs when livestock consume treated plants or when they come in direct contact through carelessness and accidents. Very young calves have been killed by doses of 44 mg/kg, and the minimum toxic dose for cattle is ~88 mg/kg. Cattle fed chlordane at 25 ppm of their diet for 56 days showed 19 ppm in their fat at the end of the feeding. Topical emulsions and suspensions have been used safely on dogs at concentrations up to 0.25%, provided freshly diluted materials were used; dry powders up to 5% have been safe. The no effect level in dogs in a 2-yr feeding study was 3 mg/kg. Pigeons and Leghorn cockerels and pullets suffered no effects after 1-2 mo exposure to vapors emanating from chlordane-treated surfaces.

Dieldrin is not a registered pesticide in the USA. Residues limit its application, and it is one of the most toxic chlorinated hydrocarbon insecticides. Young dairy calves are poisoned by 8.8 mg/kg body wt, PO, but tolerate 4. 4 mg/kg, while adult cattle tolerate 8.8 mg/kg and are poisoned by 22 mg/kg. Pigs tolerate 22 mg/kg and are poisoned by 44 mg/kg. Horses are poisoned by 22 mg/kg. Because of its effectiveness against insect pests on crops and pasture and the low dosage per acre, dieldrin is not likely to poison livestock grazing the treated areas. Diets containing 25 ppm of dieldrin have been fed to cattle and sheep for 16 wk without harmful effects other than residues in fat, which are slow to disappear. Great care must be exercised in marketing animals that have grazed treated areas or consumed products from previously treated areas. There is a zero tolerance level for residues in edible tissues.

Heptachlor is not currently registered in the USA and is not recommended for use on livestock in the USA. Because it is very effective against certain plant-feeding insects, it is encountered from time to time in some geographic areas grazed by livestock. Young dairy calves tolerate dosages as high as 13 mg/kg body wt but are poisoned by 22 mg/kg. Sheep tolerate 22 mg/kg but are poisoned by 40 mg/kg. Diets containing 60 ppm of heptachlor have been fed to cattle for 16 wk without harmful effects other than residues in fat. Heptachlor is converted to heptachlor epoxide by animals and stored in body fat. For this reason, a specific analysis performed for heptachlor usually yields negative results, while that for epoxide is positive.

Methoxychlor is one of the safest chlorinated hydrocarbon insecticides and one of the few with active registration in the USA. Young dairy calves tolerate 265 mg/kg body wt; 500 mg/kg is mildly toxic. While 1 g/kg produces rather severe poisoning in young calves, sheep are not affected. One dog was given 990 mg/kg daily for 30 days without showing signs. Six applications to cattle of a 0.5% spray at 3-wk intervals produces fat residues of 2.4 ppm; ~0.4 ppm of methoxychlor is found in milk 1 day after spraying a cow with a 0. 5% concentration. Methoxychlor sprays are not approved for use on animals producing milk for human consumption. Cattle and sheep store essentially no methoxychlor when fed 25 ppm in the total diet for 112 days. If methoxychlor is used as recommended, the established tolerance in fat will not be exceeded. Commercial products are available for garden, orchard, and field crops and for horses and ponies.

Numerous reports suggest that methoxychlor has negative reproductive effects in laboratory animal experiments, but this has not been seen in the field.

Toxaphene is no longer under active registration in the USA. It has been used with reasonable safety if recommendations were followed, but it can cause poisoning when applied or ingested in excessive quantities. Dogs and cats are particularly susceptible. Young calves have been poisoned by 1% toxaphene sprays, while all other farm animals except poultry can withstand 1% or more as sprays or dips. Chickens have been poisoned by dipping in 0.1% emulsions, and turkeys have been poisoned by spraying with 0.5% material. Toxaphene is primarily an acute toxicant and does not persist long in the tissues. Adult cattle have been mildly intoxicated by 4% sprays and severely affected by 8%. Adult cattle have been poisoned from being dipped in emulsions that contained only 0.5% toxaphene (an amount ordinarily safe) because the emulsions had begun to break down, allowing the fine droplets to coalesce into larger droplets that readily adhere to the hair of cattle. The resultant dosage becomes equivalent to that obtained by spray treatments of much higher concentrations. Toxaphene is lethal to young calves at 8.8 mg/kg body wt but not at 4.4 mg/kg. The minimum toxic dose for cattle is ~33 mg/kg, and for sheep between 22 and 33 mg/kg. Spraying Hereford cattle 12 times at 2-wk intervals with 0.5% toxaphene produced a maximum residue of 8 ppm in fat. Cattle fed 10 ppm of toxaphene in the diet for 30 days had no detectable toxaphene tissue residues, while steers fed 100 ppm for 112 days stored only 40 ppm in their fat.

Clinical Findings

The chlorinated hydrocarbon insecticides are general CNS stimulants. They produce a great variety of signs—the most obvious are neuromuscular tremors and convulsions—and there may be obvious behavioral changes common to other poisonings and CNS infections. Body temperature may be very high. Affected animals are generally first noted to be more alert or apprehensive. Muscle fasciculation occurs, becoming visible in the facial region and extending backward until the whole body is involved. Large doses of DDT, DDD, and methoxychlor cause progressive involvement leading to trembling or shivering, followed by convulsions and death. With the other chlorinated hydrocarbons, the muscular twitchings are followed by convulsions, usually without the intermediate trembling. Convulsions may be continuous, clonic, or tonic lasting from a few seconds to several hours, or intermittent and leading to the animal becoming comatose. High fever may accompany convulsions, particularly in warm environments.

Behavioral changes such as abnormal postures (e.g., resting the sternum on the ground while remaining upright in the rear, keeping the head down between the forelegs, "head pressing" against a wall or fence, or continual chewing movements) may be seen. Occasionally, an affected animal becomes belligerent and attacks other animals, people, or moving objects. Vocalisation is common. Some animals are depressed, almost oblivious to their surroundings, and do not eat or drink; they may last longer than those showing more violent symptoms. Usually, there is a copious flow of thick saliva and urinary incontinence. In certain cases, the clinical signs alternate, with the animal first being extremely excited, then severely depressed. The severity of the signs seen at a given time is not a sure prognostic index. Some animals have only a single convulsion and die, while others suffer innumerable convulsions but subsequently recover. Animals showing acute excitability often have a fever >106°F (41°C). The signs of poisoning by these insecticides are highly suggestive but not diagnostic; other poisons and encephalitis or meningitis must be considered.

Signs of acute intoxication by chlordane in birds are nervous chirping, excitability, collapse on hocks or side, and mucous exudates in the nasal passages. Signs of subacute and chronic intoxication are molting, dehydration and cyanosis of the comb, weight loss, and cessation of egg production.

Lesions

If death has occurred suddenly, there may be nothing more than cyanosis. More definite lesions occur as the duration of intoxication increases. Usually, there is congestion of various organs (particularly the lungs, liver, and kidneys) and a blanched appearance of all organs if the body temperature was high before death. The heart generally stops in systole, and there may be many hemorrhages of varying size on the epicardium. The appearance of the heart and lungs may suggest a peracute pneumonia and, if the animal was affected for more than a few hours, there may be pulmonary edema. The trachea and bronchi may contain a blood-tinged froth. In many cases, the CSF volume is excessive, and the brain and spinal cord frequently are congested and edematous.

Diagnosis

Chemical analysis of brain, liver, kidney, fat, and stomach or rumen contents is necessary to confirm the poisoning. The suspected source, if identified, should also be analysed. Brain levels of the insecticide are the most useful. Whole blood, serum, and urine from live animals may be analysed to evaluate exposure in the rest of the herd or flock. In food animal poisoning, if exposure is more than just the animals visibly affected, fat biopsies from survivors may be necessary to estimate the potential residue.

Treatment

There are no known specific antidotes. When exposure is by spraying, dipping, or dusting, a thorough bathing without irritating the skin (no brushes), using detergents and copious quantities of cool water is recommended. If exposure is by ingestion, gastric lavage and saline purgatives are indicated. The use of digestible oils such as corn oil is contraindicated; however, heavy-grade mineral oil plus a purgative hastens the removal of the chemical from the intestine. Activated charcoal appears to be useful in preventing absorption from the GI tract. When signs are excitatory, a sedative anticonvulsant such as a barbiturate or diazepam is indicated. Anything in the environment that stresses the animal—noise, handling etc—should be reduced or removed if possible. If the animal shows marked depression, anorexia, and dehydration, therapy should be directed toward rehydration and nourishment either IV or by stomach tube. Residues in exposed animals may be reduced by giving a slurry of activated charcoal or providing charcoal in feed. Feeding phenobarbital, 5 g/day, may hasten residue removal.

Examples of Organochlorines

DDT

Chemistry

— Dichloro-diphenyl-trichloroethane (DDT); insoluble in water.

— Not to be used on livestock or premises where livestock are housed.

Metabolism in animals

— Poorly absorbed from the skin as powder or in water suspension.

a. An oily vehicle increases absorption of DDT

b. Poorly absorbed from the GI tract

c. Fator fat solvents in the GItract increase absorption of DDT

— Distributes to all tissues, but selectively distributes to fat. Will store in fat over a period of time and reach levels higher than the level in the ration. Is cumulative.

— Partly biotrans formed by the liver.

— Excreted by kidney both free and in metabolites.

— Excreted by mammary gland in the butterfat of milk

Toxicity

— DDT has a relatively wide margin of safety under common uses because little is absorbed into the blood.

– Order of decreasing species-susceptibility to DDT toxicity:

1. Rodents	6. Monkey
2. Cat	7. Swine
3. Dog	8. Horse
4. Rabbit	9. Cow
5. Guinea pig	10. Sheep
11. Goat	

– Young animals are especially susceptible.

– Fasted animals are especially susceptible.

Toxic reactions:

1. Stimulation of CNS produce tremors, in coordinated walk, convulsions, coma, respiratory failure and eventually death from respiratory paralysis.
2. Sensory nerve is most sensitive; nerve ganglia are least sensitive.
3. Produces a change in the permeability of the nerve membrane.
4. Produces a prolongation of the falling phase of nerve action potential(i. e., negative after potential). 5. High body temperature.
6. Liver damage by high doses.

Treatment of toxicity:

1. Use a CNS depressant such as barbiturate anesthesia. Use with care.
2. Remove the source of exposure.

To reduce a body load of DDT, which is particularly useful in lactating dairy cows, administer:

1. Phenobarbital in the feed. This speeds liver biotransformation of DDT via enzyme induction.
2. Activated charcoal traps DDT and its metabolites in the in the GI tract for excretion with feces. Not greatly effective.

Analogs of DDT:

Methoxychlor is one of the important analogs of DDT. It is less toxic, has little tendency to accumulate in body fat and there is little secretion into milk.

Cyclodienes

These are more complex chemically than DDT. They are very good insecticides. Many of them are synthesized by what is referred to as DielsAlder reaction. Chlordeneis not an insecticide by itself. It is important as a precursor of chlordane.

Chlorination of chlordene to 68 to 69% gives chlordane which is a mixture of compounds. This mixture has three components; (1) betachlordane, (2) alfa-chlordane, and (3) heptachlor. Beta-chlordane is a cis isomer and is usually the active component. The other compounds of cyclodiene group include aldrin and dieldrin. Toxaphene has a cyclic structure but it is different from cyclodienes in being a simple molecule.

Chlordane: It is a dark brown viscous liquid and is soluble in organic solvents, insoluble in water. Its toxicity varies from preparation to preparation. The acute toxicity of chlordane is slightly less than DDT, the average single oral lethal dose being about 200-300 mg/kg for rats, rabbits, and dogs. Sheep are much more sensitive. The minimum oral toxic dose for young calves is about 25 mg/kg. The chronic toxicity of chlordane is considerably higher in animals like rabbits, sheep, goats and cattle.

Heptachlor: It is usually prepared in the form of waxy solid and is very stable and is a broad spectrum insecticide. The oral dose is of the order of 100 mg/kg. Its epoxide, heptachlor epoxide, is about ten times more toxic (orally) to dairy calves than the parent compound.

Aldrin: This is one of the most toxic of this group of insecticides. The single oral lethal dose is about 40 mg per kg in rats and slightly more in rabbits and dogs. For young calves the minimum toxic dose is about 5 mg per kg. It also has a high level of chronic toxicity. Isodrin is an isomer of aldrin and is much more toxic, the single oral lethal dose being 12-17 mg/kg.

Dieldrin: It is rather less acutely and chronically toxic than aldrin. The average single oral lethal dose for all species is 50-90 mg/kg. For one to two-week calves the single oral toxic dose is about 10-20 mg/kg. It is used as a seed dressing and is reported that wildbirds eating the treated seeds are very susceptible to dieldrin. Endrin is the isomer of dieldrin, the single oral lethal dose is about 10-12 mg/kg. Endrin together with lindane, aldrin and dieldrin has been found to be effective as a systemic acaricide in cattle. Also, it is used for the control of cotton insect.

Toxaphene: It is also a mixture of compounds and is obtained by chlorinating camphene. Dogs seem to be particularly susceptible to the acute action of toxaphene. The oral lethal dose is about 20-40 mg/kg. In young calves, oral dose of about 5 mg/kg produced toxic symptoms. Chickens appear to be relatively resistant. Chronic toxicity is relatively low. Strobane is very similar to toxaphene and is used in control of soil inhabiting insects. Endosulfan and Telodrin are compounds related to cyclodienes.

Mode of action

In general they have high degree of toxicity for most insects; topical toxicity to mammals is not very high. They are broad spectrum insecticides. They are nerve poisons but specific action is unknown. They seem to work on CNS. They all produce similar symptoms and that is why they tend to be regarded as having the same mode of action. The symptoms include tremors, convulsions and paralysis.

Hexachlorocyclohexanes

These compounds are related to cyclodienes and are formed by chlorination of benzene in presence of UV light. It is a mixture of compounds of 5 isomers which have lost the aromatic character of the ring. Alfa-isomer of hexachlorocyclohexane (HCH) is the most common(+80%). Gamma-isomerconstitutes about 10-15% in the crude mixture. Gamma-isomerwaspurified and called lindane which has insecticidal properties. In the literature, it is wrongly called benzene hexachloride. Benzenehexa-chloride (BHC) is used as a fungicide.

Lindane: It is odorless, white crystalline solid, stable, and is soluble in organic solvents. Lindane (gamma-isomer of HCH) has acute toxic effect greater than other isomers. The average single oral lethal dose of HCH (12% gamma-isomer) is said to have about 1gm/kg. The minimum toxic dose of lindane was found to be 5 mg/ kg in baby calves, and 25 mg in older cattle and sheep. Young animals are more susceptible to HCH. It is excreted in milk.

Mode of action

The mode of action of lindane and its isomers is not well understood, some say it apparently attacks the ganglia of the nervous system, while others claim that it is a neurotoxic agent whose action is similar to that of DDT. In acute toxicity, hypersensitivity, tremors and convulsions are seen. Chronic exposure results liver enlargement in mammals.

Mirex and Kepone

Mirex has been used extensively in the south eastern U. S. for control of fire ant. Dietary feeding of mirex to rats resulted in hepatocellular carcinoma. It is degraded to kepone in body. Kepone is more toxic than mirex and is known to cause tremors, liver injury and reproductive dysfunction in exposed population.

BOTANICAL INSECTICIDES

The most commonly used insecticides of natural origin are pyrethrins, rotenone and nicotine. All are characterized by very low stability, i. e., a short time of action. Pyrethrins are among the oldest insecticides and were most used during the inter war period. Their action is prompt, and affect the insects by contact. Pyrethrin dust or extract is obtained from the flowers of Chrysanthemum cinerariaefolium, which contain 0. 5-3% of active component, comprising esters of chrysanthemum dicarboxylic acid with ketoalcohols pyrethrolone and cinerolone.

Most insecticides derived from plants (eg, derris [rotenone] and pyrethrum) have traditionally been considered safe for use on animals.

Pyrethrins

This is a closely related group of naturally occurring compounds that are the active insecticidal ingredients of pyrethrum. Pyrethrum is extracted from the flowers of Chrysanthemum cinerariaefolium and has been an effective insecticide for many years. Synergists, such as piperonyl butoxide, sesamex, piperonyl cyclonene, etc, are added to increase stability and effectiveness. This is accomplished by inhibiting mixed function oxidases, enzymes that destroy pyrethrum; unfortunately, this also potentiates mammalian toxicity.

Pyrethroids: These are synthetic derivatives of natural pyrethrins and include allethrin, cypermethrin, decamethrin, fenvalerate, fluvalinate, permethrin, and tetramethrin. Generally, these compounds are more effective and less toxic to mammals than natural pyrethrins; they appear to be not well absorbed from the skin (however, allergic manifestations through skin contact and inhalation are common in humans). Mildly affected animals as well as those in early stages of toxicosis often show hypersalivation, vomiting, diarrhea, mild tremors, hyperexcitability, or depression. This syndrome may be confused with organophosphate or carbamate toxicosis. More severely affected animals can have hyperthermia, hypothermia, dyspnea, severe tremors, disorientation, and seizures. Death is due to respiratory failure. Clinical signs usually begin within a few hours of exposure, but the onset may be altered by the rate of dermal absorption or the timing of grooming behavior.

Generally, treatment is not required after ingestion of a dilute pyrethrin or pyrethroid preparations. Because the chief hazard may be the solvent, induction of emesis may be contraindicated. A slurry of activated charcoal at 2-8 g/kg may be administered, followed by a saline cathartic (magnesium or sodium sulfate [10% solution] at 0. 5 mg/kg). Vegetable oils and fats, which promote the intestinal absorption of pyrethrum, should be avoided. If dermal exposure occurs, the animal should be bathed with a mild detergent and cool water. The area should be washed very gently so as not to stimulate the circulation and enhance skin absorption. Initial assessment of the animal's respiratory and cardiovascular integrity is important. Further treatment involves symptomatic and supportive care. Seizures should be controlled with either diazepam (administered to effect at 0. 2-2 mg/kg, IV) or methocarbamol (55-220 mg/kg, IV, not exceeding 200 mg/min). Phenobarbital or pentobarbital (IV), to effect, can be used if diazepam or methocarbamol are too short acting.

d-Limonene: This is used for the control of fleas on cats and for other insect pests. Adult fleas and eggs appear to be most sensitive to d-limonene, which is more effective if combined with piperonyl butoxide. At recommended dosages, the solution containing d-limonene appears to be safe, but increasing the concentration 5-10 fold in sprays or dips increases the severity of toxic signs, which include salivation, muscle tremors, ataxia, and hypothermia. The inclusion of piperonyl butoxide in the formulation potentiates the toxicity in cats. Allergies have also been reported in people in contact with d-limonene, and it appears to increase dermal absorption of some chemicals.

Nicotine

Nicotine is an alkaloid contained in different species of tobacco. It is a colorless, oily liquid, soluble in water and in many organic solvents with which it usually mixes in any ratio. Its reaction is basic. Nicotine rapidly takes on a brown colour when exposed to the air and gives off the smell of tobacco. It is one of the oldest insecticidal preparations and is often used for aphid control in horticulture. Its residual action is short, three days at the most, due to its high volatility. Nicotine is absorbed by the mucous membranes and intact skin, and excreted in milk.

Etiology of Poisoning

Animals are mostly poisoned by nicotine when bathed in, or washed with, tobacco-leafdecoction; nowadays the commonest cause is inexpert use of nicotine preparations for plant protection. However, ingestion of a large amount of dry tobacco may also be the cause of poisoning, since animals devour it with pleasure.

Toxicity

Nicotinoids are not particularly toxic to insects, e. g., LD50 of nicotine in insect is 300-600 mg/kg. But for animals it is extremely toxic. In laboratory animals the oral LD50 is 24 mg/kg in the mouse and 55 mg/kg in the rat. The minimum lethal dose of nicotine for the dog and cat is 20 to 100 mg; 100-300 mg for horse and 100-200 mg for sheep. Poisoning in the animals almost invariably results from the improper use of the 40% solution of nicotine sulfate.

Symptoms

Nicotinoids act on CNS, primarily on the ganglia. Low concentration produces excitation, rapid respiration, salivation, irritation, diarrhea, vomiting, convulsions and death. Poisoned animals may die within 15-30 minutes in heavy spasms of the respiratory muscles. The symptoms of poisoning vary with the mode of penetration of the poison into the body. Tympany, colic and diarrhea prevail in the early stages. Inhalation of nicotine vapour may kill poultry within a few minutes.

Post-mortem findings

Necropsy of animals which have died from oral poisoning reveals acute hemorrhagicgastroenteritis. The contents of the digestive tract smell of tobacco. In dead animals poisoned by the absorption of nicotine through the skin, dissection reveals only hemorrhages in the serous tissues and hyperemia of the lungs and brain.

Treatment

Cases of acute nicotine poisoning hardly afford a favourable prognosis. Nicotine must be washed from the body surface with water if it has got into the body through the skin. Stomach lavage is recommended if the animal is to be saved after oral poisoning. Tannin is a suitable antidote, and the administration of a large quantity of strong tea or some caffeine is recommended. Artificial respiration, oxygen inhalation and lobeline administration may be tried when the animals show depression of the CNS.

REFERENCES

Colin, M. E.; Bonmatin, J. M.; Moineau, I., et al. 2004. "A method to quantify and analyze the foraging activity of honey bees: Relevance to the sublethal effects induced by systemic insecticides". *Archives of Environmental Contamination and Toxicology*. Volume: 47 Issue: 3 Pages: 387-395

Oldroyd BP. 2007. "What's Killing American Honey Bees"? *PLoS Biology* 5(6): e168 doi:10.1371/journal.pbio.0050168) Retrieved on 2007-05-17.

Palmer, WE, Bromley, PT, and Brandenburg, RL. 2007. *Wildlife & pesticides— Peanuts*. North Carolina Cooperative Extension Service.

3

Herbicides, Fungicides and Rodenticides

HERBICIDES

Herbicides are used routinely to control noxious plants. Most of these chemicals, particularly the more recently developed synthetic organic herbicides, are quite selective for specific plants and have low toxicity for mammals; other less selective compounds (e.g, arsenicals, chlorates, dinitrophenols) are more toxic to animals. Most toxicity problems in animals result from exposure to excessive quantities of herbicides because of improper or careless use or disposal of containers. When used properly, problems are rare.

Vegetation treated with herbicides at proper rates normally will not be hazardous to animals, including humans. Particularly after the herbicides have dried on the vegetation, only small amounts can be dislodged. When herbicide applications have been excessive, damage to lawns, crops, or other foliage is often evident.

The residue potential for most of these agents is low. However, the possibility of residues should be explored if significant exposure of food-producing animals occurs. The time recommended before treated vegetation is grazed or used as animal feed is available for a number of products.

Some of the more commonly used herbicides are discussed below. More specific information is available on the label and from the manufacturer, cooperative extension service, or poison control center. In addition, selected information on herbicides available for use on common field, vegetable, and fruit crops in the USA and Canada is included as a guideline for common toxicologic concerns. These include the toxicity of a chemical relative to other herbicides (acute toxicity, LD50), the amount an animal can be exposed to without being affected (no effect level, NOEL), and the likelihood of problems caused by dermal contact (dermal LD50, eye and skin irritation). These chemicals are used widely in food crop production and are an important source of environmental exposure to avian and aquatic species, both wild and domesticated.

Herbicide poisoning is a rare finding in veterinary practice. With few exceptions, it is only when animals gain direct access to the product that acute poisoning occurs. Acute signs usually will not lead to a diagnosis, although acute GI signs are frequent. All common differential diagnoses should be excluded in animals showing signs of a sudden onset of disease or sudden death. The case history is critical. Sickness following feeding, spraying of pastures or crops adjacent to pastures, a change in housing, or direct exposure may lead to a tentative diagnosis of herbicide poisoning. Frequently, the nature of exposure is hard to identify because of storage of herbicides in mis- or unlabeled containers. Unidentified spillage of liquid from containers or powder from broken bags near a feed source, or visual confusion with a dietary ingredient or supplement, may cause the exposure. Once a putative chemical source has been identified, an animal poison control center should be contacted for information on treatments, laboratory tests, and likely outcome.

Chronic disease caused by herbicides is even more difficult to diagnose. It may include a history of herbicide use in proximity to the animals or animal feed or water source, or a gradual change in the animals' performance or behavior over a period of weeks, months, or even years. Occasionally, it involves manufacture or storage of herbicides nearby. Samples of possible sources (ie, contaminated feed and water) for residue analysis, as well as tissues from exposed animals taken at necropsy, are essential. Months or even years may be required to successfully identify a problem of chronic exposure.

If poisoning is suspected, the first step in management is to halt further exposure. Animals should be separated from any possible source before attempting to stabilise and support them. If there are life-threatening signs, efforts to stabilise animals by general mitigation methods should be started. Any treatments undertaken should make a clear improvement in the most affected animals, as the physical act of handling and treatment, although logical, may make their condition worse. Specific antidotal treatments, when available, may help to confirm the diagnosis. As time permits, a more detailed history and investigation should be completed. The owner should be made aware of the need for full disclosure of facts in order to successfully determine the source of poisoning, eg, unapproved use or failure to properly store a chemical.

Inorganic Herbicides

Arsenicals

The use of inorganic arsenicals (sodium arsenite and arsenic trioxide) as herbicides has been reduced greatly because of livestock losses, environmental persistence, and their association with carcinogenesis. Sodium arsenate and chromic copper arsenate do not have active EPA registration. Arsenic derivatives continue to be available in other parts of the world in wood preservatives and insecticide formulations. These compounds can be hazardous to animals when used as recommended. Ruminants (even deer) are apparently attracted to and lick plants poisoned with arsenite.

The highly soluble organic arsenicals (methane arsonate, methyl arsonic acid) can concentrate in pools in toxic quantities after a rain has washed them from recently treated plants. Arsenicals are used as desiccants or defoliants on cotton, and residues of cotton harvest fed to cattle may contain toxic amounts of arsenic. Signs and lesions caused by organic arsenical herbicides resemble those of inorganic arsenical poisoning. Single toxic oral doses for cattle and sheep are 22-55 mg/kg body wt. Poisoning may be expected from smaller doses if consumed on successive days. Dimercaprol (3 mg/kg for large animals, and 2.5-5 mg/kg for small animals, IM, every 4-6 hr) is the recommended therapy. Sodium thiosulfate also has been used (20-30 g, PO in ~300 mL of water for cattle; one-fourth this dose for sheep); however, a rationale for its use is not established, and it may be unrewarding.

Ammonium Sulfamate

Ammonium sulfamate currently has no active EPA registration in the USA. It is used to kill brush and poison ivy. Ruminants apparently can metabolise this chemical to some extent and, in some studies, exposed animals made better gains than did controls. However, sudden deaths have occurred in cattle and deer that consumed treated plants. Large doses (>1.5 g/kg body wt) induce ammonia poisoning in ruminants. Treatment is designed to lower rumen pH by dilution with copious amounts of water to which weak acetic acid (vinegar) has been added.

Borax

Borax has been used as a herbicide, an insecticide, and a soil sterilant. It is toxic to animals if consumed in moderate to large doses (>0.5 g/kg). Poisoning has not been reported when borax was used properly but has occurred when it was accidentally added to livestock feed and when borax powder was scattered in the open for cockroach control. Principal signs of acute poisoning are diarrhea, rapid prostration, and perhaps convulsions. An effective antidote is not known. Balanced electrolyte fluid therapy with supportive care is indicated.

Sodium Chlorate

This is now seldom used as a herbicide but remains registered. Treated plants and contaminated clothing are highly combustible and constitute fire hazards. In addition, many cases of chlorate poisoning of livestock have occurred both from ingestion of treated plants and from accidental consumption of feed to which it was mistakenly added as salt. Cattle sometimes are attracted to foliage treated with sodium chlorate. Considerable quantities must be consumed before signs of toxicity appear. The minimum lethal dose is 1.1 g/kg body wt for cattle, 1.54-2.86 g/kg for sheep, and 5. 06 g/kg for poultry. Ingestion results in hemolysis of RBC and conversion of Hgb to methemoglobin.

Treatment with methylene blue (10 mg/kg) must be repeated frequently because, unlike the nitrites, the chlorate ion is not inactivated during the conversion of Hgb to methemoglobin and is capable of producing an unlimited quantity of methemoglobin as long as it is present in the body. Blood transfusions may reduce some of the tissue anoxia caused by methemoglobin; isotonic saline can hasten elimination of the chlorate ion. Mineral oil containing 1% sodium thiosulfate will inhibit further absorption of chlorate in monogastric animals.

Organic Herbicides

Organic herbicides are plant growth regulators, and some members of this group are more toxic than others. Hemolysis, methemoglobinemia, and immunotoxicity have occurred after experimental exposure to propanil. The half-life in catfish is >15 days. Major organic herbicides are:

- Bipyridyl Compounds or Quaternary Ammonium Herbicides (diquat, paraquat)
- Carbamate and Thiocarbamate Compounds (terbucarb, asulam, carboxazole, EPTC, pebulate, triallate, vernolate, butylate, thiobencarb)
- Aromatic/Benzoic Acid Compounds (chloramben, dicamba)
- Phenoxyacetic and Phenoxybutyric Compounds (2, 4-D [2-4-dichlorophenoxyacetic acid], 2, 4, 5-T [2, 4, 5-trichlorophenoxyacetic acid], 2, 4-DB, MCPA)
- Dinitrophenolic Compounds (dinoseb, binapacryl, DNOC)
- Organophosphate Compounds (glyphosate, bensulide)
- Triazolopyrimidine Compounds (bromacil, terbacil)
- Phenyl or Substituted Urea Compounds (diuron, fenuron, linuron, monolinuron)
- Polycyclic Alkanoic Acids or Aryloxypheno-xypropionic Compounds (diclofop, fenoxaprop, fenthiaprop, fluazifop, haloxyfop)
- Triazinylsulfonylurea or Sulfonylurea Compounds (chlorsulfuron, sulfometuron, ethametsulfuron, chloremuron)

— Triazine, Methylthiotriazine, Triazinone Compounds (atrazine, cyanazine, prometryn, metribuzin, simazine)

Bipyridyl Compounds

The bipyridyl compounds are nonvolatile desiccant herbicides used at rather low rates of 2 oz/acre (150 mL/hectare). These compounds act rapidly, are inactivated on soil contact, and rapidly decompose in light. They produce toxic effects in the tissues of exposed animals by development of free radicals. Tissues can be irritated after contact (eg, mouth lesions after recent spraying of pastures). Skin irritation and corneal opacity occur on external exposure to these chemicals, and inhalation is dangerous. Animals, including humans, have died as a result of drinking from contaminated containers.

Paraquat and diquat have somewhat different mechanisms of action. Diquat exerts most of its harmful effects in the GI tract. Animals drinking from an old diquat container showed anorexia, gastritis, GI distension, and severe loss of water into the lumen of the GI tract. Signs of renal impairment, CNS excitement, and convulsions occur in severely affected individuals. Lung lesions are uncommon.

Paraquat has a biphasic toxic action after ingestion. Immediate effects include excitement, convulsions or depression and incoordination, gastroenteritis with anorexia, and possibly renal involvement and respiratory difficulty.

Eye, nasal, and skin irritation can be caused by direct contact, followed within days to 2 wk by pulmonary lesions as a result of lipid-membrane peroxidation and thus destruction of the type I alveolar pneumocytes. This is reflected in progressive respiratory distress and is evident on necropsy as pulmonary edema, hyaline membrane deposition, and alveolar fibrosis. Toxicity of paraquat is enhanced by deficiency of vitamin E or selenium, oxygen, and low tissue activity of glutathione peroxidase.

Due to slow absorption of these chemicals, intensive oral administration of adsorbants in large quantities and cathartics is advised. Bentonite or Fuller's earth is preferred, but activated charcoal will suffice. In conjunction with supportive therapy, eg, vitamin E and selenium, excretion is accelerated by forced diuresis induced by mannitol and furosemide. Oxygen therapy should not be used, and some suggest only 15% oxygen in inspired air.

Carbamate and Thiocarbamate Compounds

These herbicides are moderately toxic; however, they are used at low concentrations, and poisoning problems would not be expected from normal use. Massive overdosage, as seen with accidental exposure, produces symptoms similar to the insecticide carbamates, with lack of appetite, depression, respiratory difficulty, mouth watering, diarrhea, weakness, and seizures. Thiobencarb has induced toxic neuropathies in neonatal and adult laboratory rats. It appears to increase permeability of the blood-brain barrier.

Aromatic/Benzoic Acid Compounds

The herbicides in this group have a low order of toxicity to domestic animals, and poisoning after normal use has not been reported. Environmental persistence and toxicity to wildlife is also low for this group. The signs and lesions are similar to those described for the phenoxyacetic compounds.

Phenoxyacetic and Phenoxybutyric Compounds

These acids and their salts and esters are commonly used to control undesirable plants. As a group, they are essentially nontoxic to animals exposed to properly treated forage. When large doses are fed experimentally, general depression, anorexia, weight loss, tenseness, and muscular weakness (particularly of the hindquarters) are noted. Large doses in cattle may interfere with rumen function. Dogs may develop myotonia, ataxia, posterior weakness, vomiting, diarrhea, and metabolic acidosis. Even large doses, up to 2 g/kg, have not been shown to leave residues in the fat of animals. These compounds are plant growth regulators, and treatment may result in increased palatability of some poisonous plants as well as increased nitrate and cyanide content.

The use of 2, 4, 5-T was curtailed because extremely toxic contaminants, collectively called dioxins (TCDD and HCDD), were found in technical grade material. The 2, 3, 7, 8-TCDD is considered carcinogenic, mutagenic, teratogenic, fetotoxic, and able to cause reproductive damage and other toxic effects. Although manufacturing methods have reduced the level of the contaminants, use of this herbicide is very limited worldwide. Its EPA registration was canceled and it is no longer manufactured in the USA.

Dinitrophenolic Compounds

The old 2-4 dinitrophenol and dinitrocresol compounds were highly toxic to all classes of animals (eg, LD50 of 20-56 mg/kg body wt). Poisoning can occur if animals are sprayed accidentally or have immediate access to forage that has been sprayed, because these compounds are readily absorbed through skin or lungs. Dinitrophenolic herbicides markedly increase oxygen consumption and deplete glycogen reserves. Clinical signs include fever, dyspnea, acidosis, tachycardia, and convulsions, followed by coma and death with a rapid onset of rigor mortis. Cataracts can occur in animals with chronic dinitrophenol intoxication. Exposure to dinitro compounds may cause yellow staining of the skin, conjunctiva, or hair. An effective antidote is not known. Affected animals should be cooled and sedated to help control hyperthermia. Phenothiazine tranquilizers are contraindicated; however, diazepam can be used to calm the animal. Atropine sulfate, aspirin, and antipyretics should not be used. Administration of intravenous (IV) drug of large doses of carbohydrate solutions and parenteral vitamin A may be useful. If toxic amounts of one of these is ingested and the animal is alert, emetics should be administered in animals that readily vomit (e.g., not horses); if the animal is depressed, gastric lavage should be performed. Treatment with activated charcoal should follow.

Organophosphate Compounds

These are widely used herbicides with low toxicity, although fish and pond life have been killed experimentally. Sprayed forage appears to be preferred by cattle for 5-7 days after application and causes little or no problem. Acute LD50 in rats is >5.6 g/kg.

A few dogs and cats show eye, skin, and upper respiratory tract signs when exposed during or subsequent to an application to weeds or grass. Nausea, vomiting, staggering, and hindleg weakness have been seen in dogs and cats that were exposed to fresh chemical on treated foliage. The signs usually disappear when exposure ceases, and minimal symptomatic treatment is needed. Washing the chemical off the skin, evacuating the stomach, and tranquilising the animal are usually sufficient. Massive exposure with acute signs due to accidental contact should be handled as an organophosphate poisoning.

Bensulide, listed as a plant growth regulator, has an oral LD50 in rats of 271-770 mg/kg, in dogs the lethal dose is ~200 g/kg. The most prominent clinical sign is anorexia, but other signs are similar to 2, 4-D poisoning.

Triazolopyrimidine Compounds

These compounds can cause mild toxic signs at levels of 50 mg/kg body wt in sheep, 250 mg/kg in cattle, and 500 mg/kg in poultry when given daily for 8-10 doses. Signs include bloat, incoordination, depression, and anorexia. Application rates of ~5 lb/acre (5. 6 kg/hectare) can be hazardous, especially for sheep, but no field cases of toxicity have been reported.

Phenyl or Substituted Urea Compounds

Exposure to toxic amounts of these herbicides is unlikely with recommended application and handling of containers. Signs and lesions are similar to those described for the phenoxyacetic herbicides. The substituted urea herbicides induce hepatic microsomal enzymes and may alter metabolism of other xenobiotic agents. Altered calcium metabolism and bone morphology have been seen in laboratory animals.

Polycyclic Alkanoic Acids

Members of this group that are approved as herbicides are of moderately low toxicity with acute oral LD50 doses from 950 mg/kg to >4, 000 mg/kg. (Haloxyfop-methyl is an exception and has an LD50 in male rats of ~400 mg/kg.) They tend to be more toxic if exposure is dermal. The dermal LD50 of diclofop in rabbits is only 180 mg/kg.

Triazinylsulfonylurea or Sulfonylurea Compounds

Toxicity in this group appears to be quite low. The oral acute LD50 in rats is in the range of 4, 000-5, 000 mg/kg. The dermal acute LD50 in rabbits is ~2, 000 mg/kg.

Triazine, Methylthiotriazine, Triazinone Compounds

Although these herbicides are widely used, incidents of poisoning are uncommon. Occasionally, accidental exposure of animals to large dosages (eg, open containers, spills) can cause toxic effects and even death. (Doses of 500 mg of simazine/kg or 30 mg of atrazine/kg for 36-60 days were lethal to sheep.) Generally, single doses >100-200 mg/kg body wt can be detrimental; repeat administration may reduce the toxic dose to <100 mg/kg body wt. Deaths have been reported in sheep and horses grazing triazine-treated pastures 1-7 days after spraying. Cumulative effects are not evident. The signs and lesions are similar to those described for the phenoxyacetic compounds.

The oral LD50 of metribuzin is 2, 200 mg/kg in rats and 500-1, 000 mg/kg in birds. No harmful effects were apparent when it was fed to dogs at 100 ppm in the diet.

FUNGICIDES

Fungicides are chemical substances used to combat parasitic fungi. Many fungi may be responsible for diseases of cultivated plants, thus reducing yields and causing damage to stores of grain, foodstuffs and industrial raw materials (wood, leather and others).

Fungicides destroy fungi by a fungicidal or fungistatic effect (the latter only arrests the growth and development of fungi without killing them). Fungicides are used in agriculture for the protection of growing plants and also for the prevention of fungus diseases in seeds. Fungicidal compounds used in seed treatments are known as seed dressings or disinfectants.

In selecting which fungicides to use, as with any pesticides, due thought should be given not only to the desired effect, i. e., fungicidal action, but also to all undesirable side-effects, such as possibilities of poisoning in man and animals, impairment of the biological balance of nature, accumulation of poisonous substances in the soil, etc.

There are at least 250 different types of fungicides. They include copper compounds, sulfur preparations, inorganic and organic derivatives of mercury and miscellaneous organic compounds. The main hazard to live stock from fungicides is likely toarise from their useasseed-dressing for the protection of stored grain, potatoes, etc., and there are number of reported cases of poisoning in horses, cattle, pigs and poultry caused by feeding of treated grain.

Many of the carriers or solvents for fungicides are in them- selves toxic. Carbon disulfide, carbontetrachloride, ethylene dibromide, formaldehyde, petroleum ethers, and low molecular weight hydrocarbons may serve as a carrier for fungicides. Animals housed close to the storage of treated grain may suffer from the vapors of these volatile compounds. Toxicological implications of some of the fungicides are discussed below.

Copper Fungicides

Until recently, copper compounds were the most widely used fungicides. Nowadays they are being gradually replaced by organic fungicides. The oldest preparation of this group is cupric sulfate pentahydrate. It is also used as a constituent of spray mixtures. Copper oxychloride is contained in preparations used mainly for the spraying of farm crops. Cupric sulphate is used mainly for algae control in lakes and as a wood preservative.

Mercurial Fungicides

These compounds are important as seed dressings but may also be used for spraying field crops. Of the inorganic mercury compounds, mercuric chloride, $HgCl_2$, and mercurous chloride (calomel), Hg_2Cl_2, were used in the past, though now they have been replaced by organic mercury compounds.

Phenylmercuric chloride is a constituent of preparations used as dry seed dressings. It is a solid substance, insoluble in water, with a high fungicidal effect, good stability in air, and good adhesive properties. Its oral LD50 for the rat is 20-50 mg/kg. Phenyl mercuric acetate is a constituent of a number of seed-dressings (Germisan), all having a similar effect and toxi- city. Its oral LD50 for rat is between 60 and 100 mg/kg. Ethyl mercuric chloride, C_2H_5-Hg-Cl, is the active agent of a dryseed-dressing preparation which is more toxic than the phenyl mercuric chloride preparations.

These seed-dressings mentioned above are often combined with other fungicides(benzenehexachloride)or insecticides, either chlorinated (e.g., lindane)or organophosphorous (e.g., disyston).

Etiology of poisoning

Farm animals are poisoned if fed treated grain. Mercurial fungicides are now widely used as seed dressings, and frequently give rise to poisoning, particularly in pigs. Wild birds (pigeons, pheasants, etc.) are often poisoned in spring in fields sown with disinfected seeds.

Course of poisoning

Pigs fed disinfected grain for over a long period showed vision disturbances, anorexia, normal to subnormal body temperature and locomotor disturbances. Deaths occurred within a week of development of the first symptoms. Hematuria and intense diarrhea are frequent symptoms of poisoning, and the feces are blood-stained. Nervous symptoms, timidity, tremor and paresis occur when the condition is protracted.

Poultry may develop necrotic inflammation of the mucous membranes of the crop and stomach. There is intense diarrhea with offensively smelling, bloodstained feces. Central nervous system lesions appear as in coordination of movement, dizziness and muscu-lartremors. General weakness becomes paralysis. Kidney function is also impaired.

Post-mortem findings

Necropsy reveals damage of different intensity in the digestive tract from congestion to necrotic peeling of the mucous membranes. Further, the kidneys are enlarged and congested; parenchymatous degeneration of the liver and degenerative changes of the cerebral tissue also occur.

Treatment

Activated charcoal may be used. Sodium thio- sulphate may be given orally or intravenously. Proteins should be given in large quantities. Infusion of saline is recommended for more rapid elimination of the poison from the body. Antibiotics should also be administered to prevent secondary infection. Dimercaprol may be used therapeutically in cases of mercury poisoning.

Fungicides Containing Sulfur

Preparations containing elementary sulfur are among the oldest fungicides. Wet sulfur preparations, applicable as sprays, are the most widely used. These are powders or pastes containing a suspension of sulfur and usually referred to as colloidal sulfur. These preparations are practically non-toxic for animals.

Carbamate Fungicides

The carbamate fungicides are all derivatives of dithiocarbamic acid (NH_2-CS_2-H). These fungicides are widely used and have low toxicity.

Zineb (Zincethylene-bis-dithiocarbamate). It is a stable compound, insoluble in water which decomposes in an acid medium. Its oral LD50 is 5,200 mg/kg.

Maneb (Manganese ethylene-bis-dithiocarbamate). There is little difference between maneb and zineb, either in their physical and chemical properties or in their toxicity.

Ziram (Zinc N, N-dimethyl dithiocarbamate). Ziram is insoluble in water and has a low toxicity. The oral is 500-1400 mg/kg.

Thiram (Tetramethylthiuram disulphide). It is insoluble in water and has low toxicity. Its oral LD50 for the rat is 780-865 mg/kg and for the rabbit 210 mg/kg. It is a widely used fungicide and may also be used as a seed-dressing. Tentofiftyppm of thiram in diets fedtolayinghens caused as light increase, and 100-200 ppm a considerable increase, in the proportion of soft shelled or otherwise abnormal eggs. Chickens fed on mixtures containing 40 ppm of thiram were weak. Goslings fed diets containing 150 ppm lost weight and had deformed legs. However, young male turkeys withstood 200 ppm in their diet.

Pentachlorophenol (PCP)

In addition to its use as a fungicide, pentachlorophenol and its salts enjoy a wide range of applications. These include the following:

- Fungicide and/or bactericide in the processing of cellulose products starches, adhesives, leather, oils, paints and rubber.
- Rug shampoos and textiles to control mildew.
- Food processing plants to control mold and slime.
- Mothproofing of fabrics (pentachlorophenyl laurate).
- Construction and lumber for mold and termite control;
- Control power post beetles and wood boring insects.
- Herbicide and preharvest desiccant.

- Fungicide on seeds and bulbs (SPERGON).
- Molluscacide-snail intermediate host of human schistosomes.
- Processing aid in manufacture of polyvinyl chloride emulsion polymers.
- Manufacture of closure-sealing gaskets for food containers (not to exceed 0.05 percent by weight).
- Wood preservative in wooden crates for packaging raw agriculture products (not to exceed 50 ppm).

Pentachlorophenol is toxic and is absorbed by the skin. Its minimum single lethal oral dose is 120 mg per kg in sheep and 140 mg/kg in calves. The minimum toxic dose is 28 mg/kg for sheep.

In the majority of species, the minimum lethal dose ranges from 40 to 200 mg/kg, depending on the sex, age and condition of the animals as well as on the mode of administration and on the solvent used. Pentachlorophenol has a cumulative effect.

The clinical symptoms of percutaneous poisoning appear as erythema, dermatitis and acne. Hyperkeratosis develops as a result of continued contact of the skin with the preparation. Oral poisoning leads to general weakness, laboured breathing, increased body temperature, gastritis and enteritis. Further, kidney and liver function is impaired. Death generally occurs within 24 hrs, followed by rigor mortis within a few minutes. Hyperkeratosis also develops in cases of chronic poisoning, combined with damage to the tissue of the liver, kidneys and heart. Poisoned animals are very weak and emaciated. At necropsy, gastroenteritis, hepaitis and kidney damage are evident.

The treatment is symptomatic. It is necessary to eliminate the source of poisoning.

Dinitroorthocresol (DNOC)

This compound is a by-product of the dye industry. It is used as a fungicide, insecticide, wood preservative, and herbicide.

Absorption may be either oral, respiratory, or percutaneous. Dinitroderivatives produce uncoupling of oxidative phosphorylation resulting in increased oxidative processes with energy converted to heat instead of ATP. Clinically, this is manifested as fever, acidosis, and damage to myocardium. The toxic effects are potentiated by increased environmental temperature. The LD50 for dogs and swine is approximately 50 mg/kg.

Hyperpyrexia, dyspnea, early rigormortis, and yellow discoloration of the organs should suggest dinitrocresolor dinitrophenol as possible etiologic agents. Whole blood levels in excess of 10 mg/100 ml dinitrocresol correlates with poisoning. Presence of beta-carotene in blood may interfere with this test.

Treatment

Administer gastric lavage for oral exposure, using 5 percent sodium bicarbonate and activated charcoal. Catharsis with sodium sulfate is also indicated. Paraffin oil (but not castor oil) may be used because the dinitrocresol is fat soluble, butthe paraffin oil is not absorbed. Keeping the patient cool(e.g., with ice packs) is helpful and administration of thiouracilto slow the metabolic rate may be indicated.

Benzenehexachloride (BHC)

BHC, also known as hexachlorobenzene or HCH, is used as a fungicidal agent in the treatment of many seeds including grains. Also, it is a constituent of many disinfectants. Industrially, it is used in the manufacture of PCP. Exists as a contaminant of pentachloronitrobenzene, as oil fumigant used in cotton fields.

BHC causes severe skin manifestations including photosensitivity, permanent loss of hair and skin atrophy. Consumption of wheat that had been prepared for planting by treating with BHC has been reported to have caused mass poisoning in humans with the main symptoms being photosensititzation and porphyrinuria. Its oral LD50 value for rat is 1300-3500 mg/kg.

Captan

Captan is one of the widely used organic fungicides. Its oral toxicity to mammals is quite low. Its oral LD50 value for rat is 1-9 gm/kg. However, it is highly toxic intraperitoneally.

Others

Benomyl is a new carbamate fungicide that does not have a metal ion in its moiety. Its oral LD50 value for rats is greater than 10 g/kg.

Triphenyltinacetate (Fentin) and triphenyltinoxide (Du-ter) are the organic tin compounds used as fungicides. These compounds are soluble in fats and are absorbed percutaneously. Triphenyltinoxide irritates the skin and mucous membranes. Clinical signs of poisoning by this compound set in some time after absorption whereas those of triphenyltinacetate occur very soon. The function of the central nervous system is impaired. The symptoms of poisoning are similar to those of mercurial fungicide poisoning. The oral LD50 of triphenyltinacetate for the rat is 136-238 mg/kg, whereas the LD50 of triphenyltinoxide for the mouse is 550 mg/kg.

Mycotoxic Diseases

Acute or chronic toxicoses can result from exposure to feed or bedding contaminated with toxins that may be produced during growth of various saprophytic or phytopathogenic fungi or molds on cereals, hay, straw, pastures, or any other fodder. A few principles characterise mycotoxic diseases: 1) the cause may not be immediately identified; 2) they are not transmissible from one animal to another; 3) treatment with drugs or antibiotics has little effect on the course of the disease; 4) outbreaks are usually seasonal because particular climatic sequences may favor fungal growth and toxin production; 5) study indicates specific association with a particular feed; and 6) although large numbers of fungi found on examination of feedstuff does not necessarily indicate that toxin production has occurred.

Confirmation of diagnosis of mycotoxic disease requires a combination of information. Detection of fungal spores alone, even at high concentrations, is not sufficient for diagnosis; fungal spores or even mold growth may be present without formation of mycotoxins. Especially important in diagnosis is the presence of a disease documented to be caused by a known mycotoxin, combined with detection of the mycotoxin in either feedstuffs or animal tissues.

Sometimes more than one mycotoxin may be present in feedstuffs, and their different toxicologic properties may cause clinical signs and lesions that are not consistent with those seen when animals are dosed experimentally with pure, single mycotoxins. Several mycotoxins are immunosuppressive, which may allow viruses, bacteria, or parasites to create a secondary disease that is more obvious than the primary.

In reaching a diagnosis of mycotoxicosis characterised by reduced feed intake, reproductive failure, or increased infectious disease due to immunosuppression, differential diagnoses must be carefully established and eliminated by a combination of thorough clinical and historical evaluation, examination of production records, and close attention to appropriate diagnostic testing.

There are no specific antidotes for mycotoxins; removal of the source of the toxin (ie, the moldy feedstuff) eliminates further exposure. The absorption of some mycotoxins (eg, aflatoxin) has been effectively prevented by aluminosilicate. If financial circumstances do not allow for disposal of the moldy feed, it can be blended with unspoiled feed just before feeding to reduce the toxin concentration or fed to less susceptible species. When contaminated feed is blended with good feed, care must be taken to prevent further mold growth by the toxigenic contaminants. This may be accomplished by thorough drying or by addition of organic acids (eg, propionic acid) to prevent mold growth.

Aflatoxicosis

Aflatoxins are produced by toxigenic strains of Aspergillus flavus and A parasiticus on peanuts, soybeans, corn (maize), and other cereals either in the field or during storage when moisture content and temperatures are sufficiently high for mold growth. Usually, this means consistent day and night temperatures >70°F. The toxic response and disease in mammals and poultry varies in relation to species, sex, age, nutritional status, and the duration of intake and level of aflatoxins in the ration. Earlier recognised disease outbreaks called "moldy corn toxicosis", "poultry hemorrhagic syndrome" and "Aspergillus toxicosis" may have been caused by aflatoxins.

Aflatoxicosis occurs in many parts of the world and affects growing poultry (especially ducklings and turkey poults), young pigs, pregnant sows, calves, and dogs. Adult cattle, sheep, and goats are relatively resistant to the acute form of the disease but are susceptible if toxic diets are fed over long periods. Experimentally, all species of animals tested have shown some degree of susceptibility. Dietary levels of aflatoxin (in ppb) generally tolerated are =50 in young poultry, =100 in adult poultry, £50 in weaner pigs, =200 in finishing pigs, <100 in calves, and <300 in cattle. Dietary levels as low as 10-20 ppb may result in measurable metabolites of aflatoxin (aflatoxin M1 and M2) being excreted in milk; feedstuffs that contain aflatoxins should not be fed to dairy cows.

Aflatoxins bind to macromolecules, especially nucleic acids and nucleoproteins. Their toxic effects include mutagenesis due to alkylation of nuclear DNA, carcinogenesis, teratogenesis, reduced protein synthesis, and immunosuppression. Reduced protein synthesis results in reduced production of essential metabolic enzymes and structural proteins for growth. The liver is the principal organ affected. High doses of aflatoxins result in severe hepatocellular necrosis; prolonged low dosages result in reduced growth rate and liver enlargement.

Clinical Findings

In acute outbreaks, deaths occur after a short period of inappetence. Subacute outbreaks are more usual, and unthriftiness, weakness, anorexia, and sudden deaths can occur. Generally, aflatoxin concentrations in feed >1, 000 ppb are associated with acute aflatoxicosis. Frequently, there is a high incidence of concurrent infectious disease, often respiratory, that responds poorly to the usual chemotherapy.

Lesions

In acute cases, there are widespread hemorrhages and icterus. The liver is the major target organ. Microscopically, the liver shows marked fatty accumulations and massive centrilobular necrosis and hemorrhage. In subacute cases, the hepatic changes are not so pronounced, but the liver is somewhat enlarged and firmer than usual. There may be edema of the gallbladder. Microscopically, the liver shows proliferation and fibrosis of the bile ductules; the hepatocytes and their nuclei (megalocytosis) are enlarged. The GI mucosa may show glandular atrophy and associated inflammation. In the kidneys, there may be tubular degeneration and regeneration. Prolonged feeding of low concentrations of aflatoxins may result in diffuse liver fibrosis (cirrhosis) and carcinoma of the bile ducts or liver.

Diagnosis

Disease history, necropsy findings, and microscopic examination of the liver should indicate the nature of the hepatotoxin, but hepatic changes are somewhat similar in Senecio poisoning. The presence and levels of aflatoxins in the feed should be determined. Aflatoxin M1 can be detected in urine or kidney or in milk of lactating animals if toxin intakes are high.

Control

Contaminated feeds can be avoided by monitoring batches for aflatoxin content. Young, newly weaned, pregnant, and lactating animals require special protection from suspected toxic feeds. Dilution with noncontaminated feedstuff is one possibility. Ammoniation of grain reduces contamination but is not currently approved for use in food animals.

Hydrated sodium calcium aluminosilicates (HSCAS) have shown promise in reducing the effects of aflatoxin when fed to pigs or poultry; at 10 lb/ton (5 kg/tonne), they provided substantial protection against dietary aflatoxin. HSCAS reduced, but did not eliminate, residues of aflatoxin M1 in milk from dairy cows fed aflatoxin B1.

Ergotism

This worldwide disease of farm animals results from continued ingestion of sclerotia of the parasitic fungus Claviceps purpurea, which replaces the grain or seed of rye and other small grains or forage plants, such as the bromes, bluegrasses, and ryegrasses. The hard, black, elongated sclerotia may contain varying quantities of ergot alkaloids, of which ergotamine and ergonovine (ergometrine) are pharmacologically most important. Cattle, pigs, sheep, and poultry are involved in sporadic outbreaks, and most species are susceptible.

Etiology

Ergot causes vasoconstriction by direct action on the muscles of the arterioles, and repeated dosages injure the vascular endothelium. These actions initially reduce blood flow and eventually lead to complete stasis with terminal necrosis of the extremities due to thrombosis. A cold environment predisposes the extremities to gangrene. In addition, ergot has a potent oxytocic action and also causes stimulation of the CNS, followed by depression. Ergot alkaloids inhibit pituitary release of prolactin in many mammalian species, with failure of both mammary development in late gestation and delayed initiation of milk secretion, resulting in agalactia at parturition.

Clinical Findings and Lesions

Cattle may be affected by eating ergotised hay or grain or occasionally by grazing seeded pastures that are infested with ergot. Lameness, the first sign, may appear 2-6 wk or more after initial ingestion, depending on the concentration of alkaloids in the ergot and the quantity of ergot in the feed. Hindlimbs are affected before forelimbs, but the extent of involvement of a limb and the number of limbs affected depends on the daily intake of ergot. Body temperature and pulse and respiration rates are increased. Epidemic hyperthermia and hypersalivation may also occur in cattle poisoned with C purpurea.

Associated with the lameness are swelling and tenderness of the fetlock joint and pastern. Within ~1 wk, sensation is lost in the affected part, an indented line appears at the limit of normal tissue, and dry gangrene affects the distal part. Eventually, one or both claws or any part of the limbs up to the hock or knee may be sloughed. In a similar way, the tip of the tail or ears may become necrotic and slough. Exposed skin areas, such as teats and udder, appear unusually pale or anemic. Abortion is not seen.

The most consistent lesions at necropsy are in the skin and subcutaneous parts of the extremities. The skin is normal to the indented line, but beyond, it is cyanotic and hardened in advanced cases. Subcutaneous hemorrhage and some edema occur proximal to the necrotic area.

In pigs, ingestion of ergot-infested grains may result in reduced feed intake and reduced weight gain. If fed to pregnant sows, ergotised grains result in lack of udder development with agalactia at parturition, and the piglets born may be smaller than normal. Most of the litter die within a few days due to starvation. No other clinical signs or lesions are seen.

Clinical signs in sheep are similar to those in cattle. Additionally, the mouth may be ulcerated, and marked intestinal inflammation may be seen at necropsy. A convulsive syndrome has been associated with ergotism in sheep.

Diagnosis

Diagnosis is based on finding the causative fungus (ergot sclerotia) in grains, hay, or pastures provided to livestock showing signs of ergotism. Ergot alkaloids may be extracted and detected in suspect ground grain meals.

Identical signs and lesions of lameness, and sloughing of the hooves and tips of ears and tail, are seen in fescue foot in cattle grazing in winter on tall fescue grass infected with an endophyte fungus, in which the ergot alkaloid ergovaline is considered a major toxic principle. In gilts and sows, lactation failure not associated with ergot alkaloids is prevalent and must be differentiated from prolactin inhibition due to ergot.

Control

Ergotism can be controlled by an immediate change to an ergot-free diet. Under pasture feeding conditions, frequent grazing or topping of pastures prone to ergot infestation during the summer months reduces flower-head production and helps control the disease. Grain that contains even small amounts of ergot should not be fed to pregnant or lactating sows.

Estrogenism and Vulvovaginitis

Fusarium spp molds are extremely common and often contaminate growing plants and stored feeds. Corn (maize), wheat, and barley are commonly contaminated. In moderate climates under humid weather conditions, F graminearum may produce zearalenone, one of the resorcyclic acid lactones (RAL). Zearalenone (formerly called F2 toxin) is a potent nonsteroidal estrogen and is the only known mycotoxin with primarily estrogenic effects. Often, zearalenone is produced concurrently with deoxynivalenol. Depending on the ratio of these 2 mycotoxins, signs of reduced feed intake or reproductive dysfunction may predominate, but presence of deoxynivalenol may limit exposure to zearalenone, thus reducing its practical effect.

Zearalenone binds to receptors for estradiol-17-b, and this complex binds to estradiol sites on DNA. Specific RNA synthesis leads to signs of estrogenism. Zearalenone is a weak estrogen with potency 2-4 times less than estradiol. Under controlled administration, zearalanol, a closely related RAL, is widely used in cattle as an anabolic agent.

Estrogenism due to zearalenone was first clinically recognised as vulvovaginitis in prepubertal gilts fed moldy corn (maize), but zearalenone is occasionally reported as a disease-causing agent in sporadic outbreaks in dairy cattle, sheep, chickens, and turkeys. High dietary concentrations are required to produce disease in cattle and sheep, and extremely high dosages are required to affect poultry.

Etiology

Zearalenone has been detected in corn, oats, barley, wheat, and sorghum (both fresh and stored); in rations compounded for cattle and pigs; in corn ensiled at the green stage; and rarely in hay. It has been detected occasionally in samples from pastures in temperate climates at levels thought to be sufficient to cause reproductive failure of grazing herbivores.

Clinical Findings

The condition cannot be distinguished from excessive estrogen administration. Physical and behavioral signs of estrus are induced in young gilts by as little as 1 ppm dietary zearalenone. In pigs, zearalenone primarily affects weaned and prepubertal gilts, causing hyperemia and enlargement of the vulva. There is hypertrophy of the mammary glands and uterus, with occasional prolapse of the uterus in severe cases. In multiparous sows, signs include diminished fertility, anestrus, reduced litter size, smaller offspring, and probably fetal resorption. Constant estrus or pseudopregnancy may be seen.

Zearalenone causes reproductive toxicosis in sexually mature sows by inhibiting secretion and release of follicle-stimulating hormone (FSH) resulting in arrest of preovulatory ovarian follicle maturation. Reproductive effects in sexually mature sows depend on time of consumption. Zearalenone fed at 3-10 ppm on days 12-14 of the estrous cycle in open gilts results in retention of the corpora lutea and prolonged anestrus (pseudopregnancy) for up to 40-60 days. Zearalenone fed at =30 ppm in early gestation (7-10 days post-mating) may prevent implantation and cause early embryonic death.

In cattle, dietary concentrations >10 ppm may cause reproductive dysfunction in dairy heifers, while mature cows may tolerate up to 20 ppm. Clinical signs include weight loss, vaginal discharge, nymphomania, uterine hypertrophy, and in pregnant heifers, abortion 1-3 mo after conception—usually followed by multiple returns to service.

Young males, both swine and cattle, may become infertile, with atrophy of the testes.

Ewes may show reduced reproductive performance (reduced ovulation rates and numbers of fertilised ova, and markedly increased duration of estrus) and abortion or premature live births.

Lesions

Lesions in pigs include ovarian atrophy and follicular atresia, uterine edema, cellular hypertrophy in all layers of the uterus, and a cystic appearance in degenerative endometrial glands. The mammary glands show ductal hyperplasia and epithelial proliferation. Squamous metaplasia is seen in the cervix and vagina.

Diagnosis

This is based on reproductive performance in the herd or flock, clinical signs, and history of diet-related occurrence. Chemical analysis of suspect feed for zearalenone and careful examination of reproductive organs at necropsy are required. As a bioassay, virgin prepubertal mice fed diets or extracts of zearalenone-contaminated feed demonstrate enlarged uteri and vaginal cornification typical of estrogens.

Differential diagnoses include reproductive tract infections and other causes of impaired fertility such as diethylstilbestrol in the diet of housed stock. In grazing herbivores, especially sheep, the plant estrogens (eg, isoflavones associated with some varieties of subterranean and red clovers, and coumestans in certain fodders [eg, alfalfa]) should be considered.

Control

Unless stock are severely or chronically affected, usually reproductive functions recover and signs regress 1-4 wk after intake of zearalenone stops. However, multiparous sows may remain anestrous up to 8-10 wk.

Management of swine with hyperestrogenism should include changing the grain immediately. Signs should stop within 1 wk. Animals should be treated symptomatically for vaginal or rectal prolapse and physical damage to external genitalia. For sexually mature sows with anestrus, one 10-mg dose of prostaglandin F2a, or two 5-mg doses on successive days, has corrected anestrus caused by retained corpora. Alfalfa and alfalfa meal fed to swine at 25% of the ration may reduce absorption and increase fecal excretion of zearalenone, but this is often not considered practical. Bentonite added to contaminated diets has been generally ineffective against zearalenone.

Facial Eczema

In this mycotoxic disease of grazing livestock, the toxic liver injury commonly results in photodynamic dermatitis. In sheep, the face is the only site of the body that is readily exposed to ultraviolet light, hence the common name. The disease is most common in New Zealand but also occurs in Australia, France, South Africa, several South American countries, and probably North America. Sheep, cattle, and farmed deer of all ages can contract the disease, but it is most severe in young animals.

Etiology and Pathogenesis

Sporidesmins are secondary metabolites of the saprophytic fungus Pithomyces chartarum, which grows on dead pasture litter. The warm ground temperatures and high humidity required for rapid growth of this fungus restrict disease occurrence to hot summer and autumn periods shortly after warm rains. By observing weather conditions and estimating toxic spore numbers on pastures, danger periods can be predicted and farmers alerted.

The sporidesmins are excreted via the biliary system, in which they produce severe cholangitis and pericholangitis as a result of tissue necrosis. Biliary obstruction may be seen, which restricts excretion of bile pigments and results in jaundice. Similarly, failure to excrete phylloerythrin in bile leads to photosensitisation.

Previous ingestion of toxic spores causes potentiation, thus a succession of small intakes of the spores can lead to subsequent severe outbreaks.

Clinical Findings, Lesions, and Diagnosis

Few signs are apparent until photosensitisation and jaundice appear ~10-14 days after intake of the toxins. Animals frantically seek shade. Even short exposure to the sun rapidly produces the typical erythema and edema of photodermatitis in unpigmented skin. The animals suffer considerably, and deaths occur from one to several weeks after photodermatitis appears.

Characteristic liver and bile duct lesions are seen in all affected animals whether photosensitised or not. In acute cases showing photodermatitis, livers are initially enlarged, icteric, and have a marked lobular pattern. Later, there is atrophy and marked fibrosis. The shape is distorted, and large nodules of regenerated tissue appear on the surface. In subclinical cases, livers often develop extensive areas in which the tissue is depressed and shrunken below the normal contour, which distorts and roughens the capsule. Generally, these areas are associated with fibrosis and thickening of corresponding bile ducts. The bladder mucosa commonly shows hemorrhagic or bile-pigment-stained ulcerative erosions with circumscribed edema.

The clinical signs together with characteristic liver lesions are pathognomonic. In live animals, high levels of hepatic enzymes may reflect the extensive injury to the liver.

Control

To minimise intake of pasture litter and toxic spores, short grazing should be avoided. Other feedstuffs should be fed during danger periods; encouraging clover dominance in pastures helps to provide a milieu unsuited to growth and sporulation of P chartarum on litter.

The application of benzimidazole fungicides to pastures considerably restricts the buildup of P chartarum spores and reduces pasture toxicity. A pasture area calculated at 1 acre (0. 45 hectare)/15 cows or 100 sheep should be sprayed in midsummer with a suspension of thiabendazole. When danger periods of fungal activity are predicted, animals should be allowed only on the sprayed areas. The fungicide is effective within 4 days after spraying, provided that no more than 1 in. (2. 5 cm) of rain falls within 24 hr during the 4-day period. After this time, heavy rainfall does little to reduce the effectiveness of spraying because the thiabendazole becomes incorporated within the plants. Pastures will then remain safe for ~6 wk, after which spraying should be repeated to ensure protection over the entire dangerous season.

Sheep and cattle can be protected from the effects of sporidesmin if given adequate amounts of zinc. Zinc may be administered by drenching with zinc oxide slurry, by spraying pastures with zinc oxide, or by adding zinc sulfate to drinking water. Sheep may be selectively bred for natural resistance to the toxic effects of sporidesmin. The heritable trait for resistance is high. Ram sires are now being selected in stud and commercial flocks for resistance either by natural field challenge or by low-level, controlled dosage of ram lambs with sporidesmin.

Fescue Lameness

Fescue lameness, which resembles ergot poisoning, is believed to be caused by ergot alkaloids, especially ergovaline, in tall fescue (Festuca arundinacea). It begins with lameness in one or both hindfeet and may progress to necrosis of the distal part of the affected limb(s). The tail and ears also may be affected independently of the lameness. In addition to gangrene of these extremities, animals may show loss of body mass, an arched back, and a rough coat. Outbreaks have been confirmed in cattle and similar lesions have been reported in sheep.

Tall fescue is a cool-season perennial grass adapted to a wide range of soil and climatic conditions; it is used in Australia and New Zealand for stabilizing the banks of watercourses. It is the predominant pasture grass in the transition zone in the eastern and central USA. Fescue lameness has been reported in Kentucky, Tennessee, Florida, California, Colorado, and Missouri, as well as in New Zealand, Australia, and Italy. The causative toxic substance has actions similar to those produced by sclerotia of Clàviceps purpurea. However, ergot poisoning is not the cause of fescue lameness. Ergotism is most prevalent in late summer when the seed heads of grass mature. Fescue lameness is most common in late fall and winter and has been reproduced in cattle by feeding dried fescue free of seed heads and ergot. Two fungi from toxic pastures have been implicated in fescue lameness. The clavicipitaceous endophyte fungus Acremonium coenophialum can synthesise ergot alkaloids in culture. The ergot alkaloid ergovaline has been detected in toxic fescue and is strongly implicated in some of the fescue toxicosis syndromes. However, the complete etiology of fescue foot remains unresolved.

Some reports indicate an increased incidence of fescue lameness as plants age and after severe droughts. Strains of tall fescue vary in their toxicity (eg, Kentucky-31 is more toxic than Fawn) due to variation in infection level with the fungus and to high variability within a strain. In some Kentucky-31 fescues, infection levels cannot be detected. High nitrogen applications appear to enhance the toxicity. Susceptibility of cattle is subject to individual variation. Low environmental temperature is thought to exacerbate the lesions of fescue lameness; however, high temperatures increase the severity of a toxic problem known as epidemic hyperthermia or "summer syndrome", in which a high proportion of a herd of cattle exhibits hypersalivation and hyperthermia. It appears that the toxin is a vasoconstrictor that induces hyperthermia in hot weather and results in cold extremities during cold weather. Another cause of this is poisoning with *C. purpurea* (ergot alkaloids).

Erythema and swelling of the coronary region occur, and cattle are alert but lose weight and may be seen "paddling" or weight-shifting. The back is slightly arched, and knuckling of a hind pastern may be an initial sign. There is progressive lameness, anorexia, depression, and later, dry gangrene of the distal limbs (hindlimbs first). Signs usually develop within 10-21 days after turnout into a fescue-contaminated pasture in fall. A period of frost tends to increase the incidence.

Summer Fescue Toxicosis

This warm season condition is characterised by reduced feed intake and weight gains or milk production. The toxin(s) affects cattle, sheep, and horses during the summer when they are grazing or being fed tall fescue forage or seed contaminated with the endophytic fungus Acremonium coenophialum. The severity of the condition varies from field to field and year to year.

Signs other than reduced performance, which may appear within 1-2 wk after fescue feeding is started, include fever, tachypnea, rough coat, lower serum prolactin levels, and excessive salivation. The animals seek wet spots or shade. Lowered reproductive performance also has been reported. Agalactia has been reported for both horses and cattle. Thickened placentas, delayed parturition, birth of weak foals, and agalactia have been reported in horses. The severity increases when environmental temperatures are >75-80°F (24-27°C) and if high nitrogen fertilizer has been applied to the grass. For control, toxic tall fescue pastures must be destroyed and reseeded with seed that does not contain endophytic fungus because transfer of the fungus from plant to plant is primarily, if not solely, through infected seed. Not using pastures during hot weather, diluting tall fescue pastures with interseeded legumes, clipping pastures to reduce seed formation, or offering other feedstuffs helps reduce severity.

Fumonisin Toxicosis

Equine leukoencephalomalacia is a mycotoxic disease of the CNS that affects horses, mules, and donkeys. It occurs sporadically in North and South America, South Africa, Europe, and China. It is associated with the feeding of moldy corn (maize), usually over a period of several weeks. Fumonisins are produced worldwide primarily by Fusarium moniliforme Sheldon and F proliferatum. Conditions favoring fumonisin production appear to include a period of drought during the growing season with subsequent cool, moist conditions during pollination and kernel formation. Three toxins produced by the fungi have been classified as fumonisin B1 (FB1), B2 (FB2), and B3 (FB3). Current evidence suggests that FB1 and FB2 are of similar toxicity, whereas FB3 is relatively nontoxic. Major health effects are observed in Equidae and swine.

Signs in Equidae include apathy, drowsiness, pharyngeal paralysis, blindness, circling, staggering, and recumbency. The clinical course is usually 1-2 days but may be as short as several hours or as long as several weeks. Icterus may be present if the liver is involved. The characteristic lesion is liquefactive necrosis of the white matter of the cerebrum. The necrosis is usually unilateral but may be asymmetrically bilateral. Some horses may have hepatic necrosis similar to that seen in aflatoxicosis. Horses may develop leukoencephalomalacia from prolonged exposure to as little as 8-10 ppm fumonisins in the diet.

Fumonisins have also been reported to cause acute epidemics of disease in weanling or adult pigs, characterised by pulmonary edema and hydrothorax. Porcine pulmonary edema (PPE) is usually an acute, fatal disease and appears to be caused by pulmonary hypertension with transudation of fluids in the thorax resulting in interstitial pulmonary edema and hydrothorax. Acute PPE results after consumption of fumonisins for 3-6 days at dietary concentrations >100 ppm. Morbidity within a herd may be >50%, and mortality among affected pigs ranges from 50 to 100%. Signs include acute onset of dyspnea, cyanosis of mucous membranes, weakness, recumbency, and death, often within 24 hr after the first clinical signs. Affected sows in late gestation that survive acute PPE may abort within 2-3 days, presumably as a result of fetal anoxia.

The biochemical mechanism of action for PPE or liver toxicosis is believed to be due to the ability of fumonisins to interrupt sphingolipid synthesis in many animal species. Cattle, sheep, and poultry are considerably less susceptible to fumonisins than are horses or swine. Cattle and sheep tolerate fumonisin concentrations of 100 ppm with little effect. Dietary concentrations of 200 ppm cause inappetence, weight loss, and mild liver damage. Poultry are affected by concentrations >200-400 ppm and may develop inappetence, weight loss, and skeletal abnormalities. No treatment is available. Avoidance of moldy corn is the only prevention, although this is difficult because it may not be grossly moldy or it may be contained in a mixed feed. However, most of the toxin is present in broken kernels or small, poorly formed kernels. Therefore, cleaning grain to remove the screenings markedly reduces fumonisin concentration. Corn suspected of containing fumonisins should not be given to horses.

Mycotoxic Lupinosis

Lupines (Lupinus spp) cause 2 distinct forms of poisoning in livestock—lupine poisoning and lupinosis. The former is a nervous syndrome caused by alkaloids present in bitter lupines; the latter is a mycotoxic disease characterised by liver injury and jaundice, which results mainly from the feeding of sweet lupines. Lupinosis is important in Australia and South Africa and also has been reported from New Zealand and Europe. There is increasing use of sweet lupines, either as forage crops or through feeding of their residues after grain harvest, as strategic feed for sheep in Mediterranean climate zones. Sheep, and occasionally cattle and horses, are affected, and pigs are also susceptible.

Etiology and Pathogenesis:

The causal fungus is Phomopsis leptostromiformis, which causes Phomopsis stem-blight, especially in white and yellow lupines; blue varieties are resistant. It produces sunken, linear stem lesions that contain black, stromatic masses, and it also affects the pods and seeds. The fungus is also a saprophyte and grows well on dead lupine material (e.g., haulm, pods, stubble) under favorable conditions. It produces phomopsins as secondary metabolites on infected lupine material, especially after rain. Clinical changes are mainly attributable to toxic hepatocyte injury, which causes mitotic arrest in metaphase, isolated cell necrosis, and hepatic enzyme leakage, with loss of metabolic and excretory function.

Clinical Findings, Lesions, and Diagnosis:

Early signs in sheep and cattle are inappetence and listlessness. Complete anorexia and jaundice follow, and ketosis is common. Cattle may show lacrimation and salivation. Sheep may become photosensitive. In acute outbreaks, deaths occur in 2-14 days. In acute disease, icterus is marked. Livers are enlarged, orange-yellow, and fatty. More chronic cases show bronze- or tan-colored livers that are firm, contracted in size, and fibrotic. Copious amounts of transudates may be found in the abdominal and thoracic cavities and in the pericardial sac. Feeding of moldy lupine material, together with clinical signs and increased levels of serum liver enzymes, strongly indicate lupinosis.

Control

Frequent surveillance of sheep and of lupine fodder material for characteristic black spot fungal infestation, especially after rains, is advised. The utilisation of lupine cultivars, bred and developed for resistance to *P. leptostromiformis* is advocated. Oral doses of zinc (=0. 5 g/day) have protected sheep against liver injury induced by phomopsins.

Paspalum Staggers

This incoordination results from eating paspalum grasses infested by *Claviceps paspali.* The life cycle of this fungus is similar to that of *C. purpurea.* The yellow-gray sclerotia, which mature in the seed heads in autumn, are round, roughened, and 2-4 mm in diameter. Ingestion of sclerotia causes nervous signs in cattle most commonly, but horses and sheep also are susceptible. Guinea pigs can be affected experimentally. The toxicity is not ascribed to ergot alkaloids; the toxic principles are thought to be paspalinine and paspalitrem A and B, tremorgenic compounds from the sclerotia.

A sufficiently large single dose causes signs that persist for several days. Animals display continuous trembling of the large muscle groups; movements are jerky and incoordinated. If they attempt to run, the animals fall over in awkward positions. Affected animals may be belligerent and dangerous to approach or handle. After prolonged exposure, condition is lost and complete paralysis can occur. The time of onset of signs depends on the degree of the infestation of seed heads and the grazing habits of the animals. Experimentally, early signs appear in cattle after ~100 g/day of sclerotia has been administered for >2 days. Although the mature ergots are toxic, they are most dangerous just when they are maturing to the hard, black (sclerotic) stage.

Recovery follows removal of the animals to feed not contaminated with sclerotia of *C. paspali*. Animals are less affected if left alone and provided readily available nutritious forages. Care should be taken to prevent accidental access to ponds or rough terrain where accidental trauma or drowning could occur. Topping of the pasture to remove affected seed heads has been effective in control.

Slaframine Toxicosis

Trifolium pratense (red clover) may become infected with the fungus Rhizoctonia leguminocola (black patch disease), especially in wet, cool years. Rarely, other legumes (white clover, alsike, alfalfa) may be infected. Slaframine is an indolizidine alkaloid recognised as the toxic principle, and it is stable in dried hay and probably in silage. Horses are highly sensitive to slaframine, but clinical cases occur in cattle as well. Profuse salivation (salivary syndrome) develops within hours after first consumption of contaminated hay; signs also include mild lacrimation, diarrhea, mild bloat, and frequent urination. Morbidity can be high, but death is not expected, and removal of contaminated hay allows recovery and return of appetite within 24-48 hr. A related alkaloid, swainsonine, produced by *R. leguminicola,* has caused a lysosomal storage disease from prolonged exposure, but its importance in the salivary syndrome is not confirmed. Diagnosis is tentatively based on recognition of the characteristic clinical signs and the presence of "black patch" on the forages. Chemical detection of slaframine or swainsonine in forages helps to confirm the diagnosis. There is no specific antidote to slaframine toxicosis, although atropine may control at least some of the prominent salivary and GI signs. Removal of animals from the contaminated hay is essential. Prevention of Rhizoctonia infection of clovers has been difficult. Some clover varieties may be relatively resistant to black patch disease. Reduced usage of red clover for forages or dilution with other feeds is helpful.

Trichothecene Toxicosis

The trichothecene mycotoxins are a group of closely related secondary metabolic products of several families of imperfect, saprophytic, or plant pathogenic fungi such as Fusarium, Trichothecium, Myrothecium, Cephalosporium, Stachybotrys, Trichodesma, Cylindrocarpon, and Verticimonosporium spp. On the basis of molecular structure, the trichothecenes are classed as nonmacrocyclic (eg, deoxynivalenol [DON] or vomitoxin, T-2 toxin, diacetoxyscirpenol, and others) or macrocyclic (satratoxin, roridin, verrucarin).

The trichothecene mycotoxins are highly toxic at the subcellular, cellular, and organic system level. They swiftly penetrate cell lipid bilayers, thus allowing access to DNA, RNA, and cellular organelles. Trichothecenes inhibit protein synthesis by affecting polyribosomes to interfere with the initiation phase of protein synthesis. At the subcellular level, these toxins inhibit protein synthesis and covalently bond to sulfhydryl groups.

Trichothecene mycotoxins are generally cytotoxic to most cells, including neoplastic cells; they are not mutagenic. Toxicity of the trichothecenes is based on direct cytotoxicity and is often referred to as a radiomimetic effect (eg, bone marrow hypoplasia, gastroenteritis, diarrhea, hemorrhages). The cutaneous cytotoxicity that follows administration of these compounds is a nonspecific, acute, necrotising process with minimal inflammation of both the epidermis and dermis. Stomatitis, hyperkeratosis with ulceration of the esophageal portion of the gastric mucosa, and necrosis of the GI tract have been seen after ingestion of trichothecenes.

Given in sublethal toxic doses via any route, the trichothecenes are highly immunosuppressive in mammals; however, longterm feeding of high levels of T-2 toxin does not seem to activate latent viral or bacterial infections. The main immunosuppressive effect of the trichothecenes is at the level of the T-suppressor cell, but the toxins may affect function of helper T cells, B cells, or macrophages, or the interaction among these cells.

Hemorrhagic diathesis may occur after thrombocytopenia or defective intrinsic or extrinsic coagulation pathways. It appears that hemorrhage results from depression of clotting factors, thrombocytopenia, inhibition of platelet function, or possibly a combination of these.

Refusal to consume contaminated feedstuff is the typical sign, which limits development of other signs. If no other food is offered, animals may eat reluctantly, but in some instances, excessive salivation and vomiting may occur. In the past, the ability to cause vomiting had been ascribed to DON only, hence the common name, vomitoxin. However, other members of the trichothecene family also can induce vomiting. Feed refusal caused by DON is a learned response known as taste aversion. It may be related to neurochemical changes in serotonin, dopamine, and 5-hydroxyindoleacetic acid. Feed refusal response to vomitoxin varies widely among species. DON in swine causes conditioned taste aversion, and swine would be expected to recognise new flavors (eg, flavoring agents) added to DON-containing feed and thus develop aversion to the new taste as well. Provision of uncontaminated feed usually leads to resumption of eating within 1-2 days.

In swine, reduced feed intake may occur at dietary concentrations as low as 1 ppm, and refusal may be complete at 10 ppm. Ruminants generally will readily consume up to 10 ppm dietary vomitoxin, and poultry may tolerate as much as 100 ppm. Horses may accept as much as 35-45 ppm dietary DON without feed refusal or adverse clinical effects. Related effects of weight loss, hypoproteinemia, and weakness may follow prolonged feed refusal. There is little credible evidence that vomitoxin causes reproductive dysfunction in domestic animals.

Irritation of the skin and mucous membranes and gastroenteritis are another set of signs typical of trichothecene toxicosis. Hemorrhagic diathesis can occur, and the radiomimetic injury (damage to dividing cells) is expressed as lymphopenia or pancytopenia. Paresis, seizures, and paralysis occur in almost all species. Eventually, hypotension may lead to death. Many of the severe effects described for experimental trichothecene toxicosis are due to dosing by gavage. From a practical perspective, high concentrations of trichothecenes often cause feed refusal and therefore are self-limiting as a toxic problem.

Due to the immunosuppressive action of trichothecenes, secondary bacterial, viral, or parasitic infections may mask the primary injury. The lymphatic organs are smaller than normal and may be difficult to find on necropsy. Although no specific name has been given to most nonmacrocyclic trichothecene-related diseases, the term fusariotoxicosis is often used. Some other names used are moldy corn poisoning in cattle, bean hull poisoning of horses, and feed refusal and emetic syndrome in pigs. A condition in chickens, referred to as "rickets in broilers," is also thought to be caused by trichothecenes. Macrocyclic trichothecene-related diseases have received a number of specific names. The best known is stachybotryotoxicosis of horses, cattle, sheep, pigs, and poultry, first diagnosed in the former USSR but occurring also in Europe and South Africa. Cutaneous and mucocutaneous lesions, panleukopenia, nervous signs, and abortions have been seen. Death may occur in 2-12 days. Myrotheciotoxicosis and dendrodochiotoxicosis have been reported from the former USSR and New Zealand. The signs resemble those of stachybotryotoxicosis, but death may occur in 1-5 days.

Diagnosis

Because the clinical signs are nonspecific, or masked by secondary infections and disease, diagnosis is difficult. Analysis of feed is often costly and time consuming but ideally should be attempted. Interim measures are carefully examining feedstuff for signs of mold growth or caking of feed particles and switching to an alternative feed supply. Change of feed supply often results in immediate improvement and thus may provide one more clue that the original feed was contaminated.

Control

Symptomatic treatment and feeding of uncontaminated feed are recommended. Steroidal anti-shock and anti-inflammatory agents, such as methylprednisolone, prednisolone, and dexamethasone, have been used successfully in experimental trials. Poultry and cattle are more tolerant of trichothecenes than are pigs.

RODENTICIDES

Rodenticidesarepesticidalcompounds that are used to destroy rodents particularly mice, field mice, rats and sewer rats. These rodents cause potential widespread destruction of food and fiber. The greatest losses are suffered through damage to farm crops, stored foodstuffs and feed stuffs, various industrial goods, equipments, etc. Apart from this, with some rodents, there is always arisk of spreading infectious diseases (bubanic plague, leptospirosis, etc.) to man and animals. This is especially serious when there is their over population. Therefore, there has been always a demand for strong and effective rodenticides to control rodents and to prevent losses caused by them. Unfortunately, many rodenticides are equally toxic to man and animals. In some cases, the rodenticidal selectivity of these compounds is based on peculiar physiology of rodents. For example, the rodenticide ANTU is a strong emetic and as a result it will be less toxic to cats and dogs but more toxic to rodents.

Since rodenticides can be used in baits and placed in in accessible places, their likelihood of becoming widespread contaminants of the environment is much less than that of insecticides and herbicides. Therefore, toxicologic problems posed by rodenticides are primarily ones of acute accidental or suicidal ingestion. Poisoning of domestic animals may be malicious. Animals may consume baits set out for rodents or may possibly eat dead (poisoned) rodents. Sometimes deranged persons may distribute meat or bones covered with rodenticides throughout a neighborhood.

Rodenticides should be selectively toxic for the rodents and non-toxic for man and farm animals. There is no rodenticide, now in use, which fully meets this requirement. Experience in toxicological practice shows that the poisoning off arm and domestic animals by rodenticidal preparations occurs very frequently. Considerable progress has been made in the use of rodenticides, from inorganic compounds to synthetic organic substances which have many advantages over those used formerly. The group of inorganic preparations used in the past includes arsenictrioxide, sodium hydrogen arsenite, barium carbonate, elementary phosphorus and fluorine compounds (sodium fluorosilicate). Thallous sulphate and zinc phosphide are still in use. The organic compounds used asrodenticides are coumar in preparations(which have an anticoagulant action), alphanaphthylthio urea, sodium fluoroacetate, preparations from the sea onion, strychnine and some others.

Anticoagulant Rodenticides

Potentially dangerous to all mammals and birds, anticoagulant rodenticides are the most frequent cause of poisoning in pets. Pets and wildlife may be poisoned directly from baits or indirectly by consumption of poisoned rodents. Intoxications in domestic animals have resulted from contamination of feed with anticoagulant concentrate, malicious use of these chemicals, and feed mixed in equipment used to prepare rodent bait. All anticoagulants have the basic coumarin or indanedione nucleus. The "first-generation" anticoagulants (warfarin, pindone, coumafuryl, coumachlor, isovaleryl indanedione, and others less frequently used) require multiple feedings to result in toxicity. The "intermediate" anticoagulants (chlorophacinone and in particular diphacinone) require fewer feedings than "first-generation" chemicals, and thus are more toxic to nontarget species. The "second-generation" anticoagulants (brodifacoum and bromadiolone) are highly toxic to nontarget species (dogs, cats, and potentially livestock) after a single feeding.

The anticoagulants antagonise vitamin K, which interferes with the normal synthesis of coagulation proteins (factors I, II, VII, IX, and X) in the liver; thus, adequate amounts are not available to convert prothrombin into thrombin. A latent period, dependent on species, dose, and activity, is required, during which clotting factors already present are used up. New products have a longer biologic half-life and therefore prolonged effects (which require prolonged treatment). For example, the half-life in canine plasma of warfarin is 15 hr, diphacinone is 5 days, and bromadiolone is 6 days, with maximum effects estimated at 12-15 days. Brodifacoum may continue to be detectable in serum for up to 24 days. Clinical signs generally reflect some manifestation of hemorrhage, including anemia, hematomas, melena, hemothorax, hyphema, epistaxis, hemoptysis, and hematuria. Signs dependent on hemorrhage, such as weakness, ataxia, colic, and polypnea, may be seen. Depression and anorexia occur in all species even before bleeding occurs.

Anticoagulant rodenticide toxicosis is usually diagnosed based on history of ingestion of the substance. Differential diagnoses when massive hemorrhage is encountered include disseminated intravascular coagulation, congenital factor deficiencies, von Willebrand's disease, platelet deficiencies, and canine ehrlichiosis. A prolonged prothrombin, partial thromboplastin, or thrombin time in the presence of normal fibrinogen, fibrin degradation products, and platelet counts is strongly suggestive of anticoagulant rodenticide toxicosis, as is a positive therapeutic response to vitamin K1.

Vitamin K1 is antidotal. Recommended dosages vary from 0.25-2.5 mg/kg in warfarin (coumarin) exposure, to 2.5-5 mg/kg in the case of long-acting rodenticide intoxication (diphacinone, brodifacoum, bromadiolone). Vitamin K1 is administered SC (with the smallest possible needle to minimise hemorrhage) in several locations to speed absorption. Administration of vitamin K1 is contraindicated, as anaphylaxis may occasionally result. The oral form of K1 may be used daily after the first day, commonly at the same level as the loading dose (divided bid). Fresh or frozen plasma (9 mL/kg) or whole blood (20 mL/kg) IV is required to replace needed clotting factors and RBC if bleeding is severe. One week of vitamin K1 treatment is usually sufficient for first-generation anticoagulants. For intermediate and second-generation anticoagulants or if anticoagulant type is unknown, treatment should continue for 2-4 wk to control longterm effects. Administration of oral vitamin K1 with a fat-containing ration, such as canned dog food, increases its bioavailability 4-5 times as compared with vitamin K1 given PO alone. Coagulation should be monitored weekly until values remain normal for 5-6 days after cessation of therapy. Vitamin K3 given as a feed supplement is ineffective in the treatment of anticoagulant rodenticide toxicosis. Additional supportive therapy may be indicated, including thoracocentesis (to relieve dyspnea due to hemothorax) and supplemental oxygen if needed.

ANTU (a-Naphthylthiourea)

ANTU causes local gastric irritation; when absorbed, it increases permeability of the lung capillaries in all animals, although species variability in dose response is marked. Properties of ANTU, when compared with those of warfarin, have led to near abandonment of its use. Dogs and pigs are occasionally poisoned; ruminants are resistant. Animals with an empty stomach readily vomit after ingestion of ANTU;

however, food in the stomach decreases the stimulation to vomit, and fatal quantities may be absorbed. Signs include vomiting, hypersalivation, coughing, and dyspnea. Animals prefer to sit. Severe pulmonary edema, moist rales, and cyanosis are present. Dependent signs include weakness; ataxia; rapid, weak pulse; and subnormal temperature. Death from hypoxia may occur within 2-4 hr of ingestion, while animals that survive 12 hr may recover.

The lesions are suggestive. The most striking findings are pulmonary edema and hydrothorax. Hyperemia of the tracheal mucosa; mild to moderate gastroenteritis; marked hyperemia of the kidneys; and a pale, mottled liver are found in most cases. Tissue for chemical analysis must be obtained within 24 hr. Emetics should be used only if respiratory distress is not evident. Prognosis is grave when severe respiratory signs occur. Agents providing sulfhydryl groups, eg, n-amyl mercaptan, sodium thiosulfate (10% solution), or n-acetylcysteine are beneficial. Positive-pressure oxygen therapy, an osmotic diuretic (e.g., mannitol), and atropine (0.02-0.25 mg/kg) may relieve the pulmonary edema.

Bromethalin

This nonanticoagulant, single-dose rodenticide is a neurotoxin that appears to uncouple oxidative phosphorylation in the CNS. CSF pressure increases, which places pressure on nerve axons and results in decreased conduction of nerve impulses, paralysis, and death. In dogs, a dose of 1.67 mg/kg is toxic, and 2.5 mg/kg (25 g of bait/kg body wt) is lethal. Bromethalin can cause either an acute or a chronic syndrome. The acute effects follow consumption of =5 mg/kg bromethalin. Signs, which include hyperexcitability, muscle tremors, grand mal seizures, hindlimb hyperreflexia, CNS depression, and death, may appear ~10 hr after ingestion. Chronic effects are seen with lower dosages and may appear 24-86 hr after ingestion. This syndrome is characterised by vomiting, depression, ataxia, tremors, and lateral recumbency. The effects may be reversible if exposure to bromethalin is discontinued. Bromethalin toxicosis should be considered when cerebral edema or posterior paralysis is present. Treatment should be directed at blocking absorption from the gut and reducing cerebral edema. Use of mannitol as an osmotic diuretic and corticosteroids have been suggested but have shown little effect in dogs poisoned by bromethalin. Use of activated charcoal for several days may improve the recovery rate.

Cholecalciferol

Although this rodenticide was introduced with claims that it was less toxic to nontarget species than to rodents, clinical experience has shown that rodenticides containing cholecalciferol are a significant health threat to dogs and cats. Cholecalciferol produces hypercalcemia, which results in systemic calcification of soft tissue, leading to renal failure, cardiac abnormalities, hypertension, CNS depression, and GI upset.

Signs generally develop within 18-36 hr of ingestion and can include depression, anorexia, polyuria, and polydipsia. As serum calcium concentrations increase, clinical signs become more severe. Serum calcium concentrations >16 mg/dL are not uncommon. GI smooth muscle excitability decreases and is manifest by anorexia, vomiting, and constipation. Hematemesis and hemorrhagic diarrhea may develop as a result of dystrophic calcification of the GI tract and should not lead to a misdiagnosis of anticoagulant rodenticide toxicosis. Loss of renal concentrating ability is a direct result of hypercalcemia. As hypercalcemia persists, mineralisation of the kidneys results in progressive renal insufficiency.

Diagnosis is based on history of ingestion, clinical signs, and hypercalcemia. Other causes of hypercalcemia, such as hyperparathyroidism, normal juvenile hypercalcemia, paraneoplastic hypercalcemia, hemoconcentration (hyperproteinemia), and diffuse osteoporosis should be ruled out. Gross lesions associated with hypercalcemia include pitted, mottled kidneys; diffuse hemorrhage of the GI mucosa; and roughened, raised plaques on the great vessels and on the surface of the lungs and abdominal viscera. Recommended therapy includes gastric evacuation, generally followed by administration of activated charcoal at 2-8 g/kg body wt in a water slurry. Calciuresis is accomplished with 0. 9% sodium chloride solution and administration of furosemide (initial bolus of 5 mg/kg, IV, followed by a constant rate infusion of 5 mg/kg/hr) and corticosteroids (prednisolone, 1-2 mg/kg, bid). Furosemide and prednisolone should be continued for 2-4 wk, and the serum calcium concentration monitored at 24 hr, 48 hr, and 2 wk after cessation of treatment. Additionally, calcitonin may be used at 4-6 IU/kg, SC, every 2-3 hr, until the serum calcium stabilizes at <12 mg/dL.

The use of calcium chelators such as Na-EDTA has been used in severe cases, but this use is experimental and requires close monitoring of blood calcium to prevent hypocalcemia. The dose of prednisolone should be tapered if it is administered for >2 wk to prevent acute adrenocortical insufficiency. Continuous peritoneal dialysis may be considered if the animal is in renal failure. A low-calcium diet should be provided in all cases of significant exposure to cholecalciferol rodenticides.

Metaldehyde

This polymer of acetaldehyde is used as a snail or slug bait, to which dogs and livestock may be exposed. Toxic effects are due to absorption of limited acetaldehyde from metaldehyde hydrolysis in the stomach, but primarily to the metaldehyde itself. Signs range from salivation and vomiting to anxiety and incoordination with muscle tremors, fasciculations, and hyperesthesia leading to continuous muscle spasms, prostration, and death. Generally, the muscle spasms are not initiated by external stimuli, but excessive muscular activity is common, often producing high body temperatures. Differential diagnoses include strychnine poisoning and anticholinesterase insecticide toxicity. The finding of metaldehyde bait or pellets in the vomitus and the possible odor of acetaldehyde from stomach contents or on the animal's breath may assist in diagnosis.

Treatment is most effective if initiated early. Further toxicant absorption should be prevented by induced emesis, gastric lavage, and oral dosing with activated charcoal. Hyperesthesia and muscle activity may be controlled with diazepam at 2-5 mg, IV, or light barbiturate anesthesia and muscle relaxants as needed. IV fluid therapy with lactated Ringer's solution or 5% glucose should be aggressive to promote toxin excretion and to combat dehydration and the acidosis induced by the excessive muscle activity. Continuous supportive care is important. Prognosis is heavily determined by the exposure dose, but if death does not occur earlier, animals poisoned by metaldehyde may show clinical improvement 24-36 hr after initial onset of signs.

Phosphorus

In its white (or yellow) form, phosphorus is hazardous to all domestic animals and is locally corrosive and hepatotoxic when absorbed. Phosphorus is infrequently used as a rodenticide today, but dogs occasionally become exposed through ingestion of fireworks that contain white phosphorus. The onset of signs of poisoning is sudden. Early signs include vomiting, severe diarrhea (often hemorrhagic), colic, and a garlic-like odor to the breath. Apparent recovery can occur up to 4 days after ingestion, but additional signs of acute liver damage may develop, including hemorrhages, abdominal pain, and icterus. Hepatic encephalopathy is followed by convulsions and death. Lesions include severe gastroenteritis; fatty liver; multiple hemorrhages; and black, tarry blood that fails to clot. Body tissues and fluids may be phosphorescent, and the gastric contents have a garlic odor. Death is due to hepatic and renal failure.

Prognosis is grave unless treatment is instituted early. A 1% solution of copper sulfate is an effective emetic and also forms a nonabsorbable copper phosphide complex. Gastric lavage with a 0.01-0.1% potassium permanganate solution or a 0.2-0.4% copper sulfate solution should be followed by activated charcoal adsorbent and 30 min later by a saline cathartic. Any fat in the diet must be avoided for 3-4 days or longer because fats favor additional absorption of phosphorus. Mineral oil orally has been recommended because it dissolves phosphorus and prevents absorption.

Red Squill

This rodenticide is a cardiac glycoside derived from the plant Urginea maritima. It is of limited current use. Because rats are incapable of vomiting, red squill is more toxic to that species. It is unpalatable to domestic animals but, when eaten, usually induces vomiting in dogs and cats. Large quantities are required for toxicity in farm animals. It is considered relatively safe, but dogs, cats, and pigs have been poisoned. Signs are vomiting, ataxia, and hyperesthesia followed by paralysis, depression, or convulsions. Bradycardia and cardiac arrhythmias may end in cardiac arrest. The clinical course seldom is longer than 24-36 hr. Treatment consists of supportive therapy and evacuation of the GI tract using gastric lavage and saline cathartics. Atropine sulfate SC at 6- to 8-hr intervals may prevent cardiac arrest. Phenytoin at 35 mg/kg, tid, should be given to dogs to suppress arrhythmias.

Sodium Monofluoroacetate (1080)

1080 is a colorless, odorless, tasteless, water-soluble chemical that is highly toxic (0.1-8 mg/kg) to all animals, including humans. Its use is restricted to certain commercial applications. Fluoroacetate is metabolised to fluorocitrate, which blocks the tricarboxylic acid cycle—a mechanism necessary for cellular energy production. It causes toxic effects by overstimulating the CNS, resulting in death by convulsions, and by causing alteration of cardiac function that results in myocardial depression, cardiac arrhythmias, ventricular fibrillation, and circulatory collapse. CNS stimulation is the main effect in dogs, while the cardiac effects predominate in horses, sheep, goats, and chickens. Pigs and cats appear about equally affected by both.

A characteristic lag phase of =30 min after ingestion occurs before the onset of nervousness and restlessness. Marked depression and weakness follow in all species except dogs and pigs. Affected animals rapidly become prostrate, and the pulse is weak and 2-3 times normal rate. Death is due to cardiac failure. Usually, dogs and pigs rapidly develop tetanic convulsions similar to those of strychnine poisoning. Many exhibit severe pain. Vomiting is prominent in pigs. Dogs usually have urinary and fecal incontinence and exhibit frenzied running. The course is rapid; affected animals die within hours after signs appear. Few animals that develop marked signs recover. Congestion of organs, cyanosis, subepicardial hemorrhages, and a heart stopped in diastole are common necropsy findings. Emetics are contraindicated if clinical signs are present. Gastric lavage and adsorbents (activated charcoal, 0.5 g/kg) are recommended. Prognosis is grave if clinical signs are severe. Barbiturates are preferred for controlling seizures. Glyceryl monoacetate (monacetin) has been used with inconsistent results as a competitive antagonist of fluoroacetate.

Thallium Sulfate

This general cellular poison can affect all species of animals. It has been banned for use as a rodenticide. Onset of clinical signs may be delayed 1-3 days and, although all body systems are affected, the most prominent signs are of the GI, respiratory, integumentary, and nervous systems. Signs include gastroenteritis (occasionally hemorrhagic), abdominal pain, dyspnea, blindness, fever, conjunctivitis, gingivitis, and tremors or seizures. After 4-5 days and an apparent recovery, or after repeated small doses, a chronic dermatitis characterised by alopecia, erythema, and hyperkeratosis occurs. Necrosis of many tissues is a common necropsy finding. Treatment of the acute phase of thallium poisoning includes emetics, gastric lavage with a 1% sodium iodide solution, and administration of 10% sodium iodide. Diphenylthiocarbazone (dithizone, 70 mg/kg, PO, tid) is antidotal but must be given within 24 hr of exposure. At the same time and for 14 days thereafter, Prussian blue 100 mg/kg should be given bid in oral aqueous suspension to stop enterohepatic recirculation of the thallium and to enhance its excretion in the feces. Symptomatic treatment of the diarrhea and convulsions is needed with particular attention to fluid and electrolyte balance, nutrient needs, prevention of secondary infection, and good nursing care.

Zinc Phosphide and Aluminum Phosphide

Zinc phosphide has been used extensively around farms and barns because affected rats tend to die in the open. Toxicity is due to liberation of phosphine gas at the acid pH in the stomach. The gas results in direct GI tract irritation along with cardiovascular collapse. The toxic dose is ~40 mg/kg, and onset is rapid in animals with a full stomach. Clinical signs include vomiting, abdominal pain, and aimless running and howling, followed by depression, dyspnea, and convulsions (which may resemble those seen in strychnine or fluoroacetate poisoning). Death is due to respiratory arrest. The odor of acetylene is present in vomitus or stomach contents. Less frequent lesions include visceral congestion and pulmonary edema. Diagnosis is based on history of exposure to zinc phosphide, suggestive clinical signs, and detection of zinc phosphide in stomach contents. Zinc levels in the blood, liver, and kidneys may be increased. Treatment must include supportive therapy, calcium gluconate, and appropriate fluids to reduce acidosis. Sodium bicarbonate (in cattle, 2-4 L of 5%), PO, to neutralise stomach acidity is recommended.

REFERENCES

Nelson, Lewis H.; Flomenbaum, Neal; Goldfrank, Lewis R.; Hoffman, Robert Louis; Howland, Mary Deems; Neal A. Lewin. 2006. *Goldfrank's toxicologic emergencies*. New York: McGraw-Hill, Medical Pub. Division.

Richards IS. 2008. *Principles and Practice of Toxicology in Public Health*. Jones and Bartlett Publisher, Sudbury Massachusetts.

4

Toxicology of Metals

Metals, their salts and alloys are an integral part of civilization. They are also intrinsic in nature and many metals are utilized by biologic systems for essential functions. Certain metals perform essential roles in metabolism and synthesis of body constituents. The hallmark of many metals is that they may be required for life or health in small amounts but are toxic if intake is excessive. Metals commonly characterized as both essential and relatively toxic in mammals include chromium, cobalt, copper, iron, magnesium, manganese, molybdenum, selenium, strontium, and zinc. Metal toxicosis, when it occurs, is often due either to redistribution of the metal in the environment or a change in chemical form of the metal.

Redistribution of metals in the environment accounts for access of animals and man to toxic elements not normally available. Industrial sources such as mining contributes dust or tailings which can contaminate air, forages, or waterways. Mining operations involving lead, arsenic, zinc or molybdenum have been associated with livestock toxicosis in the past. Processing of metals by smelting or roasting can eventually settling on forages for livestock or being inhaled directly. Municiple sewage accounts for redistribution of metals used in commerce and industry back into waterways or sewage sludge. Of most concern from this source has been cadmium, copper, molybdenum, nickel, and zinc. Power generation serves as a source of metals redistribution in the environment. Coal burning contributes cadmium, mercury and arsenic to the environment.

Commercial sources of metals provide further distributions of sometimes concentrated amounts of metals with direct access to livestock or pets. Pesticides, medications, paint, and automotive products provide sources of lead, arsenic, selenium, cadmium, mercury, tin, zinc, and copper which may either significantly add to the body burden of animals or in some cases induce toxicosis.

Change in chemical form is an important aspect of the toxicology of metals. Metals are able to undergo oxidation-reduction reactions resulting in characteristic valence changes. Changes in valence may alter assimilation, toxicity, or excretion. For example, elemental mercury is assimilated approximately ten times faster than divalent mercury. Divalent forms of mercury bind to tissue protein resulting in increased toxicity compared to elemental mercury. Trivalent chromium is an essential element for life and health, while hexavalent chromium is not utilized but is toxic. Arsenic occurs commonly in the environment as pentavalent arsenic which is relatively nontoxic. Commercial products, as pesticides, commonly employ trivalent arsenicals which are much more toxic than the naturally occuring forms.

Metals can form carbon metal bonds and this combination may alter the distribution and toxicity of the metal. Common examples are mercury and lead which are generally much more readily absorbed in their organo metallic state and may be rapidly distributed to susceptible organs.

Heavy metals can form reversible complexes with organic ligands in the process of chelation. The ligand supplies at least one pair of non bonded electrons which can provide a reversible complex that may alter abxorption, transport, or excretion of metals. For example lead may be concentrated as a complex in bile which serves as an excretory mechanism. Proteins such as metallothionein serve as transport molecules for metals. This may alter the availability of the metal as well as the delivery of metals to specific organs. For example, the mercuty protein complex taken into renal tubular cells by endocytosis may dissociate within the cell leaving unbound mercury to function as a toxicant.

CHARACTERISTICS OF METAL POISONS

Toxic metals may be cumulative and store in definite tissue locations. Storage organs may be discrete such as bone which stores high concentrations of lead, or diffuse as with plasma proteins or skin and hair. Although metals may be cumulative storage is not always equated with toxicosis. This is because some storage sites are toxicologically inert. Lead stored in bone is considered removed from active toxicologic functions as is arsenic accumulated in hair. However, these storage sites may serve as a reservoir for toxicosis if physiologic or pathologic changes induce rapid mobilization. Prolonged acidosis, for example, could release increased amounts of lead stored in bone thus raising levels of available lead in the blood.

Route of exposure may be important in modifying toxicosis. Oral exposure could modify toxicosis in many ways. Concurrent intake of other minerals or foods may serve to reduce absorption of certain heavy metals. Plant phytates may bind lead and reduce its absorption of certain heavy metals. Plant phytates may bind lead and reduce its absorption. High sulfates can alter the net absorption of copper. The respiratory route exposes animals to fumes which may be rapidly and nearly completely absorbed. Susceptibility to dermal absorption of metals may be increased when the metal is organically bound, such as methyl mercury or tetraethyl lead.

Metals or their salts may induce tissue damage and alter metabolism or synthesis of essential molecules. Metal salts such as mercuric chloride or ferric compounds may have astringent or fixative effects resulting in direct damage to mucous membranes. Metallic compounds can bind to enzymes, membrane proteins, or other essential structural proteins.

Metal imbalances or interactions are common. Metals may complex with one another or with the same protein molecule resulting in altered toxicity. Metal toxicity may be enhanced by nutrient deficiencies. Lead toxicity has been enhanced by deficiencies of calcium, phosphate, iron and zinc. Conversely nutritional deficiencies have been induced by excessive intake of certain metals. For example, molybdenum toxicosis in cattle results in copper deficiency as excessive copper elimination is promoted by high molybdenum intake. Excessive calcium intake by swine increases dietary requiremints for zinc in order to prevent the nutritional disease perakeratosis. Providing elevated amounts of certain nutrients may also reduce metal toxicity. High dietary calcium and zinc have reduced lead toxicity in experimental animals and horses respectively. Elevated selenium levels protect against mercury toxicosis by allowing sequestration of merqueryand selenium in tissues in an apparently unavailable form.

Organic and inorganic forms of metals may result in marked variation in expression of toxicity. Organomercurials result in clinical signs and lesions commonly affecting the central nervous system while inorganic mercuty results in acute gastroenteritis and renal damage.

Absorption of metals from the gastrointestinal tract is generally low (less than 10%) and metals often form insoluble complexes with dietary components such as sulfates, oxalates, phytates, or other naturally occuring chelates. In some cases toxic metals such as lead may compete with a carrier site such as the calcium transport system. Low molecular weight organic acids and amino acids may solublize such as occurs when acetic acid and lead form highly soluble lead acetate.

Several detoxication pathways are available for metals. As mentioned earlier insoluble precipitates may form in the gastrointestinal tract thus preventing absorption. Non toxic complexes may form in blood, particularly involving phosphates, citrates, bicarbonates, red cell membrane, and serum proteins. Particulate metals entering the respiratory tract may be phagocytized by macrophages with eventual movement to lymphatics or return to the pharynx via tracheal and bronchial cilia and mucus. Storage may occur at inert depots, such as bone.

Organic ligands (EDTA, penicillamine) administered to animals allows formation of a polar complex which is readily filtered and excreted via the kidney. Metals may also by detoxified by combination with nonessential cell constituents. Metallothionein is a protein component of liver and kidney which is readily filtered and excreted via the kidney. Metals may also be detoxified by combination with nonessential cell constituents.

Metallothionein is a protein component of liver and kidney which can bind various heavy metals such as cadmiun, zinc, copper, lead, and mercury. Inclusion bodies consisting of metal-protein complexes may form at intercellular locations thus removing the metal from active sites. Metals may also combine with sulfhydryl containing natural detoxicants such as reduced glutathione.

Acute heavy metal poisoning of livestock and pets occurs less frequently today than in the past. Increasing awareness of metal toxicosis by veterinarians and the public has resulted in better control of classic toxicologic agents sich as lead, arsenic, mercury, and thallium. Intentional feed additives such as copper, arsenic, and mercury. Occational isolated incidents of over exposure from any of these sources can occur. The veterinarian should be constantly aware of those situations which can contribute to unusual heavy metal burdens or toxic exposure. Recently concern for heavy metals has been focused on low level accumulation and subtle effects such as birth defects, carcinogenesis and impaired immune performance. The role of food animals as accumulators of metal residues in the food chain has been questioned. Livestock (dairy cattle, swine, and chickens) chronically exposed to subtoxic amounts of lead and cadmium did not accumulate appreciable amounts in milk, meat, or eggs. Most accumulation occured in liver and kidney with cadmium accumulation greater than lead.

LEAD POISONING

In veterinary medicine, lead poisoning is most common in dogs and cattle. Lead poisoning in other species is limited by reduced accessibility, more selective eating habits, or lower susceptibility. In cattle, many cases are associated with seeding and harvesting activities when used oil and battery disposal from machinery is handled improperly. Other sources of lead include paint, linoleum, grease, lead weights, lead shot, and contaminated foliage growing near smelters or along roadsides. Lead poisoning is also encountered in urban environments, and renovation of old houses that have been painted with lead-based paint has been associated with lead poisoning in small animals and children.

Pathogenesis

Absorbed lead enters the blood and soft tissues and eventually redistributes to the bone. The degree of absorption and retention is influenced by dietary factors such as calcium or iron levels. In ruminants, particulate lead lodged in the reticulum slowly dissolves and releases significant quantities of lead. Lead has a profound effect on sulfhydryl-containing enzymes, the thiol content of erythrocytes, antioxidant defenses, and tissues rich in mitochondria, which is reflected in the clinical syndrome. In addition to the cerebellar hemorrhage and edema associated with capillary damage, lead is also irritating, immunosuppressive, gametotoxic, teratogenic, nephrotoxic, and toxic to the hematopoietic system.

Clinical Findings

Acute lead poisoning is more common in young animals. The prominent clinical signs are associated with the GI and nervous systems. In cattle, signs that appear within 24-48 hr of exposure include ataxia, blindness, salivation, spastic twitching of eyelids, jaw champing, bruxism, muscle tremors, and convulsions.

Subacute lead poisoning, usually seen in sheep or older cattle, is characterized by anorexia, rumen stasis, colic, dullness, and transient constipation, frequently followed by diarrhea, blindness, head pressing, bruxism, hyperesthesia, and incoordination. Chronic lead poisoning, which is occasionally seen in cattle, may produce a syndrome that has many features in common with acute or subacute lead poisoning.

GI abnormalities, including anorexia, colic, emesis, and diarrhea or constipation, may be seen in dogs. Anxiety, hysterical barking, jaw champing, salivation, blindness, ataxia, muscle spasms, opisthotonos, and convulsions may develop. CNS depression rather than CNS excitation may be evident in some dogs. In horses, lead poisoning usually produces a chronic syndrome characterized by weight loss, depression, weakness, colic, diarrhea, laryngeal or pharyngeal paralysis (roaring), and dysphagia that frequently results in aspiration pneumonia.

In avian species, anorexia, ataxia, loss of condition, wing and leg weakness, and anemia are the most notable signs.

Lesions

Animals that die from acute lead poisoning may have few observable gross lesions. Oil or flakes of paint or battery may be evident in the GI tract. The caustic action of lead salts causes gastroenteritis. In the nervous system, edema, congestion of the cerebral cortex, and flattening of the cortical gyri are present. Histologically, endothelial swelling, laminar cortical necrosis, and edema of the white matter may be evident. Tubular necrosis and degeneration and intranuclear acid-fast inclusion bodies may be seen in the kidneys. Osteoporosis has been described in lambs. Placentitis and accumulation of lead in the fetus may result in abortion.

Diagnosis

Lead levels in various tissues may be useful to evaluate excessive accumulation and to reflect the level or duration of exposure, severity, and prognosis and the success of treatment. Concentrations of lead in the blood at 0. 35 ppm, liver at 10 ppm, or kidney cortex at 10 ppm are consistent with a diagnosis of lead poisoning in most species.

Hematologic abnormalities, which may be indicative but not confirmatory of lead poisoning, include anemia, anisocytosis, poikilocytosis, polychromasia, basophilic stippling, metarubricytosis, and hypochromia. Blood or urinary d-aminolevulinic acid and free erythrocyte protoporphyrin levels are sensitive indicators of lead exposure but may not be reliable indicators of clinical disease. Radiologic examination may be useful to determine the magnitude of lead exposure.

Lead poisoning may be confused with other diseases that cause nervous or GI abnormalities. In cattle, such diseases may include polioencephalomalacia, nervous coccidiosis, tetanus, hypovitaminosis A, hypomagnesemic tetany, nervous acetonemia, arsenic or mercury poisoning, brain abscess or neoplasia, rabies, listeriosis, and Haemophilus infections.

In dogs, rabies, distemper, and hepatitis may appear similar to lead poisoning.

Treatment

If tissue damage is extensive, particularly to the nervous system, treatment may not be successful. In livestock, calcium disodium edetate (Ca-EDTA) is given IV or SC (110 mg/kg/day) divided into 2 treatments daily for 3 days; this treatment should be repeated 2 days later. In dogs, a similar dose divided into 4 treatments/day is administered SC in 5% dextrose for 2-5 days. After a 1-wk rest period, an additional 5-day treatment may be required if clinical signs persist. No approved veterinary product containing Ca-EDTA is commercially available at present.

Thiamine (2-4 mg/kg/day SC) alleviates clinical manifestations and reduces tissue deposition of lead. Combined Ca-EDTA and thiamine treatment appears to produce the most beneficial response.

d-Penicillamine can be administered PO to dogs (110 mg/kg/day) for 2 wk. However, undesirable side effects such as emesis and anorexia have been associated with this treatment. d-Penicillamine is not recommended for livestock. Succimer (meso 2, 3-dimercaptosuccinic acid, DMSA) is a chelating agent that has proven to be effective in dogs (10 mg/kg, PO, tid for 10 days) and is also useful in birds. Fewer side effects have been associated with DMSA as compared with Ca-EDTA.

Cathartics such as magnesium sulfate (400 mg/kg, PO) or a rumenotomy may be useful to remove lead from the GI tract. Barbiturates or tranquilizers may be indicated to control convulsions. Chelation therapy, in combination with antioxidant treatment, may limit oxidative damage associated with acute lead poisoning. Antioxidants such as n-acetylcysteine (50 mg/kg, PO, sid) have been used in combination with DMSA.

Mobilization of lead at parturition, excretion of lead into milk, and lengthy withdrawal times in food-producing animals raise considerable controversy regarding the rationale for treatment from both public health and animal management perspectives.

MERCURY POISONING

Mercury exists in a variety of organic and inorganic forms. The replacement of commercial mercurial compounds, including antiseptics (eg, mercurochrome), diuretics, and fungicides by other agents has decreased the likelihood of mercurial toxicosis; however, the possibility of exposure to environmental sources of organic methylmercury exists.

Inorganic Mercurials

These include the volatile elemental form of mercury (used in thermometers) and the salted forms (mercuric chloride [sublimate] and mercurous chloride [calomel]). Ingested inorganic mercury is poorly absorbed and low in toxicity. Large amounts of these mercurials are corrosive and may produce vomiting, diarrhea, and colic. Renal damage also occurs, with polydipsia and anuria in severe cases. In rare cases of chronic inorganic mercurial poisoning, the CNS effects resemble those of organic mercury poisoning. Mercury vapor from elemental mercury produces corrosive bronchitis and interstitial pneumonia and, if not fatal, may lead to neurologic signs as do organic forms.

Emesis followed by initiation of chelation therapy is recommended after acute oral ingestion. Oral administration of sodium thiosulfate to bind mercury still in the gut may be beneficial.

Organic Mercury

Inorganic mercury is converted to the organic alkyl forms, methylmercury and ethylmercury, by microorganisms in the sediment of rivers, lakes, and seas. Marine life accumulate the most toxic form, methylmercury, and fish must be monitored for contamination. There are reports of commercial cat food causing severe neurologic disturbances in cats fed an exclusive tuna diet for 7-11 mo.

The organic mercurials are absorbed via all routes and bioaccumulate in the brain and to some extent in the kidneys and muscle. Aryl mercurials (eg, phenylmercury fungicide) are slightly less toxic and less prone to bioaccumulation. Animals poisoned by organic mercury exhibit CNS stimulation and locomotor abnormalities after a lengthy latent period (weeks).

Signs may include blindness, excitation, abnormal behavior and chewing, incoordination, and convulsions. Cats show hindleg rigidity, hypermetria, cerebellar ataxia, and tremors. Mercury is also a mutagen, teratogen, and a carcinogen, and is embryocidal. Differential diagnoses include conditions with tremors and ataxia as predominant signs, such as ingestion of other metals and insecticides and cerebellar lesions due to trauma or feline parvovirus.

Histologic lesions include degeneration of neurons and perivascular cuffing in the cerebrocortical gray matter, cerebellar atrophy of the granular layer, and damage to Purkinje cells. Laboratory diagnosis must differentiate between normal concentrations of mercury in tissue (especially whole blood, kidney, and brain) and feed (<1 ppm) and concentrations associated with poisoning.

Neurologic signs may be irreversible once they develop. Chelation therapy with dimercaprol (3 mg/kg body wt, IM, every 4 hr for the first 2 days, qid on the third day, and bid for the next 10 days or until recovery is complete) has been beneficial. When available, the water soluble, less toxic analog of dimercaprol, 2, 3-dimercaptosuccinic acid, is the chelator of choice for organic mercury poisoning. Penicillamine (15-50 mg/kg, PO) may be used only after the gut is free of ingested mercury and renal function has been established.

COPPER POISONING

Acute or chronic copper poisoning is encountered in most parts of the world. Sheep are affected most often, although other species are also susceptible. In various breeds of dogs, especially Bedlington Terriers, an inherited sensitivity to copper toxicosis similar to Wilson's disease in humans has been identified.

Acute poisoning is usually seen after accidental administration of excessive amounts of soluble copper salts, which may be present in anthelmintic drenches, mineral mixes, or improperly formulated rations. Many factors that alter copper metabolism influence chronic copper poisoning by enhancing the absorption or retention of copper. Low levels of molybdenum or sulfate in the diet are important examples.

Primary chronic poisoning is seen most commonly in sheep when excessive amounts of copper are ingested over a prolonged period. The toxicosis remains subclinical until the copper that is stored in the liver is released in massive amounts. Blood copper concentrations increase suddenly, causing lipid peroxidation and intravascular hemolysis. The hemolytic crisis may be precipitated by many factors, including transportation, pregnancy, lactation, strenuous exercise, or a deteriorating plane of nutrition.

Phytogenous and hepatogenous factors influence secondary chronic copper poisoning. Phytogenous chronic poisoning is seen after ingestion of plants, such as subterranean clover (*Trifolium subterraneum*), that produce a mineral imbalance and result in excessive copper retention. The plants that are not hepatotoxic contain normal amounts of copper and low levels of molybdenum. The ingestion of plants such as Heliotropium europaeum or Senecio spp (Plants Poisonous to Animals) for several months may cause hepatogenous chronic copper poisoning. These plants contain hepatotoxic alkaloids, which result in retention of excessive copper in the liver.

Acute poisoning may follow intakes of 20-100 mg of copper/kg in sheep and young calves and of 200-800 mg/kg in mature cattle. Chronic poisoning of sheep may occur with daily intakes of 3. 5 mg of copper/kg when grazing pastures that contain 15-20 ppm (dry matter) of copper and low levels of molybdenum.

Clinical disease may occur in sheep that ingest cattle rations, which normally contain higher levels of copper, or when their water is supplied via copper plumbing; cattle are more resistant to copper poisoning than sheep, and thus are not affected in these instances. Young calves or sheep injected with soluble forms of copper may develop acute clinical signs of toxicity. Copper is used as a feed additive for pigs at 125-250 ppm; levels >250 ppm are dangerous—although as for sheep, other factors may be protective, eg, high levels of protein, zinc, or iron. Chronic copper toxicosis is more apt to occur with low dietary intake of molybdenum and sulfur. Reduced formation of copper molybdate or copper sulfide complexes in tissues impairs the excretion of copper in urine or feces.

Clinical Findings

Acute copper poisoning causes severe gastroenteritis characterized by abdominal pain, diarrhea, anorexia, dehydration, and shock. Hemolysis and hemoglobinuria may develop after 3 days if the animal survives the GI disturbances. The sudden onset of clinical signs in chronic copper poisoning is associated with the hemolytic crisis. Affected animals exhibit depression, weakness, recumbency, rumen stasis, anorexia, thirst, dyspnea, pale mucous membranes, hemoglobinuria, and jaundice. Several days or weeks before the hemolytic crisis, liver enzymes, including ALT and AST, are usually increased. During the hemolytic crisis, methemoglobinemia, hemoglobinemia, and decreases in PCV and blood glutathione are usually seen.

In camelid species such as alpacas or llamas, no hemolytic crisis is observed, although extensive liver necrosis remains a predominant sign. Morbid animals often die within 1-2 days. Herd morbidity is often <5%, although usually >75% of affected animals die. Losses may continue for several months after the dietary problem has been rectified. Severe hepatic insufficiency is responsible for early deaths. Animals that survive the acute episode may die of subsequent renal failure.

Lesions

Acute copper poisoning produces severe gastroenteritis with erosions and ulcerations in the abomasum of ruminants. Icterus develops in animals that survive >24 hr. Tissues discolored by icterus and methemoglobin are characteristic of chronic poisoning. Swollen, gunmetal-colored kidneys, port-wine-colored urine, and an enlarged spleen with dark brown-black parenchyma are manifestations of the hemolytic crisis. The liver is enlarged and friable. Histologically, there is centrilobular hepatic and renal tubular necrosis.

Diagnosis

Evidence of blue-green ingesta and increased fecal (8, 000-10, 000 ppm) and kidney (>15 ppm, wet wt) copper levels are considered significant in acute copper poisoning. In chronic poisoning, blood and liver copper concentrations are increased during the hemolytic period. Blood levels often rise to 5-20 μg/mL, as compared with normal levels of ~1 μg/mL. Liver concentrations >150 ppm (wet wt) are significant in sheep. The concentration of copper in the tissue must be determined to eliminate other causes of hemolytic disease.

Treatment and Control

Often, treatment is not successful. GI sedatives and symptomatic treatment for shock may be useful in acute toxicity. Penicillamine (50 mg/kg, PO, sid, for 6 days) or calcium versenate may be useful if administered in the early stages of disease. Experimentally, ammonium tetrathiomolybdate (15 mg/kg, IV, on alternate days) is effective for the treatment and prevention of copper poisoning. Daily administration of ammonium molybdate (100 mg) and sodium sulfate (1 g) reduces losses in affected lambs. Dietary supplementation with zinc acetate (250 ppm) may be useful to reduce the absorption of copper. Plant eradication or reducing access to plants that cause phytogenous or hepatogenous copper poisoning is desirable. Primary chronic or phytogenous poisoning may be prevented by top-dressing pastures with 1 oz of molybdenum per acre (70 g/hectare) in the form of molybdenized superphosphate or by molybdenum supplementation or restriction of copper intake.

ZINC TOXICOSIS

Zinc is an essential trace metal that plays an important role in many biologic processes. It is ubiquitous in nature and exists in many forms. The ingestion of some forms leads to creation of toxic zinc salts in the acidic gastric environment. Zinc toxicity has been documented in humans as well as in a wide range of large, small, exotic, and wild animals. It is seen commonly in pet dogs, possibly because of a higher degree of dietary indiscretion and greater levels of exposure to zinc-containing substances. Common sources of zinc include batteries, automotive parts, paints, zinc-oxide creams, herbal supplements, zippers, board-game pieces, screws and nuts on pet carriers, and the coating on galvanized metals such as pipes and cookware. One of the most well known sources of zinc that causes toxicity following ingestion is the USA Lincoln penny. Some pennies minted during 1983, and all pennies minted since, are 97. 5% zinc by weight.

Pathogenesis

The low pH in the stomach causes the formation of soluble zinc salts. These are absorbed from the duodenum and rapidly distributed to the liver, kidneys, prostate, muscles, bones, and pancreas. Zinc salts have direct irritant and corrosive effects on tissue, interfere with the metabolism of other ions such as copper, calcium, and iron, and inhibit erythrocyte production and function. The mechanisms by which zinc exerts these toxic effects are not completely understood. The median lethal dose (LD50) of zinc salts in cases of acute toxicity has been reported to be ~100 mg/kg. Also, diets containing high levels of zinc (>2, 000 ppm) have been reported to cause chronic zinc toxicosis in large animals.

Clinical Signs and Lesions

Clinical signs vary based on the duration and degree of exposure. Signs progress from anorexia and vomiting to more advanced symptoms such as diarrhea, lethargy, icterus, shock, intravascular hemolysis, hemoglobinuria, cardiac arrhythmias, and seizures.

Large animals often show decreases in weight gain and milk production, and lameness has been reported in foals secondary to epiphyseal swelling. Major histopathologic findings include hepatocellular centrolobular necrosis with hemosiderosis and vacuolar degeneration, renal tubular necrosis with hemoglobin casts, and pancreatic duct necrosis with fibrosis of the interlobular fat.

Diagnosis

Radiodense material is easily seen on radiographs of the GI tract in animals with zinc-containing foreign bodies. Changes in the CBC, chemistry profile, urinalysis, and coagulation profile reflect the degree of toxicity to various organ systems. The hemogram typically reveals a regenerative hemolytic anemia characterized by changes in erythrocyte morphology.

The leukogram often shows a neutrophilic leukocytosis secondary to stress, pancreatitis, and a regenerative bone marrow. Serum chemistry changes that are seen secondary to hepatic damage include elevations in bilirubin, the transaminases, and alkaline phosphatase. As zinc accumulates in the pancreas, increases in amylase and lipase can be seen following pancreatitis and pancreatic necrosis.

Glomerular damage and renal tubular epithelial necrosis result in elevations in BUN, creatinine, amylase, and urine protein. Hemoglobinuria can be differentiated from hematuria during urinalysis; the urine color will not clear after centrifugation in the presence of hemoglobinuria. Prolongation of prothrombin time and activated partial thromboplastin time can result from toxic effects on the synthesis or function of coagulation factors.

The hematologic and clinical findings in animals with zinc toxicosis are similar to the changes in animals with immune-mediated hemolytic anemia (IMHA). Misdiagnosis of a primary autoimmune disorder can lead to the inappropriate use of immunosuppressive drugs. Zinc toxicosis can cause the direct antiglobulin test (direct Coombs' test) to be positive in the absence of a primary autoimmune disorder. The direct Coombs' test is therefore not reliable when differentiating between zinc intoxication and IMHA.

Definitive diagnosis of zinc poisoning is achieved by measuring zinc levels in blood or other tissue. In dogs and cats, the normal serum zinc level is 0. 7-2 μg/mL. Serum samples can be submitted in green-top heparinized tubes or in royal blue-top trace element tubes. Methods for quantifying zinc levels from saliva and hair have not been validated in domestic animals, and measuring zinc in urine is unreliable because elimination of zinc through the kidneys is variable.

Differential diagnoses should include any infectious, toxic, immune-mediated, neoplastic, genetic, or other medical disorder characterized by clinical signs and laboratory test results similar to those seen in cases of zinc toxicity. These include IMHA, hypophosphatemia, splenic torsion, babesiosis, ehrlichiosis, heartworm disease, leptospirosis, hemobartonellosis, feline leukemia infection, hemangiosarcoma, lymphosarcoma, phosphofructokinase or pyruvate-kinase deficiency, and toxicity from acetaminophen, naphthalene, paradichlorobenzene, Allium, lead, or copper.

Treatment and Prevention

After stabilizing the animal with fluids, oxygen, and blood products as necessary, removal of the source of zinc as early as possible is paramount. This often requires surgery or endoscopy. Inducing emesis to remove chronic gastric zinc foreign bodies is typically not rewarding because zinc objects often adhere to the gastric mucosa.

Diuresis with a balanced crystalloid solution is indicated to promote renal excretion of zinc and prevent hemoglobinuric nephrosis.

There is debate regarding the necessity of chelation therapy in cases of zinc toxicosis. Animals can recover from zinc intoxication following only supportive care and removal of the source. However, chelation therapy enhances elimination of zinc and thus may accelerate recovery. Calcium disodium ethylenediaminetetraacetate (Ca-EDTA) successfully chelates zinc when given at 100 mg/kg/day IV or SC for 3 days (diluted and divided into 4 doses), but may exacerbate zinc-induced nephrotoxicity. Although they have been used to treat animals with zinc toxicity, d-penicillamine and dimercaprol (British antilewisite) have not been specifically validated for this purpose. Reported doses are 110 mg/kg/day for 7-14 days for d-penicillamine, and 3-6 mg/kg tid for 3-5 days for dimercaprol. Chelation therapy with any of these agents should be monitored with serial serum zinc levels to help determine the appropriate duration of treatment.

If diagnosed early and treated aggressively, the outcome is often favorable for animals with zinc toxicosis. Eliminating sources of zinc from the environment is essential in preventing recurrence.

MOLYBDENUM POISONING

Molybdenum is an essential micronutrient that forms molybdenoenzymes, which are necessary for the health of all animals. In ruminants, the dietary intake of excessive molybdenum causes, in part, a secondary hypocuprosis. Toxicosis due to massive doses of molybdenum is rare. Domestic ruminants are much more susceptible to molybdenum toxicity than nonruminants. The resistance of other species is at least 10 times that of cattle and sheep.

The metabolism of copper, molybdenum, and inorganic sulfate is a complex and incompletely understood interrelationship. It appears that the ruminal interaction of molybdates and sulfides gives rise to thiomolybdates (mono-, di-, tri-, and tetrathiomolybdates). Copper reacts with thiomolybdates (primarily tri-and tetrathiomolybdates) in the rumen to form an insoluble complex that is poorly absorbed. On this basis, tetrathiomolybdate is used in treating and preventing copper toxicity in sheep. Some thiomolybdates are absorbed and decrease blood copper availability and also appear to directly inhibit copper-dependent enzymes.

Therefore, the susceptibility of ruminants to molybdenum toxicity depends on a number of factors:

1) copper content of the diet and intake of the animal—tolerance to molybdenum toxicity decreases as the content and intake of copper decrease;
2) the inorganic sulfate content of the diet—high dietary sulfate with low copper exacerbates the condition, while low dietary sulfate causes high blood molybdenum levels due to decreased excretion;
3) chemical form of the molybdenum—water-soluble molybdenum in growing herbage is most toxic, while curing decreases toxicity;
4) presence of certain sulfur-containing amino acids;
5) species of animal—cattle are less tolerant than sheep;
6) age—young animals are more susceptible;
7) season of year—plants concentrate molybdenum beginning in spring (maximum level reached in fall); and
8) botanic composition of the pasture—legumes take up more of the element than other plant species.

Molybdenum toxicity associated with copper deficiency has been seen in areas with peat or muck soils, where plants grow in alkaline sloughs (e.g., western USA), as a result of industrial contamination (mining and metal alloy production), where excess molybdenum-containing fertilizer has been applied, and where applications of lime appeared to increase plant molybdenum uptake.

In the diet of cattle, copper:molybdenum ratios of 6:1 are considered ideal; 2:1-3:1, borderline; and <2:1, toxic. Dietary molybdenum of >10 ppm can cause toxicity regardless of copper intake; as little as 1 ppm may be hazardous if copper content is <5 ppm (dry-weight basis). Mixing errors may occur; concentrations above 1, 000 mg/kg (as sodium molybdate) cause growth retardation while concentrations of 2,000-4,000 mg/kg cause death within 40 days.

Clinical Findings and Diagnosis

Most of the clinical signs attributed to molybdenum toxicity arise from impaired copper metabolism and are the same as those produced by simple copper deficiency. Molybdenum toxicity in cattle is characterized by persistent, severe scouring with passage of liquid feces full of gas bubbles.

Depigmentation, resulting in fading of the hair coat, is most noticeable in black animals and especially around the eyes, which gives a spectacled appearance. Other signs include unthriftiness, anemia, emaciation, joint pain (lameness), osteoporosis, and decreased fertility. Effects on reproduction, particularly in heifers, include delayed puberty, decreased weight at puberty, and reduced conception rates.

It appears that fertility is uniquely vulnerable to the effects of molybdenum or thiomolybdates and alone responds indirectly to copper acting as an antidote. Some studies have suggested that relatively low levels of molybdenum may exert these direct effects on certain metabolic processes, particularly reproduction, independent of alterations in copper metabolism. Sheep, and young animals in particular, show stiffness of the back and legs with a reluctance to rise (called enzootic ataxia in Australia). Joint and skeletal lesions appear to be due to defects in development of connective tissue and growth plates. Clinical signs appear within 1-2 wk of grazing affected pasture.

In molybdenum toxicity, low copper levels in blood and tissue and the occurrence of clinical signs of copper deficiency in cattle are poorly correlated. A provisional diagnosis can be made if the diarrhea stops within a few days of oral dosing with copper sulfate; the diagnosis is further supported if other causes of diarrhea and unthriftiness (including GI parasites) are ruled out. Diagnosis is confirmed by demonstrating abnormal concentrations of molybdenum and copper in blood or liver and by a high dietary intake of molybdenum relative to copper.

The disease may be confused with many other enteritides and is commonly mistaken for internal parasitism, especially in young cattle. In pastured animals, it is not uncommon for the diseases to occur simultaneously.

Effects in cattle and sheep poisoned with massive concentrations of molybdenum are unlike the chronic induced copper deficiency described above. Cattle lose appetite within 3 days and deaths begin to occur within 1 wk and continue for months after exposure ends. Animals appear lethargic, display hind limb ataxia that progresses to involve the front limbs, salivate profusely, and produce scant, mucoid feces. The molybdenum is toxic to hepatocytes and renal tubular epithelial cells, producing periacinar to massive hepatic necrosis and nephrosis.

Prevention and Treatment

Signs of severe acute toxicosis are reversed by providing copper sulfate in the diet. In areas where the molybdenum content of the forage is <5 ppm, the use of 1% copper sulfate ($CuSO_4 \cdot 5H_2O$) in salt has provided satisfactory control of molybdenosis. With higher levels of molybdenum, 2% copper sulfate has been successful; up to 5% has been used in a few regions where the molybdenum levels are very high. In areas where, for various reasons, cattle do not consume mineral supplements, the required copper may be supplied as a drench given weekly, as parenterally administered repository copper preparations, or as a top-dressing to the pasture. Copper glycinate injectable has been used successfully as an adjunct to therapy.

ARSENIC POISONING

Arsenic poisoning in animals is caused by several different types of inorganic and organic arsenical compounds. Toxicity varies with factors such as oxidation state of the arsenic, solubility, species of animal involved, and duration of exposure. Therefore, the toxic effects produced by phenylarsonic feed additives and other inorganic and organic compounds must be distinguished.

Inorganic Arsenicals

These include arsenic trioxide, arsenic pentoxide, sodium and potassium arsenate, sodium and potassium arsenite, and lead or calcium arsenate. Trivalent arsenicals, also known as arsenites, are more soluble and therefore more toxic than the pentavalents or arsenate compounds. The lethal oral dose of sodium arsenite in most species is from 1-25 mg/kg. Cats may be more sensitive. Arsenates (pentavalents) are 5-10 times less toxic than arsenites. Poisoning is now relatively infrequent due to decreased use of these compounds as pesticides, ant baits, and wood preservatives. Arsenites are used to some extent as dips for tick control. Lead arsenate is sometimes used as a taeniacide in sheep.

Toxicokinetics and Mechanism of Action

Soluble forms of arsenic compounds are well absorbed orally. Following absorption, most of the arsenic is bound to RBC; it distributes to several tissues, with the highest levels found in liver, kidneys, heart, and lungs. In subchronic or chronic exposures, arsenic accumulates in skin, nails, hooves, sweat glands, and hair. The majority of the absorbed arsenic is excreted in the urine as inorganic arsenic or in methylated form. The mechanism of action of arsenic toxicosis varies with the type of arsenical compound. Generally, tissues that are rich in oxidative enzymes such as the GI tract, liver, kidneys, lungs, endothelium, and epidermis are considered more vulnerable to arsenic damage. Trivalent inorganic and aliphatic organic arsenic compounds exert their toxicity by interacting with sulfhydryl enzymes, resulting in disruption of cellular metabolism. Arsenate can uncouple oxidation and phosphorylation.

Clinical Findings

Poisoning is usually acute with major effects on the GI tract and cardiovascular system. Arsenic has a direct effect on the capillaries, causing damage to microvascular integrity, transudation of plasma, loss of blood, and hypovolemic shock. Profuse watery diarrhea, sometimes tinged with blood, is characteristic, as are severe colic, dehydration, weakness, depression, weak pulse, and cardiovascular collapse. The onset is rapid, and signs are usually seen within a few hours (or up to 24 hr). The course may run from hours to several weeks depending on the quantity ingested. In peracute poisoning, animals may simply be found dead.

Lesions

In peracute toxicosis, no significant lesions may be seen. Inflammation and reddening of GI mucosa (local or diffuse) may be seen followed by edema, rupture of blood vessels and necrosis of epithelial and subepithelial tissue. Necrosis may progress to perforation of the gastric or intestinal wall. GI contents are often fluid, foul smelling, and blood tinged; they may contain shreds of epithelial tissue. There is diffuse inflammation of the liver, kidneys, and other visceral organs. The liver may have fatty degeneration and necrosis, and the kidneys have tubular damage. In cases of cutaneous exposure, the skin may exhibit necrosis and be dry or leathery.

Diagnosis

Chemical determination of arsenic in tissues (liver or kidney) or stomach contents provides confirmation. Liver and kidneys of normal animals rarely contain >1 ppm arsenic (wet wt); toxicity is associated with a concentration >3 ppm. The determination of arsenic in stomach contents is of value usually within the first 24-48 hr after ingestion. The concentration of arsenic in urine can be high for several days after ingestion. Drinking water containing >0. 25% arsenic is considered potentially toxic, especially for large animals.

Treatment

In animals with recent exposure and no clinical signs, emesis should be induced (in capable species), followed by activated charcoal with a cathartic (efficacy of charcoal in arsenic toxicosis remains to be determined) and then oral administration of GI protectants (small animals, 1-2 hr after charcoal) such as kaolin-pectin, and fluid therapy as needed. In animals already showing clinical signs, aggressive fluid therapy, blood transfusion (if needed), and administration of dimercaprol (British antilewisite, 4-7 mg/kg, IM, tid for 2-3 days or until recovery). In large animals, thioctic acid (lipoic acid or a-lipoic acid) may be used alone (50 mg/kg, IM, tid, as a 20% solution) or in combination with dimercaprol (3 mg/kg, IM, every 4 hr for the first 2 days, qid for the third day, and bid for the next 10 days or until recovery). In large animals, the efficacy of dimercaprol alone is questionable.

Sodium thiosulfate has also been used, PO, at 20-30 g in 300 mL of water in horses and cattle, one-fourth this dose in sheep and goats, and 0. 5-3 g in small animals or as a 20% solution, IV, at 30-40 mg/kg, 2-3 times/day for 3-4 days or until recovery. The water-soluble analogs of dimercaprol, 2, 3-dimercaptopropane-1-sulfonate (DMPS) and dimercaptosuccinic acid (DMSA), are considered to be less toxic and more effective and could be given orally. d-Penicillamine has been reported to be an effective arsenic chelator in humans. It has a wide margin of safety and could be used in animals at 10-50 mg/kg, PO, 3-4 times/day for 3-4 days. Supportive therapy may be of even greater value, particularly when cardiovascular collapse is imminent, and should involve IV fluids to restore blood volume and correct dehydration. Kidney and liver function should be monitored during treatment.

Organic Arsenicals

Phenylarsonic organic arsenicals are relatively less toxic than inorganic compounds or aliphatic and other aromatic organic compounds.

Aliphatic organic arsenicals include cacodylic acid and acetarsonic acid. These are generally used as stimulants in large animals, but their use is no longer common. Some aliphatic arsenicals such as monosodium methanearsonate (MSMA) and disodium methanearsonate (DSMA) are occasionally used as cotton defoliants or crabgrass killers. Persistence of MSMA or DSMA in the soil and their tendency to accumulate in plants creates a potential for arsenic poisoning, especially in grazing animals. Clinical signs, lesions, and treatment of aliphatic organic arsenicals are similar to those of inorganic arsenicals.

Aromatic organic arsenicals include trivalent phenylorganicals such as thiacetarsamide and arsphenamine for the treatment of adult heartworms in dogs and pentavalent compounds such as phenylarsonic acids and their salts. Thiacetarsamide and arsphenamine are no longer used commonly, especially since the recent introduction of melarsomine dihydrochloride.

Phenylarsonic compounds are used as feed additives to improve production in swine and poultry rations and also to treat dysentery in pigs. The 3 major compounds in this class are arsanilic acid, roxarsone (4-hydroxy-3-nitrophenylarsonic acid), and nitarsone (4-nitro-phenylarsonic acid).

Toxicosis results from an excess of arsenic-containing additives in pig or poultry diets. Severity and rapidity of onset are dose-dependent. Signs may be delayed for weeks after incorporation of 2-3 times the recommended (100 ppm) levels or may occur within days when the excess is >10 times the recommended levels. Chickens are tolerant of arsanilic acid; however, roxarsone can produce toxicosis in turkeys at only twice the recommended dose (50 ppm). Roxarsone also has a higher toxicity in pigs as compared with other phenylarsonics.

Clinical Findings and Diagnosis

The earliest sign in pigs may be a reduction in weight gain, followed by incoordination, posterior paralysis, and eventually quadriplegia. Animals remain alert and maintain good appetite. Blindness is characteristic of arsanilic acid intoxication but not of other organic arsenicals. In ruminants, phenylarsonic toxicosis is similar to inorganic arsenic poisoning. There are usually no specific lesions present in phenylarsonic poisoning. Demyelination and gliosis of peripheral nerves, the optic tract, and optic nerves are usually seen on histopathology. Analyses of feed for the presence of high levels of phenylarsonics confirm the diagnosis.

Phenylarsonic poisoning in pigs should be differentiated from salt poisoning, insecticide poisoning, and pseudorabies. In cattle, arsenic poisoning should be differentiated from other heavy metal (lead) poisoning, insecticide poisoning, and infectious diseases such as bovine viral diarrhea.

Treatment and Prognosis

There is no specific treatment, but the neurotoxic effects are usually reversible if the offending feed is withdrawn within 2-3 days of onset of ataxia. Once paralysis occurs, the nerve damage is irreversible. Blindness is also usually irreversible, but animals retain their appetite, and weight gain is good if competition for food is eliminated. Recovery may be doubtful when the exposure is long and the onset of intoxication slow.

REFERENCES

Clarkson, T. W. 1977. *Factors Involved in Heavy Metal Poisoning*. Fed. Proc. 36: 1634-1639.

Hammond, P. B. and Beliles, R. P. 1980. *Metals in Doull, J. ; Klassen, C. D. and Amdur, M. O. editors, Casarett and Doull's Toxicology: The Basic Science of Poisons*. Second edition, New York, MacMillan p 409.

Lee, D. H. K. 1973. "Biologic Effect of Metallic Contaminants—The Next Step". *Environ. Research* 6:121-131

Neatherly, M. W. and Miller W. J. 1975. "Metabolism and Toxicity of Cadmium, Mercuty, and Lead in Animals: A rewiew". *J. Diary Science* 58:1967-1982.

Pond, W. G. 1975. *Mineral Interrelationships in Nutrition: Practical Implications*. Cornell Vet. 65:441-456.

Sharma, R. P. and Street, J. C. 1980. "Public Health Aspects of Toxic Heavy Metals in Animal Feeds". *JAVMA* 177:149-153.

Ulmer, D. D. 1973. "Metals—from Provation to Pollution". *Fed. Proc.* 32:1758-1762.

5

Toxicology of Drugs

Human drugs or nutritional supplements available without a prescription are known as over-the-counter (OTC) medications. Exposures to OTC drugs in pets can be accidental or intentional. A valid client-patient-veterinarian relationship must exist for veterinarians to recommend extra-label use of these drugs to their clients. Safety of most OTC drugs has not been determined in animals, as most are not approved for veterinary use by the FDA. Veterinarians should understand the potential risks of using OTC medications and communicate them to their clients.

COLD AND COUGH MEDICATIONS

Antihistamines

Antihistamines are H1-receptor antagonists that provide symptomatic relief of allergic signs caused by histamine release, including pruritus and anaphylactic reactions. They are also used as sedatives and antiemetics. Antihistamines belong to different classes and are categorized as first- or second-generation antihistamines. First-generation antihistamines may cause adverse effects because of their cholinergic activity and ability to cross the blood-brain barrier. Second-generation antihistamines are more lipophobic than first-generation antihistamines and are thought to lack CNS and cholinergic effects at therapeutic doses. Antihistamines are often found in combination with other ingredients in many OTC cold, sinus, and allergy medications.

Chlorpheniramine is a first-generation propylamine-derivative antihistamine. Oral absorption of chlorpheniramine in dogs is rapid and complete, reaching peak plasma concentrations in 30-60 min. Chlorpheniramine maleate undergoes substantial first-pass effect. Chlorpheniramine and its metabolites are primarily excreted in urine. The recommended dose in cats and dogs is 1-2 mg and 2-8 mg respectively, PO, bid-tid. Mild clinical signs such as depression and GI upset have been reported for dosages <1 mg/kg. Significant clinical signs such as ataxia, tremors, depression or hyperactivity, hyperthermia, and seizures may be seen within 6 hr of ingestion of large amounts.

Dimenhydrinate and *diphenhydramine* are first-generation ethanolamine-derivative antihistamines. Diphenhydramine is well absorbed orally in people, but undergoes first-pass metabolism in the liver with only 40-60% of the drug reaching the systemic circulation. Peak plasma concentrations of ethanolamine-derivative antihistamines occur within 1-5 hr; elimination half-lives vary from 2.4-10 hr. A recommended dose for dimenhydrinate and diphenhydramine in cats and dogs is 4-8 mg/kg and 2-4 mg/kg, respectively. Hyperactivity or depression, hypersalivation, tachypnea, and tachycardia are the most common adverse signs reported with these antihistamines, generally within 1 hr of exposure.

Promethazine hydrochloride is an ethylamino derivative of phenothiazine and first-generation antihistamine used for the management of motion sickness. Promethazine is widely distributed in body tissues and readily crosses the placenta. Overdoses may result in CNS depression or excitation. CNS depression was reported in a dog 30 min after ingesting 1 mg/kg of promethazine.

Meclizine is a first-generation piperazine-derivative antihistamine commonly used as an antiemetic. Peak plasma concentrations occur within 2-3 hr of oral administration. Meclizine is primarily excreted as metabolites in urine, with a reported serum half-life of 6 hr. In cases involving <33 mg/kg of meclizine in dogs, only mild hyperactivity or depression has been reported.

Loratadine is a tricyclic long-acting antihistamine with selective peripheral histamine H1-receptor antagonist activity. In humans, loratadine is well absorbed orally and extensively metabolized to an active metabolite. Most of the parent drug is excreted unchanged in the urine. The mean elimination half-life in humans is 8.4 hr. Loratadine appears to have a large margin of safety in laboratory animals. No deaths were reported at oral doses up to 5 g/kg in rats and mice. In rats, mice, and monkeys, no clinical signs were observed at 10 times the maximum recommended human daily oral dose.

Treatment

Treatment of antihistamine toxicosis is primarily symptomatic and supportive. Emesis should only be considered in asymptomatic patients. Activated charcoal may be useful for recent ingestion. Cardiovascular function and body temperature should be closely monitored. Diazepam can be used to control seizures or seizure-type activity. Physostigmine is recommended to counteract the CNS anticholinergic effects of antihistamine overdoses in people, although the risk of seizures associated with this drug may limit its use.

DECONGESTANTS

Imidazoline Decongestants

The imidazoline derivatives, *oxymetazoline, xylometazoline, tetrahydrozoline,* and *naphazoline* are found in topical ophthalmic and nasal decongestants available OTC. They are generally used as topical vasoconstrictors in the nose and eyes for temporary relief of nasal congestion due to colds, hay fever or other upper respiratory allergies, or sinusitis.

Imidazolines are sympathomimetic agents, with primary effects on a-adrenergic receptors and little if any effect on ß-adrenergic receptors. Oxymetazoline is readily absorbed orally. Effects on a-receptors from systemically absorbed oxymetazoline hydrochloride may persist for up to 7 hr after a single dose. The elimination half-life in humans is 5-8 hr. It is excreted unchanged both by the kidneys (30%) and in feces (10%).

Clinical Findings

In dogs, signs of intoxication may include vomiting, bradycardia, cardiac arrhythmias, poor capillary refill time, hypotension or hypertension, panting, increased upper respiratory sounds, depression, weakness, nervousness, hyperactivity, or shaking. These signs appear within 30 min to 4 hr postexposure. In general, imidazoline decongestant exposure may affect the GI, cardiopulmonary, and nervous systems.

Treatment

Decontamination may not be practical due to the rapid absorption and onset of clinical signs. Heart rate and rhythm and blood pressure should be assessed, and an ECG obtained if needed. IV fluids should be given, along with atropine at 0.02 mg/kg, IV, if bradycardia is present. Diazepam (0.25-0.5 mg/kg, IV) can be given if CNS signs (eg, apprehension, shaking) are present. Serum electrolytes (ie, potassium, sodium, chloride) should be assessed and corrected as needed. Yohimbine, which is a specific a_2-adrenergic antagonist, can also be used at 0.1 mg/kg, IV, and repeated in 2-3 hr if needed.

Pseudoephedrine and Ephedrine

Pseudoephedrine is a sympathomimetic drug, which occurs naturally in plants of the genus Ephedra. Pseudoephedrine is a stereoisomer of ephedrine and is available as the hydrochloride or sulfate salt. Ephedrine and pseudoephedrine are common OTC medications used as nasal decongestants; these drugs are not currently affected by the

FDA ban on products containing ephedra. Both ephedrine and pseudoephedrine have α- and ß-adrenergic agonist effects.

The pharmacologic effects of the drugs are due to direct stimulation of adrenergic receptors and the release of norepinephrine. In humans, pseudoephedrine is rapidly absorbed orally. The onset of action is 15-30 min, with peak effects within 30-60 min. It is incompletely metabolized in the liver. Approximately 90% of the drug is eliminated through the kidneys. Renal excretion is accelerated in acidic urine. Elimination half-life varies between 2-21 hr, depending on urinary pH.

Clinical Findings

Pseudoephedrine and ephedrine overdose can result in mydriasis, tachycardia, hypertension, sinus arrhythmias, agitation, anxiety, hyperactivity, tremors, head bobbing, hiding, and vomiting. Clinical signs can be seen at 5-6 mg/kg and death may occur at 10-12 mg/kg.

Treatment

Treatment of pseudoephedrine toxicosis consists of decontamination, controlling the CNS and cardiovascular effects, and supportive care. Vomiting should be induced, followed by administration of activated charcoal with a cathartic. If the animal's condition contraindicates induction of emesis, a gastric lavage with a cuffed endotracheal tube should be performed.

Hyperactivity, nervousness, or seizures can be controlled with acepromazine (0.05-1.0 mg/kg, IM, IV, or SC), chlorpromazine (0.5-1.0 mg/kg, IV), phenobarbital (3-4 mg/kg, IV), or pentobarbital to effect. Diazepam should be avoided as it can exaggerate hyperactivity. Phenothiazines should be used with caution as they can lower the seizure threshold, lower blood pressure, and cause bizarre behavioral changes. Tachycardia can be controlled with propranolol at 0.02-0.04 mg/kg, IV, repeated if needed. IV fluids should be given.

Acidifying the urine with ammonium chloride (50 mg/kg, PO, qid) or ascorbic acid (20-30 mg/kg, IM or IV, tid) may enhance urinary excretion of pseudoephedrine. Acid-base status should be monitored if ammonium chloride or ascorbic acid is given. Electrolytes, heart rate and rhythm, and blood pressure should be monitored. Excessive trembling or shaking can cause myoglobinuria; if this occurs, kidney function should be monitored. Clinical signs of toxicosis can last 1-4 days. The presence of pseudoephedrine in urine can support the diagnosis.

Analgesics

Nonsteroidal Anti-inflammatory Drugs (NSAID)

NSAID are the most commonly used class of human medications in the world. Due to their widespread availability and use, acute accidental ingestion of human NSAID in dogs and cats is quite common. Ibuprofen, aspirin, and naproxen are some of the most commonly encountered NSAID in pet animals.

NSAID inhibit the enzyme cyclooxygenase (COX; also referred to as prostaglandin synthetase), blocking the production of prostaglandins (PG). It is believed that most NSAID act through COX inhibition, although they may also have other mechanisms of action.

Ibuprofen, 2-(4-isobutylphenyl) propionic acid, is used for its anti-inflammatory, antipyretic, and analgesic properties in animals and humans. It is rapidly absorbed orally in dogs with peak plasma concentrations seen in 30 min to 3 hr. Presence of food can delay absorption and the time to reach peak plasma concentration. The mean elimination half-life is ~4.6 hr. Ibuprofen is metabolized in the liver to several metabolites, which are mainly excreted in the urine within 24 hr. The major metabolic pathway is via conjugation with glucuronic acid, sometimes preceded by oxidation and hydroxylation.

Ibuprofen has been recommended in dogs at 5 mg/kg. However, prolonged use at this dosage may cause gastric ulcers and perforations. GI irritation or ulceration, GI hemorrhage, and renal damage are the most commonly reported toxic effects of ibuprofen ingestion in dogs. In addition, CNS depression, hypotension, ataxia, cardiac effects, and seizures can be seen. Ibuprofen has a narrow margin of safety in dogs. Dogs dosed with ibuprofen at 8-16 mg/kg/day, PO for 30 days showed gastric ulceration or erosions, along with other clinical signs of GI disturbances. An acute single ingestion of 100-125 mg/kg can lead to vomiting, diarrhea, nausea, abdominal pain, and anorexia. Renal failure may follow dosages of 175-300 mg/kg. CNS effects (i.e., seizures, ataxia, depression, coma) in addition to renal and GI signs can be seen at dosages >400 mg/kg. Dosages >600 mg/kg are potentially lethal in dogs.

Cats are susceptible to ibuprofen toxicosis at approximately half the dosage required to cause toxicosis in dogs. Cats are especially sensitive because they have a limited glucuronyl-conjugating capacity. Ibuprofen toxicity is more severe in ferrets than in dogs that consume similar dosages. Typical toxic effects of ibuprofen in ferrets involve the CNS, GI, and renal systems.

Aspirin (acetylsalicylic acid), the salicylate ester of acetic acid, is the prototype of salicylate drugs. It is a weak acid derived from phenol. The oral bioavailability of aspirin may vary due to differences in drug formulation. Aspirin reduces prostaglandin and thromboxane synthesis by COX inhibition. Salicylates also uncouple mitochondrial oxidative phosphorylation and inhibit specific dehydrogenases. Platelets are incapable of synthesizing new cyclooxgenase, leading to an effect on platelet aggregation.

Aspirin is rapidly absorbed from the stomach and proximal small intestine in monogastric animals. The rate of absorption depends on gastric emptying, tablet disintegration rates, and gastric pH. Peak salicylate levels are reached 0.5-3 hr after ingestion. Topically applied salicylic acid can be absorbed systemically.

Aspirin is hydrolyzed to salicylic acid by esterases in the liver and, to a lesser extent, in the GI mucosa, plasma, RBC, and synovial fluid. Salicylic acid is 50-70% protein bound, especially to albumin. Salicylic acid readily distributes to extracellular fluids and to the kidneys, liver, lungs, and heart. Salicylic acid is eliminated by hepatic conjugation with glucuronide and glycine. Renal clearance is enhanced by an alkaline urinary pH. There are significant differences in the elimination and biotransformation of salicylates among different species. Plasma half-lives vary from 1-37.6 hr in animals.

Aspirin toxicosis is usually characterized by depression, fever, hyperpnea, seizures, respiratory alkalosis, metabolic acidosis, coma, gastric irritation or ulceration, liver necrosis, or increased bleeding time. Seizures may occur as a consequence of severe intoxication, although the exact etiology is unknown.

Cats are deficient in glucuronyl transferase and have a prolonged excretion of aspirin (the half-life in cats is 37.5 hr). No clinical signs of toxicosis occurred when cats were given 25 mg/kg of aspirin every 48 hr for up to 4 wk. Dosages of 5 grains (325 mg), bid, can be lethal to cats.

Dogs tolerate aspirin better than cats; however, prolonged use can lead to the development of gastric ulcers. Dosages of 25 mg/kg, tid, of regular aspirin have caused mucosal erosions in 50% of dogs after 2 days. Gastric ulcers were seen by day 30 in 66% of dogs given aspirin at 35 mg/kg, PO, tid. Similarly, 43% of dogs given aspirin at 50 mg/kg, PO, bid, showed gastric ulcers after 5-6 wk of dosing. Acute ingestion of 450-500 mg/kg can cause GI disturbances, hyperthermia, panting, seizures, or coma. Alkalosis due to stimulation of the respiratory center can occur early in the course of intoxication. Metabolic acidosis with an elevated anion gap usually develops later.

Naproxen, a propionic acid-derivative NSAID is available OTC as an acid or the sodium salt. It is available as 200-550 mg tablets or gelcaps or as a suspension (125 mg/ 5 mL). Structurally and pharmacologically, naproxen is similar to carprofen and ibuprofen. In humans and dogs, it is used for its anti-inflammatory, analgesic, and antipyretic properties.

Oral absorption of naproxen in dogs is rapid, with peak plasma concentration reached in 0. 5-3 hr. The reported elimination half-life in dogs is 34-72 hr. Naproxen is highly protein bound (>99. 0%). In dogs, naproxen is primarily eliminated through the bile, whereas in other species, the primary route of elimination is through the kidneys. The long half-life of naproxen in dogs appears to be due to its extensive enterohepatic recirculation.

Several cases of naproxen toxicosis in dogs have been described. Dosages of 5.6-11.1 mg/kg, PO, for 3-7 days have caused melena, frequent vomiting, abdominal pain, perforating duodenal ulcer, weakness, stumbling, pale mucous membranes, regenerative anemia, neutrophilia with a left shift, increased BUN and creatinine, and decreased total protein. Acute toxicity from a single oral dose has been described at 35 mg/kg. Cats may be more sensitive to naproxen toxicity than dogs due to their limited glucuronyl-conjugating capacity.

Acetaminophen is a synthetic nonopiate derivative of p-aminophenol widely used in humans for its antipyretic and analgesic properties. Its use has largely replaced salicylates due to the reduced risk of gastric ulceration.

Acetaminophen is rapidly absorbed from the GI tract. Peak plasma concentrations are usually seen within an hour, but can be delayed with extended-release formulations. It is uniformly distributed into most body tissues. Protein binding varies from 5-20%. The metabolism of acetaminophen involves 2 major conjugation pathways in most species. Both involve cytochrome P-450 metabolism, followed by glucuronidation or sulfation.

Cats are more sensitive to acetaminophen toxicosis because they are deficient in glucuronyl transferase and therefore have limited capacity to glucuronidate this drug. In cats, acetaminophen is primarily metabolized via sulfation; when this pathway is saturated, toxic metabolites are produced. In dogs, signs of acute toxicity are usually not observed unless the dosage of acetaminophen exceeds 100 mg/kg. Clinical signs of methemoglobinemia have been reported in 3 out of 4 dogs at 200 mg/kg. Toxicity can be seen at lower dosages with repeated exposures. In cats, toxicity can occur with 10-40 mg/kg.

Methemoglobinemia and hepatotoxicity characterize acetaminophen toxicosis. Renal injury is also possible. Cats primarily develop methemoglobinemia within a few hours, followed by Heinz body formation. Methemoglobinemia makes mucous membranes brown or muddy in color, and is usually accompanied by tachycardia, hyperpnea, weakness, and lethargy. Other clinical signs of acetaminophen toxicity include depression, weakness, hyperventilation, icterus, vomiting, hypothermia, facial or paw edema, cyanosis, dyspnea, hepatic necrosis, and death. Liver necrosis is more common in dogs than in cats. Liver damage in dogs is usually seen 24-36 hr after ingestion. Centrilobular necrosis is the most common form of hepatic necrosis seen with acetaminophen toxicity.

Treatment

Treatment of NSAID toxicosis consists of early decontamination, protection of the GI tract and kidneys, and supportive care. Vomiting should be induced in recent exposures, followed by administration of activated charcoal with a cathartic. Activated charcoal can be repeated in 6-8 hr to prevent NSAID reabsorption from enterohepatic recirculation. Use of H_2-receptor antagonists (ranitidine, famotidine, cimetidine) may not prevent GI ulcers but can be useful in treating them. Omeprazole, which is a proton pump inhibitor used for inhibiting gastric acid secretions, can be used instead of an H_2-blocker at 0. 5-1.0 mg/kg, PO, sid, in dogs. Sucralfate (dog: 0.5-1 g, PO, bid-tid; cat: 0.25-0.5 tablet, PO, bid-tid) reacts with hydrochloric acid in the stomach and forms a paste-like complex that binds to the proteins in ulcers and protects them from further damage. Because sucralfate requires an acidic environment, it should be given ≥30 min before administering H_2 antagonists. Misoprostol (dog: 1-3 mg/kg, PO, tid) has recently been shown to prevent GI ulceration when used concomitantly with aspirin and other NSAID.

IV fluids should be given at a diuretic rate if the potential for renal damage exists. Alkalinization of the urine with sodium bicarbonate results in ion trapping of salicylates in kidney tubules and can increase their excretion. However, ion trapping should be used judiciously and only in cases where the acid-base balance can be monitored closely. Baseline renal function should be monitored and rechecked at 48 and 72 hr. Prognosis depends on the dose ingested and how soon the animal receives treatment following exposure.

Treatment of Acetaminophen: The objectives of treating acetaminophen toxicosis are early decontamination, prevention or treatment of methemoglobinemia and hepatic damage, and provision of supportive care. Induction of emesis is useful when performed early. This should be followed by administration of activated charcoal with a cathartic. Activated charcoal may be repeated because acetaminophen undergoes some enterohepatic recirculation.

Administration of N-acetylcysteine (NAC), a sulfur-containing amino acid, can reduce the extent of liver injury or methemoglobinemia. NAC provides sulfhydryl groups, directly binds with acetaminophen metabolites to enhance their elimination, and serves as a glutathione precursor. It is available as a 10% or 20% solution. The loading dose is 140 mg/kg of a 5% solution IV or PO (diluted in 5% dextrose or sterile water), followed by 70 mg/kg, PO, qid for generally 7 more treatments.

Vomiting can occur with oral NAC. NAC is not labeled for IV use; however, it can be administered as a slow IV (over 15-20 min) with a 0. 2 micron bacteriostatic filter. Activated charcoal and oral NAC should be administered 2 hr apart as activated charcoal could adsorb NAC. Liver enzymes should be monitored and rechecked at 24 and 48 hr. The animal should also be monitored for methemoglobinemia, Heinz body anemia, and hemolysis. Fluids and blood transfusions should be given as needed. Ascorbic acid (30 mg/kg, PO or injectable, bid-qid) may further reduce methemoglobin levels. Cimetidine (5-10 mg/kg, PO, IM, or IV), a cytochrome P-450 inhibitor, may help reduce formation of toxic metabolites and prevent liver damage.

GASTROINTESTINAL DRUGS

H_2-Receptor Antagonists

H_2-receptor antagonists are structural analogs of histamine, commonly used to treat GI ulcers, erosive gastritis, esophagitis, and gastric reflux. They act at the H_2 receptors of parietal cells to competitively inhibit histamine, reducing gastric acid secretions during basal conditions and when stimulated by food, amino acids, pentagastrin, histamine, or insulin. Cimetidine, famotidine, and ranitidine are examples of this group, also commonly referred to as H_2 blockers. These drugs are rapidly absorbed, reaching peak plasma concentrations within 1-3 hr. Ranitidine is widely distributed throughout the body. H_2 blockers are primarily metabolized in the liver. Famotidine and ranitidine are excreted in the urine as metabolites and unchanged drug, while cimetidine is eliminated in feces. The elimination half-life for all 3 drugs is ~2. 2 hr in dogs. Because cimetidine may inhibit the hepatic microsomal enzyme system, ingestion of an H_2 blocker may result in reduced metabolism of certain drugs, including ß blockers, calcium channel blockers, diazepam, metronidazole, and theophylline.

H_2 blockers have a wide margin of safety, with acute oral overdoses typically resulting in minor effects such as vomiting, diarrhea, anorexia, and dry mouth. Serious adverse effects, such as tremors, hypotension, and bradycardia, are more likely to occur with IV H_2-blocker overdoses. The minimum lethal dose of famotidine in dogs is >2 g/kg, PO, and 300 mg/kg, IV. Most exposures require only monitoring and supportive care, although massive overdoses may also warrant decontamination.

Antacids

Antacids come in pill and liquid forms, and are frequently used to treat GI upset. Common antacids include calcium carbonate, aluminum hydroxide, and magnesium hydroxide (milk of magnesia). These agents are poorly absorbed orally. Calcium- and aluminum-containing antacids generally cause constipation, while magnesium-containing antacids tend to cause diarrhea. Some products contain both aluminum and magnesium salts in an attempt to balance their constipating and laxative effects. Acute single ingestion of calcium salts may cause transient hypercalcemia, but is unlikely to be associated with significant systemic effects. Induction of emesis within 2-3 hr of exposure may be helpful in preventing severe GI upset.

Multivitamins and Iron

The common ingredients in multivitamins include: ascorbic acid (vitamin C), cyanocobalamin (vitamin B12), folic acid, thiamine (vitamin B1), riboflavin (vitamin B2), niacin (vitamin B3), biotin, pantothenic acid, pyridoxine (vitamin B6), calcium, phosphorus, iodine, iron, magnesium, copper, zinc, and vitamins A, D, and E. Among these ingredients, iron and vitamins A and D may cause significant systemic signs. Acute ingestion of other listed ingredients in companion animals can result in self-limiting GI upset (eg, vomiting, diarrhea, anorexia, lethargy). However, toxicity is typically rare in pets.

Multivitamin preparations contain varying amounts of *iron*. Unless otherwise listed, iron should be assumed to be elemental iron. Various iron salts may contain 12-48% elemental iron. Iron has direct caustic or irritant effects on the GI mucosa. It can also be a direct mitochondrial poison.

Once the iron-carrying capacity of serum has been exceeded, free iron is deposited in the liver where it damages mitochondria, leading to necrosis of periportal hepatocytes. Signs of iron toxicosis usually develop within 6 hr. Initial vomiting and diarrhea, with or without blood, may be followed by hypovolemic shock, depression, fever, acidosis, and liver failure 12-24 hr later, often with a period of apparent recovery in between. Oliguria and anuria secondary to shock-induced renal failure may also occur. Ingestion of >20 mg/kg of elemental iron generally warrants decontamination and administration of GI protectants. Additional treatment and monitoring will be necessary for patients that have ingested >60 mg/kg of elemental iron.

Milk of magnesia can complex with iron to decrease its absorption from the GI tract. Serum iron levels and the total iron binding capacity should be checked at 3 hr and again at 8-10 hr post-exposure. If serum iron is >300 mg/dL, or greater than the total iron binding capacity, chelation therapy may be needed. Desferoxamine (40 mg/kg, IM, every 4-8 hr) is a specific iron chelator and is most effective within the first 24 hr post-ingestion, before iron has been distributed from blood to tissues. Other signs should be treated symptomatically.

Even though vitamin A toxicity following consumption of large amounts of fish oil or bear's liver has been well documented, it is less likely to occur following acute ingestion of multivitamins. The amount of vitamin A needed to cause toxic effects is 10-1, 000 times the dietary requirements for most species. The vitamin A requirement for cats is 10, 000 IU/kg of diet fed, with levels up to 100, 000 IU/kg of diet considered to be safe. For dogs, the requirement is 3, 333 IU/kg of diet fed, with up to 333, 300 IU/kg of diet considered to be safe. Signs associated with acute vitamin A toxicity include general malaise, anorexia, nausea, peeling skin, weakness, tremors, convulsions, paralysis, and death.

Vitamin D is included in many calcium supplements to aid the absorption of the calcium. Most vitamins contain cholecalciferol (vitamin D3). After consumption, cholecalciferol is converted into 25-hydroxycholecalciferol (calcifediol) in the liver, which is subsequently converted to the active metabolite 1, 25-dihydroxycholecalciferol (calcitriol) in the kidneys. One IU of vitamin D3 is equivalent to 0. 025 μg of cholecalciferol. Even though the oral LD50 of cholecalciferol in dogs has been reported as 88 mg/kg, signs have been seen at dosages as low as 0. 5 mg/kg. Vomiting, depression, polyuria, polydipsia, and hyperphosphatemia may be seen within 12 hr of a significant vitamin D exposure, followed by hypercalcemia and acute renal failure 24-48 hr post-exposure. In addition to renal failure, the kidneys, heart, and GI tract may show signs of necrosis and mineralization. Initial treatment should include decontamination and assessment of baseline calcium, phosphorus, BUN, and creatinine. Multiple doses of activated charcoal with a cathartic should be administered. If clinical signs of toxicosis develop, treatment consists of saline diuresis and the use of furosemide, corticosteroids, and phosphate binders. Specific agents such as (salmon) calcitonin or pamidronate may be needed for patients that remain hypercalcemic despite symptomatic treatment. Stabilization of serum calcium may require days of treatment due to the long half-life of calcifediol (16-30 days).

TOPICAL PREPARATIONS

Zinc Oxide

Zinc oxide ointments or creams are commonly used as topical skin protectants, astringents, and bactericidal agents. Most ointments contain 10-40% zinc oxide.

Ingestion of zinc oxide-containing products usually results in gastric irritation (vomiting) and diarrhea, without the intravascular hemolysis, and liver and renal damage associated with elemental zinc ingestion. Signs are usually seen within 2-4 hr of a significant exposure. Vomiting animals should be managed symptomatically and supportively.

NUTRITIONAL SUPPLEMENTS

Ma Huang (Ephedrine) and Guarana (Caffeine)

Several herbal supplements, sold with the claim of providing weight loss and energy, contain guarana (Paullinia cupana), a natural source of caffeine, and ma huang (Ephedra sinica), a natural source of ephedrine. In humans, use of herbal supplements containing guarana and ma huang have been linked to acute hepatitis, nephrolithiasis, hypersensitivity myocarditis, and sudden death. In dogs, accidental ingestion of herbal supplements containing ma huang and guarana can have synergistic effects when ingested together and can lead to severe hyperactivity, tremors, seizures, vomiting, tachycardia, hyperthermia, and death within a few hours of exposure. The use of ephedra-containing supplements has recently been banned by the FDA.

5-Hydroxytryptophan

Several OTC herbal supplements containing 5-hydroxytryptophan (5-HTP) or Griffonia seed extracts claim to treat depression, headaches, insomnia, and obesity. Orally, 5-HTP is rapidly absorbed and constitutively converted to serotonin (5-hydroxy-tryptamine). In cases of 5-HTP overdose, excessive concentrations of serotonin at target cells (GI, CNS, cardiovascular, and respiratory systems) can lead to a serotonin-like syndrome in dogs (eg, seizures, depression, tremors, ataxia, vomiting, diarrhea, hyperthermia, transient blindness, and death). Clinical signs can develop within 4 hr after ingestion and last up to 36 hr. Treatment consists of early decontamination, control of CNS signs (diazepam, barbiturates), thermoregulation (cool water bath, fans), fluid therapy, and administration of a serotonin antagonist such as cyproheptadine (1. 1 mg/kg, PO or rectally).

TOXICITIES FROM PRESCRIPTION DRUGS

Pets commonly ingest prescription medications, from countertops, pill minders, mail-order packages, or other sources. Veterinarians can prescribe certain human drugs in animals. Safety data for human prescription drugs in certain animals species may not be available, as most are not approved for veterinary use by the FDA. A valid client-patient-veterinarian relationship must exist for veterinarians to recommend extra-label use of human prescription medications to their clients

CARDIOVASCULAR MEDICATIONS

Angiotensin-converting Enzyme (ACE) Inhibitors

Several ACE inhibitors (e.g., enalapril, captopril, lisinopril) are used therapeutically in dogs and cats. The primary concern in cases of acute ACE inhibitor overdose is usually marked hypotension. If hypotension is severe, secondary renal damage may result. Onset occurs within a few hours of exposure, depending on the agent (extended-release formulations may have a delayed onset of action). Other clinical signs of overdose may include vomiting, poor mucous membrane color, weakness, and tachycardia or bradycardia. Activated charcoal is effective in binding the drug from the GI tract if administered within 1-2 hr of ingestion. Blood pressure should be monitored and IV fluids given at twice the maintenance rate if hypotension develops. Renal function should be monitored if severe or persistent hypotension develops.

Calcium Channel Blockers

Calcium channel blockers (e.g., diltiazem, amlodipine, verapamil) inhibit movement of calcium from extracellular sites through cell membrane-based calcium channels. The most common signs seen with overdoses of calcium channel blockers are hypotension, bradycardia, GI upset, and heart block. Reflex tachycardia may develop in response to the drop in blood pressure.

Management of an acute overdose includes correcting hypotension and rhythm disturbances. In general, emesis is not recommended unless induced within minutes of witnessed ingestion—the increased vagal tone can worsen the bradycardia. Activated charcoal binds unabsorbed drug in the GI tract and is most useful in the first 1-2 hr after ingestion; if a sustained-release product was ingested, repeat doses of activated charcoal every 4-6 hr for a total of 2-4 doses can provide additional benefit. Specific therapies should be instituted based on blood pressure, heart rate, ECG, and blood chemistry profiles. IV fluids are recommended; calcium gluconate should be added if chemistries reveal hypocalcemia. Atropine (0.02-0.04 mg/kg) can be given for bradycardia; isoproterenol can be used if the ECG indicates atrioventricular block. For persistent hypotension not corrected by administration of IV fluids, dopamine (1-20 μg/kg/min) or dobutamine (2-20 μg/kg/min) can be given via continuous IV infusion. Calcium channel blockers may interact with almost any other cardioactive medication, resulting in more profound bradycardia, hypotension, and depression of cardiac contractility.

ß Blockers

Drugs in this class (e.g., propanolol, atenolol, timolol) act by competitively inhibiting catecholamine binding to ß-adrenergic receptor sites. The most common signs of overdose are bradycardia and hypotension; respiratory depression, coma, seizures, hyperkalemia, and hypoglycemia may occur. It is also possible to precipitate congestive heart failure. Significant clinical signs may arise even at therapeutic doses—no approved veterinary products are on the market.

Because of rapid absorption, emesis should only be induced within minutes of ingestion. Administration of activated charcoal should be considered if either multiple tablets or capsules or sustained-release formulation tablets are ingested. Heart rate and clinical condition should be monitored for at least 2-4 hr for the development of signs. If clinical signs do develop, blood chemistries should also be measured. Hypotension should be treated with IV fluids; atropine can be used for bradycardia. If hyperkalemia is confirmed, administration of insulin, followed by IV glucose, may drive the excess potassium back into the cells.

Diuretics

Oral diuretic agents include thiazides (eg, chlorothiazide, hydrochlorothiazide), loop diuretics such as furosemide, and potassium-sparing agents such as spironolactone (an aldosterone antagonist) and triamterene. Osmotic diuretics, administered by injection, include mannitol and urea. The most common signs of diuretic overdose include vomiting, depression, polyuria, polydipsia, and electrolyte changes. Electrolytes, especially potassium, may shift subsequent to a very large ingestion of a diuretic. Management should include monitoring hydration and electrolytes, with correction as needed.

TRANQUILIZERS AND ANTIDEPRESSANTS

Benzodiazepines

These drugs bind γ-aminobutyric acid (inhibitory neurotransmitter) receptors and are used for seizure control and as anxiolytics. While diazepam is probably best known in the veterinary field, alprazolam, chlordiazepoxide, clonazepam, lorazepam, oxazepam, and triazolam are all commonly prescribed medications. In general, all are rapidly and fairly completely absorbed, lipophilic, and highly protein bound. Metabolism is mostly by glucuronidation, so cats may be more sensitive to adverse effects. Several have active metabolites (eg, diazepam, clorazepate) and consequently have much longer duration of signs. The most common signs seen, at a wide range of dosages, are CNS depression, respiratory depression, ataxia, weakness, disorientation, nausea, and vomiting. Some animals, especially at high doses, may show CNS excitation instead of depression (paradoxical reaction), which may be followed by CNS depression. Other common signs are hypothermia, hypotension, tachycardia, muscle hypotonia, and meiosis.

Emesis can be induced if ingestion is recent and no clinical signs are present. Gastric lavage, followed by administration of activated charcoal can be performed if the ingested amount is very high. The patient should be kept warm and quiet and closely monitored for responsiveness to stimuli and adequate breathing. IV fluids will help support blood pressure. If severe respiratory depression develops, the reversal agent flumazenil can be given at a dose of 0. 01 mg/kg, slow IV, in both cats and dogs. Flumazenil has a short half-life, so it may need to be repeated. Benzodiazepines should not be used to control CNS excitation due to a paradoxical reaction. In such situations, low doses of barbiturates may be useful to control initial CNS excitation.

Antidepressants

Antidepressants fall into several classes. An overdose of almost any of them can result in development of serotonin syndrome.

Selective Serotonin Reuptake Inhibitors

This group of antidepressant agents include sertraline, fluoxetine, paroxetine, and fluvoxamine. They block the activity of serotonin receptors at presynaptic membranes and have little effect on other neurotransmitters.

Tricyclic Antidepressants

These antidepressants (e.g., amitriptyline, clomipramine, nortriptyline) are commonly used psychoactive agents. They are structurally similar to the phenothiazines, with a similar anticholinergic, adrenergic, and α-blocking properties. Following absorption, these agents are extensively bound to plasma proteins and also bind to tissue and cellular sites, including the mitochondria. Cyclic antidepressants block the amine pump and stop neuronal reuptake of norepinephrine, serotonin, and dopamine. These agents also appear to have a slight α-adrenergic blocking effect. Tricyclics may exert their major toxicity via a nonspecific membrane-stabilizing effect, similar to chlorpromazine and the ß-blockers. Tricyclics also have central and peripheral anticholinergic activity, along with antihistaminic effects. Clinical signs of toxicosis include CNS stimulation (agitation, confusion, pyrexia), cardiac arrythmias, hypertension, myoclonus, nystagmus, seizures, metabolic acidosis, urinary retention, dry mouth, mydriasis, and constipation. This may be followed by CNS depression (lethargy), ataxia, hypothermia, respiratory depression, cyanosis, hypotension, and coma.

Treatment

Emesis should be induced in cases of recent exposure if the animal is asymptomatic. This can be followed by activated charcoal (even several hours after ingestion) plus a cathartic such as sorbital or sodium sulfate (magnesium sulfate is contraindicated, as it can add to CNS depression). Diazepam can be given to control seizures. Serotonin syndrome signs should be managed as needed. Heart rate and rhythm should be monitored and cardiac arrythmias treated. Atropine should not be used to control bradycardia as it can aggravate anticholinergic effects of tricyclic antidepressants.

Serotonin Syndrome

This group of clinical signs usually includes 3 of the following features: altered mental status, agitation, myoclonus, hyperreflexia, tremors, diarrhea, incoordination, and fever. It often occurs after overdose or ingestion of substances that result in elevated free levels of serotonin, such as antidepressants or profound stimulants (eg, amphetamines, cocaine, pseudoephedrine, and ephedra). Cyproheptadine is a serotonin antagonist often used for treatment. It is available only as a tablet, but can be dissolved in a small amount of saline and administered per rectum at 1. 1 mg/kg in dogs or 2 mg/dose in cats. If there is a good response to the initial dose, it can be repeated if signs recur.

Barbiturates

Both long-acting and short-acting barbiturates may be encountered. The long-acting group includes phenobarbital, mephobarbital, and primadone—all commonly used as anticonvulsants or sedatives. The short-acting (butabarbital, pentobarbital, secobarbital) and ultra short-acting (thiamylal and thiopental) barbiturates are used mainly for induction of anesthesia and seizure control. All are readily absorbed from the gut and have extensive liver metabolism; metabolites are primarily excreted via the kidneys. The onset of clinical signs varies from 15 min to several hours, and duration can be up to several days for the long-acting class. The most common signs are sedation, ataxia, respiratory depression, coma, loss of reflexes, hypotension, and hypothermia.

Management is aimed at life support while attempting to remove unmetabolized drug from the system. Emesis should be induced if the exposure is very recent and the animal is asymptomatic. Gastric lavage while protecting the airway can remove much of the drug still in the stomach. Activated charcoal readily adsorbs barbiturates; small doses repeated every 4-6 hr can further decrease the body burden, even if overdose has resulted from use of an injectable product. IV fluids can be given to support blood pressure. Respiratory effort and effectiveness needs to be closely monitored; treatment may require a respirator. Support for maintaining body temperature may be necessary.

Sleep Aids

Zolpidem and zaleplon are the newest drugs used as sleep aids and have a mechanism of action similar to the benzodiazepines. These agents have a very rapid onset (usually <30 min) and a similarly short half-life. While the expected result from ingestion would be marked sedation, they have been associated with paradoxical excitement. Dosages as low as 0.22 mg/kg have resulted in sedation and ataxia, and dogs have developed tremors, vocalizing, and pacing at dosages as low as 0.6 mg/kg.

GI decontamination can be performed if the ingestion was recent and no signs are seen. For mild signs, keeping the pet quiet and in a safe place may suffice. If paradoxical excitement develops, symptomatic treatment should be given and will vary with the signs and their intensity. Hyperexcitation may be controlled with acepromazine or other phenothiazines. Use of valium may aggravate signs of CNS depression. Flumazenil (0. 01 mg/kg, IV) can be used if clinical signs of toxicosis are severe.

Phenothiazine Tranquilizers

The most commonly used phenothiazines in veterinary medicine are acepromazine, chlorpromazine, and promazine. In domestic animals, they are used as tranquilizers, preanesthetic agents, antiemetics, and for the treatment of CNS agitation following specific drug overdoses (amphetamines, cocaine). The most common signs of overdose are sedation, weakness, ataxia, collapse, behavioral changes, hypothermia, hypotension, tachycardia, and bradycardia.

Treatment consists of symptomatic and supportive care. Due to rapid onset of CNS signs, emesis should only be attempted in a recent exposure and should be followed by administration of activated charcoal and a cathartic. Repeated doses of activated charcoal may be helpful, especially for large ingestions. Hypotension should be treated with IV fluids. Dopamine may be used if fluid administration does not correct hypotension. Body temperature, heart rate, and blood pressure should be monitored and treated symptomatically.

Muscle Relaxants

The most commonly encountered centrally acting muscle relaxants include baclofen and cyclobenzaprine. Baclofen is rapidly absorbed orally. The onset of clinical signs of toxicosis may be <30 min to 2 hr following ingestion. The most common signs of toxicosis are vocalization, salivation, vomiting, ataxia, weakness, tremors, shaking, coma, seizures, bradycardia, hypothermia, and blood pressure abnormalities. Cyclobenzaprine, often used in management of acute muscle spasms, is almost completely absorbed after an oral dose, with peak plasma levels in 3-8 hr. It has extensive liver metabolism and undergoes enterohepatic recirculation. The most common signs seen in both dogs and cats include depression and ataxia.

Treatment of muscle relaxant overdose consists of symptomatic and supportive care. Vomiting should be induced if the exposure is recent and no clinical signs are present, followed by administration of activated charcoal. Respiratory support (ie, ventilator) should be provided if needed. Recumbent or comatose animals should be monitored for hypothemia and aspiration. IV fluids should be given as needed.

TOPICAL AGENTS

There are many topical preparations that pets ingest, often resulting in only mild gastroenteritis. For example, ingestion of most corticosteroid-containing creams or ointments usually results in only mild to moderate stomach upset, polydipsia, and polyphagia. However, ingestion of certain topical agents in pet animals, such as 5-fluorouracil and calcipotriene, can be deadly even at low doses.

5-Fluorouracil

5-Fluorouracil (5-FU) is available as an ointment (1% or 5%) or topical solution (1%, 2%, or 5%). It is used in the treatment of skin cancers and solar keratoses in humans. Most exposures result from accidental ingestion, although occasionally 5-FU is used extra-label in pets. Ingestion in dogs and cats leads to the onset of signs within a few hours. In dogs, signs have been seen at dosages as low as 8. 6 mg/kg, with the minimum lethal dose reported as 20 mg/kg. Initial signs include severe vomiting, which may progress to bloody vomiting and diarrhea. Signs often progress to severe tremors, ataxia, and seizures. In cats and dogs, 5-FU may be converted to fluorocitrate and interfere with the Kreb's cycle, which may be one cause of seizures and ataxia. Generally, 5-FU destroys rapidly dividing cells, affecting the GI tract, liver, kidneys, CNS, and bone marrow. The mortality rate among dogs ingesting 5-FU is high.

All 5-FU exposures in pets should be treated aggressively. Treatment consists primarily of symptomatic and supportive care. Emesis should be induced and the animal given activated charcoal and a cathartic if it is asymptomatic and the ingestion has occurred within 1 hr. If the animal is symptomatic (eg, vomiting or seizuring) it should be stabilized first. The GI tract should be protected with sucralfate (1 g in large dogs, 0. 5 g in small dogs, PO, tid) and inhibitors of gastric acid secretion such as cimetidine. Diazepam may be used initially to control seizures and tremors, but in severe cases it is usually not effective and other antiseizure medications such as pentobarbital (3-15 mg/kg, IV slowly to effect) or phenobarbital (3-30 mg/kg, slowly IV to effect) can be used. Constant rate infusion using diazepam or barbiturates has been recently shown to be successful in controlling severe seizures. If this also fails to control CNS signs, gas anesthetics (eg, isoflurane) and propofol (4-6 mg/kg, IV or as a continuous drip 0. 6 mg/kg/min) can be tried. IV fluids should be given and body temperature monitored. Monitoring electrolytes, serum chemistries (liver-specific enzymes and renal function), and CBC is usually required for ~2 wk. Surviving dogs may show evidence of bone marrow suppression later. For severe neutropenia in dogs, administration of filgrastim or granulocyte colony stimulating factor at 4-6 μg/kg, SC may be useful.

Calcipotriene

Calcipotriene, used to treat psoriasis in humans, is available as an ointment or cream (0. 005% or 50 μg/g). Calcipotriene is a novel structural analog of calcitriol (1, 25-dihydroxycholecalciferol), the most active metabolite of cholecalciferol (vitamin D3). Accidental ingestion of 40-60 μg/kg of calcipotriene in dogs has been associated with life-threatening hypercalcemia. Clinical signs usually occur within 24-72 hr of ingestion and include anorexia, vomiting, diarrhea, polyuria, polydipsia, depression, and weakness. Serum calcium is usually elevated within 12-24 hr and may remain above normal for weeks. This is usually accompanied by an increase in serum phosphorous concentration and calcium phosphorous product (Ca × P) and soft tissue mineralization. Acute renal failure as evidenced by elevated BUN and creatinine levels, coma, and death occur in severe or untreated cases.

Treatment of calcipotriene toxicosis involves standard decontamination (emesis induction, administration of activated charcoal and a cathartic) and reduction of serum calcium concentrations by saline diuresis, furosemide, and corticosteroids, with or without salmon calcitonin treatment. Recent reports indicate that concurrent use of pamidronate (1. 3-2 mg/kg diluted in saline and given IV over 2 hr) in dogs may be a useful adjunctive therapy. Calcipotriene toxicosis cases usually require monitoring of serum calcium, phosphorous, BUN, and creatinine for several days or even weeks. Signs of renal failure are managed with ongoing supportive fluids.

NONSTEROIDAL ANTI-INFLAMMATORY DRUGS

Carprofen

Carprofen is a proprionic acid-derived NSAID of the carbazole class approved for the relief of pain and inflammation associated with osteoarthritis and surgery in dogs.

Carprofen is well absorbed orally with peak serum levels occurring in 1-3 hr. It is metabolized in the liver primarily via glucuronidation and oxidation. Because cats are deficient in glucuronyl transferase, they are particularly sensitive to toxicosis. Most of the drug is eliminated in the feces, with some enterohepatic recirculation; 10-20% is eliminated in urine. The mean half-life in dogs is ~8 hr after oral dosing. Carprofen seems to be well tolerated by dogs. Like most other NSAID, it has the potential to adversely affect the GI, renal, and hepatic systems. Idiosyncratic hepatocellular toxicosis characterized by hepatocellular necrosis, cholestasis, anorexia, lethargy, icterus, vomiting, increased hepatic enzymes, and hyperbilirubinemia has been reported in dogs following administration of therapeutic (approved) dosages.

Etodolac

Etodolac is an indole acetic acid-derivative NSAID labeled for use in dogs to treat pain and inflammation associated with osteoarthritis. It is rapidly absorbed orally, with peak serum concentrations seen 2 hr after dosing. It is primarily eliminated through the bile. The elimination half-life is 8-12 hr. Etodolac appears to be well tolerated by dogs when used at the labeled dosage (10-15 mg/kg, PO, sid) for 1 yr. With multiple doses, clinical signs of toxicity such as GI ulcers, vomiting, diarrhea, and weight loss can be seen at 40 mg/kg. Six of 8 dogs died or became moribund due to GI ulceration at 80 mg/kg.

Deracoxib

Deracoxib has been recently approved for control of inflammation and pain associated with osteoarthritis and postoperative pain and inflammation associated with orthopedic surgery in dogs. The approved oral dose of deracoxib for the control of pain and inflammation is 1-2 mg/kg/day; the dose for postoperative orthopedic pain is 3-4 mg/kg/day, not to exceed 7 days of administration. Deracoxib is well absorbed orally. It is extensively metabolized in the liver. The majority of the parent drug and its metabolites are eliminated through the bile, with a plasma elimination half-life of ~3 hr. Deracoxib administration to healthy young dogs at 10 mg/kg for 14 days resulted in erosions and ulcers in the jejunum. At 25, 50, and 100 mg/kg for 14 days, weight loss, vomiting, and melena occurred. In a 6-mo study, dose-dependent focal renal tubular degeneration and regeneration was seen in some dogs at 6, 8, and 10 mg/kg.

TOXICITIES FROM ILLICIT AND ABUSED DRUGS

Exposures to illicit or abused drugs in pet animals can be accidental, intentional, or malicious. Occasionally, drug-sniffing dogs also ingest these substances. Due to the illegal nature of illicit or abused drugs, owners may provide inaccurate, incomplete, or misleading exposure histories. Illicit drugs are often adulterated with other pharmacologically active substances, making the diagnosis even more difficult.

In suspected cases of illicit or abused drug exposure, an attempt should be made to gather information about the animal's environment; amount of exposure; and the onset time of clinical signs and their type, severity, and duration. These questions will help include or exclude possible exposure to an illicit or abused drug. Illicit and abused drugs are often known by street names that vary from area to area. A call to a local police station, or animal or human poison control center, can be extremely helpful in identifying the illicit substance. Most human hospitals, emergency clinics, or veterinary diagnostic laboratories have illicit drug screens available and can check for the presence of illicit drugs or their metabolites in different body fluids. The presence of a parent drug or its metabolites in blood or urine may help confirm the exposure in suspect cases. Veterinarians should contact these laboratories for the types of samples needed and time required for completion.

Commonly available over-the-counter drug test kits may be helpful in ruling out a suspected case of illicit drug toxicosis. These test kits are inexpensive, efficient, and easy to use. They are designed to detect drug metabolites in the urine and can detect most commonly available illicit or recreational drugs such as amphetamines, cocaine, marijuana, opiates, and barbiturates. The sensitivities and specificities of these test kits may vary. The instructions provided with each kit should be followed carefully for best results.

Cocaine

Cocaine (benzoyl-methylecgonine) alkaloid is obtained from the leaves of the coca plant, Erythroxylon coca and E monogymnum. Some common street names for cocaine are coke, gold dust, stardust, snow, "C", white girl, white lady, baseball, and speedball (cocaine and heroin). Cocaine alkaloid from coca leaves is processed into cocaine hydrochloride salt. The salt is not suitable for smoking because heat decomposes it. The salt is then reprocessed to form cocaine alkaloid or free base (a process called free-basing or base balling), which is colorless, odorless, transparent, and more heat stable. Free base cocaine is also called crack, rock, or flake. Cocaine is cut (diluted) several times before it reaches the user. Xanthine alkaloids, local anesthetics, and decongestants are some of the most common adulterants.

Cocaine is a schedule II drug approved for human use. Its medical uses are restricted to topical administration as a local anesthetic on mucous membranes of the oral, laryngeal, and nasal cavities. Mostly, it is used as a recreational drug.

Pharmacokinetics and Toxicity

Cocaine is absorbed from most routes. Orally, it is better absorbed in an alkaline medium (ie, intestine). In humans, ~20% of an oral dose is absorbed. The reported plasma half-life is 0. 9-2. 8 hr. Cocaine is extensively metabolized by liver and plasma cholinesterases to several inactive metabolites that are primarily excreted in the urine. The acute LD50 of IV-administered cocaine hydrochloride in dogs is 13 mg/kg; the LD100 in dogs and cats is 12 mg/kg and 15 mg/kg, respectively. The oral LD50 in dogs is believed to be 2-4 times more than the IV dose.

Pathogenesis

Cocaine acts on the sympathetic division of the autonomic nervous system. It blocks the reuptake of dopamine and norepinephrine in the CNS leading to feelings of euphoria, restlessness, and increased motor activity. Cocaine can also decrease concentrations of serotonin or its metabolites. Topical use of cocaine causes vasoconstriction of small vessels. Hyperthermia in cocaine toxicosis may develop either due to increased heat production from muscular activity or due to decreased heat loss from vasoconstriction.

Clinical Findings and Diagnosis

Hyperactivity, shaking, ataxia, panting, agitation, nervousness, seizures, tachycardia, acidosis, or hyperthermia characterize cocaine toxicosis. CNS depression and coma may follow CNS excitation. Death may be due to hyperthermia, cardiac arrest, or respiratory arrest.

Diagnosis is based on a history of exposure and the presence of characteristic clinical signs. Identification of cocaine in plasma, stomach contents, or urine can confirm exposure. Differential diagnoses include amphetamines, pseudoephedrine, ephedrine, caffeine, chocolate, metaldehyde, strychnine, tremorgenic mycotoxins, lead, nicotine, permethrin (cats) and other pesticides, and encephalitis.

Treatment

The objectives of treatment are GI decontamination, stabilization of CNS and cardiovascular effects, thermoregulation, and supportive care. Animals with clinical signs should be stabilized first before attempting decontamination. Emesis can be induced in a recent exposure if the animal is asymptomatic and has the ability to guard its airway via a gag reflex. This should be followed by administration of activated charcoal with a cathartic. If the animal's condition contraindicates induction of emesis (e.g., presence of CNS signs or extreme tachycardia) a gastric lavage with a cuffed endotracheal tube to reduce the risk of aspiration should be performed. A dose of activated charcoal with a cathartic should be left in the stomach after the lavage.

Controlling the CNS signs may require use of more than one anticonvulsant. Clinical signs of CNS excitation can be controlled with diazepam. However, the effects of diazepam are short-lived and repeated administration may be needed to control signs of CNS excitation. Phenothiazine tranquilizers such as acepromazine (0.05-1.0 mg/kg, IV, IM, or SC) or chlorpromazine (0.5-1.0 mg/kg, IV or IM) usually work well to control the CNS effects. Phenothiazines should be used cautiously as they may lower the seizure threshold. If phenothiazines are ineffective, phenobarbital at 3-4 mg/kg, IV, or pentobarbital, IV to effect, could be used. If CNS signs are uncontrolled from the preceding measures, a gas anesthetic such as isoflurane may be useful.

Blood pressure, heart rate and rhythm, ECG, and body temperature should be monitored frequently and treated as needed. Propranolol at 0.02-0.06 mg/kg, IV, tid-qid or other ß-blocking agents can be used to control tachycardia. After stabilization of CNS and cardiovascular effects, IV fluids should be administered and electrolyte changes monitored and corrected as needed. Treatment and monitoring should continue until all clinical signs have resolved.

Amphetamines and Related Drugs

Amphetamines and their derivatives are CNS and cardiovascular system stimulants commonly used in humans for depression of appetite, narcolepsy, attention deficit disorder, Parkinsonism, and some behavior disorders. Some commonly encountered amphetamines or related drugs are benzphetamine, dextroamphetamine, pemoline, methylphenidate, phentermine, diethylpro-pion, phendimetrazine, methamphetamine, and phenmetrazine. Amphetamines are sold on the street with common names such as speed, bennies, or uppers. Commonly used adulterants are caffeine, ephedrine, or phenylpropanolamine.

Pharmacokinetics and Toxicity

Amphetamines are rapidly absorbed in the GI tract, reaching a peak plasma concentration in 1-2 hr. Sustained-release formulations have a delayed absorption. The plasma half-life of amphetamines depends on the urinary pH. With an alkaline pH, the half-life is 15-30 hr; with an acidic urinary pH the half-life is 8-10 hr. The acute oral LD50 of amphetamine in rats and mice is 10-30 mg/kg. In humans, deaths from metamphetamine have been reported at 1.3 mg/kg following ingestion.

Pathogenesis

Amphetamine stimulates the release of norepinephrine, affecting both α- and ß-adrenergic receptor sites. Amphetamine also stimulates catecholamine release centrally in the cerebral cortex, medullary respiratory center, and reticular activating system. It increases the amount of catecholamine at nerve endings by increasing release and inhibiting reuptake and metabolism. The neurotransmitters that are affected in the CNS are norepinephrine, dopamine, and serotonin.

Clinical Findings and Diagnosis

Clinical signs of amphetamine and cocaine toxicosis are similar and difficult to differentiate clinically. The only difference may be the longer duration of clinical signs of amphetamine toxicosis due to a longer half-life compared to cocaine. The most commonly reported signs are hyperactivity, aggression, hyperthermia, tremors, ataxia, tachycardia, hypertension, mydriasis, circling, and death.

Diagnosis is as for cocaine and relies mostly on owner knowledge of exposure. Most amphetamines and related drugs or their metabolites are detectable in the stomach contents and urine. They are difficult to detect in plasma unless large amounts have been ingested.

Treatment

Phenothiazines are preferred for controlling CNS signs in amphetamine toxicosis. Other anticonvulsants, such as diazepam, barbiturates, or isoflurane, may be used if needed. Acidifying the urine with ammonium chloride (25-50 mg/kg/day, PO, qid) or ascorbic acid (20-30 mg/kg, PO, SC, IM, or IV) may enhance amphetamine elimination in the urine. However, this should be done only if acid-base status can be monitored. Heart rate and rhythm, body temperature, and electrolytes should be monitored and treated as needed.

Marijuana (Cannabis)

Marijuana refers to a mixture of cut, dried, and ground flowers, leaves, and stems of the leafy green hemp plant Cannabis sativa. The plant grows in most tropical and temperate regions of the world. Marijuana is the principal drug produced from the hemp plant. There are several cannabinoids present in the plant resin but delta-9-tetrahydro-cannabinol (THC) is considered the most active and main psychoactive agent. The concentration of THC in marijuana varies between 1-8%. Hashish is the resin extracted from the top of the flowering plant and is higher in THC concentration than marijuana. Street names for marijuana include pot, Mary Jane, hashish, weed, grass, THC, ganja, bhang, and charas. Pure THC is available by prescription under the generic name dronabinol. A synthetic cannabinoid, nabilone, is also available. Marijuana or hashish sold on the streets may be contaminated with phencyclidine, LSD, or other drugs.

Marijuana is a schedule I controlled substance mostly used by people as a recreational drug. It is also used as an antiemetic for chemotherapy patients and to decrease intraocular pressure in glaucoma patients. Some clinicians advocate the use of dronabinol as an appetite stimulant, but the dysphoric effects of this drug outweigh any benefit of appetite stimulation.

Pharmacokinetics and Toxicity

The most common route of exposure is oral. After ingestion, THC goes through a substantial first pass effect. It is metabolized by liver microsomal hydroxylation and nonmicrosomal oxidation. In dogs, the onset of clinical signs occurs within 30-90 min and can last up to 72 hr. THC is highly lipophilic and readily distributes to the brain and other fatty tissues following absorption. The oral LD50 of pure THC in rats and mice is 666 mg/kg and 482 mg/kg, respectively. However, clinical effects of marijuana are seen at much lower doses than this.

Pathogenesis

THC is believed to act on a unique receptor in the brain that is selective for cannabinoids and is responsible for the CNS effects. Cannabinoids can enhance the formation of norepinephrine, dopamine, and serotonin.

Clinical Findings and Diagnosis

The most common signs of marijuana toxicosis are depression, ataxia, bradycardia, hypothermia, vocalization, hypersalivation, vomiting, diarrhea, urinary incontinence, seizures, and coma. Diagnosis is based on a history of exposure and typical clinical signs. THC is difficult to detect in body fluids because of the low levels found in the plasma. Urine testing in the early course of exposure may help confirm the diagnosis. Marijuana toxicosis can be confused with ethylene glycol (antifreeze, *Ethylene Glycol Toxicity: Introduction*) or ivermectin toxicosis; hypoglycemia; or benzodiazepine, barbiturate, or opioid overdose.

Treatment

Treatment consists of supportive care. The animal should be decontaminated if the exposure is recent and there are no contraindications. Comatose animals should be given IV fluids, treated for hypothermia, and rotated frequently to prevent dependent edema or decubital ulceration. Diazepam can be given for sedation or to control seizures. Treatment and monitoring should be maintained until all clinical signs have resolved (up to 72 hr in dogs).

Opiates

The term opiate initially referred to all naturally occurring alkaloids obtained from the sap of the opium poppy (Papaver somniferum). Opium sap contains morphine, codeine, and several other alkaloids. Currently, opioid refers to all drugs, natural or synthetic, that have morphine-like actions or actions that are mediated through opioid receptors. Structurally, opioids can be divided into 5 classes. Some of the common agents within each class are:

1) phenanthrenes—morphine, heroin, hydromorphone, oxymorphone, hydrocodone, codeine, and oxycodone;
2) morphinan—butorphanol;
3) diphenylheptanes—methadone and propoxyphene;
4) phenylpiperidines— meperidine, diphenoxylate, fentanyl, loperamide, and profadol; and
5) benzomorphans— pentazocine and buprenorphine.

A new synthetic opiate, tramadol, is a derivative of codeine and has become a widely used veterinary analgesic.

Opioids are used primarily for analgesia. In addition, they are also used as cough suppressants and for the treatment of diarrhea. Occasionally, opioids are also used for sedation before surgery and as a supplement to anesthesia.

Pharmacokinetics and Toxicity:

Opioids are generally well absorbed following oral, rectal, or parenteral administration. Some more lipophilic opioids are also absorbed through nasal, buccal, respiratory (heroin, fentanyl, buprenorphine), or transdermal (fentanyl) routes. For some opioids, there is variable reduction in bioavailability due to a first pass effect when given orally. Opioids generally undergo hepatic metabolism with some form of conjugation, hydrolysis, oxidation, dealkylation, or glucuronidation. Because cats are deficient in glucuronidation, the half-life of some opioids in cats may be prolonged. Following absorption, opioids are rapidly cleared from blood and stored in kidney, liver, brain, lung, spleen, skeletal muscle, and placental tissue. Most of the opioid metabolites are excreted through the kidneys.

Toxicity of opioids in animals is highly variable. In dogs, 100-200 mg/kg of morphine administered SC or IV is considered lethal. The estimated lethal dose of codeine in adult humans is 7-14 mg/kg. In infants, 2.5 mg of hydrocodone has been lethal.

Pathogenesis

The effects of opioids are due to their interaction with opiate receptors that are found in the limbic system, spinal cord, thalamus, hypothalamus, striatum, and midbrain. Opioids may be agonists, mixed agonist-antagonists, or antagonists at these receptors. Agonists bind and activate a receptor, whereas antagonists bind without causing activation.

Clinical Findings

The primary effects of opioids are on the CNS, respiratory, cardiovascular, and GI systems. Commonly reported clinical signs of toxicosis include CNS depression, drowsiness, ataxia, vomiting, seizures, miosis, coma, respiratory depression, hypotension, constipation/defecation, and death. Some animals—especially cats, horses, cattle, or swine—can show CNS excitation instead of CNS depression.

Diagnosis

Diagnosis of opioid toxicosis is based on history of exposure and the types of clinical signs (CNS and respiratory depression) present. Plasma opioid levels are usually not clinically useful. Urine may be used to determine exposure to opioids using some of the over-the-counter illicit drug kits (manufacturer's instructions should be followed). Opioid toxicosis should be differentiated from antifreeze toxicosis, ivermectin, benzodiazepines, barbiturates, marijuana, and hypoglycemia-inducing conditions.

Treatment

Clinical signs can be reversed with the opiate antagonist naloxone. The dosages in different animals are: dog and cat, 0.002-0. 04 mg/kg, IV, IM or SC; rabbit and rodent, 0.01-0.1 mg/kg, SC or IP; horse, 0.01-0.02 mg/kg, IV. Administration of naloxone should be repeated as needed because its duration of action may be shorter than the opioid being treated. Animals should be closely monitored for respiratory depression and ventilatory support provided if needed. Other signs should be treated symptomatically.

REFERENCES

Crosby, Donald G. 1998. *Environmental Toxicology and Chemistry*. New York: Oxford University Press.

Needleman, H.L. 1998. "Clair Patterson and Robert Kehoe: Two Views of Lead Toxicity." *Environmental Research* 78(2):79–85.

Ohlendorf, H.M.; Hoffman, D.J.; Daiki, M.K.; and Aldrich, T.W. 1986. "Embryonic Mortality and Abnormalities of Aquatic Birds—Apprent Impacts of Selenium from Irrigation Drainwater." *Science of the Total Environment* 52(44).

Williams, P.L.; James, R.C.; and Roberts, S.M., eds. 2000. *Principles of Toxicology: Environmental and Industrial Applications*, 2nd edition. New York: John Wiley & Sons.

6

Food Poisoning

Food poisoning usually refers to the infection of an animal or human, via food, with Salmonella organisms or with other bacteria that have similar effects. Cats are much more susceptible than dogs; in fact they can quite easily die of infection with Salmonella. This species difference is hardly surprising, when one views the evolutionary niche of each species.

Cats in the wild tend to catch and eat live prey. This means that their natural food is always fresh. Dogs rely more on 'carrion' and dead flesh. To have arrived at this capability, dogs had to acquire mechanisms that protected them from the ill-effects of eating decomposing meat. They have a very acid stomach and a ready ability to vomit food that is unacceptable, before it does harm.

Food-poisoning usually occurs through poor food hygiene in the home. A deplorable fact of modern life, however, is that raw meats, such as chicken, come to the house carrying a heavy load of food-poisoning bacteria. This is a sad comment on modern methods of husbandry, slaughter and processing. Organic chicken is much less likely to carry the organisms, since there is not the prevalence of antibiotics in the rearing system. It can, however, still be contaminated in processing plants, in which they may share facilities with other infected carcases.

Feeding pets food that we enjoy is not only wrong, it can also be fatal. There are some foodstuffs that humans relish which cause illness and death if eaten by pets. Chocolate, macadamia nuts and onions are good examples. Each of these foods contains chemicals which rarely cause problems for humans, but for dogs, these same chemicals can be deadly.

Re-heated rice can also represent a risk, if not stored and re-cooked at the correct temperature or if stored for too long. Food items that have been thawed and re-frozen can also be risky.

Assuming that there has not been a catastrophic decline in health and vitality, too rapid for any veterinary intervention, homeopathic medicine can usually very successfully rid an animal of Salmonella infection and deal with the toxic ill-effects.

In the kitchen, damp cloths and damp wooden chopping boards can not only harbour but also multiply infective bacteria. The use of disinfectants in food areas is neither effective nor wise. Disinfectant-impregnated chopping boards and cloths are not common sense, since they encourage resistant strains of bacteria and are potentially toxic in themselves. Clean and dry materials are the best defence, so hygienic washing up and excellent draining and drying techniques, before putting things away, are vital. Surfaces should be kept clean and allowed to dry thoroughly. Wooden chopping boards should be well-scrubbed and allowed to drain and dry properly.

Cat food and water dishes should be ceramic or china and should be kept very clean.

It is true that tinned or dried food does not carry this risk (unless manufacturing or packaging errors occur), making it tempting to use processed food for your cats, despite the other health penalties that may follow this policy, as opposed to feeding wholesome fresh food. Each person must make a decision, based on personal circumstance and philosophy.

INGESTION OF AVOCADO

Ingestion of avocado (Persea americana) has been associated with myocardial necrosis in mammals and birds and with sterile mastitis in lactating mammals. Cattle, goats, horses, mice, rabbits, guinea pigs, rats, sheep, budgerigars, canaries, cockatiels, ostriches, chickens, turkeys, and fish are susceptible. Caged birds appear more sensitive to the effects of avocado, while chickens and turkeys appear more resistant. A single case report exists of 2 dogs developing myocardial damage secondary to avocado ingestion.

Etiology

Ingestion of fruit, leaves, stems, and seeds of avocado has been associated with toxicosis in animals; leaves are the most toxic part. The Guatemalan varieties of avocado have been most commonly associated with toxicosis.

Purified persin at 60-100 mg/kg causes mastitis in lactating mice and doses >100 mg/kg result in myocardial necrosis. Goats develop severe mastitis when ingesting 20 g of leaves/kg, whereas 30 g of leaves/kg results in cardiac injury. Acute cardiac failure developed in sheep fed avocado leaves at 25 g/kg for 5 days; 5.5 g/kg of leaves fed for 21 days or 2.5 g/kg for 32 days caused chronic cardiac insufficiency. Budgerigars fed 1 g of avocado fruit developed agitation and feather pulling, while 8. 7 g of mashed avocado fruit resulted in death within 48 hr.

Pathogenesis

Avocado causes necrosis and hemorrhage of mammary gland epithelium of lactating mammals and myocardial necrosis in birds and mammals. The toxic principle, persin, extracted from avocado leaves has caused lesions similar to those reported in natural cases.

Clinical Findings

In lactating animals, mastitis occurs within 24 hr of exposure to avocado, accompanied by a 75% decrease in milk production. Affected mammary glands are firm, swollen, and produce watery, curdled milk. Lactation may provide a degree of protection against myocardial injury at lower doses. In nonlactating mammals, or at higher doses, myocardial insufficiency may develop within 24-48 hr of ingestion and is characterised by lethargy, respiratory distress, subcutaneous edema, cyanosis, cough, exercise intolerance, and death. Horses may develop edema of the head, tongue, and brisket. Birds develop lethargy, dyspnea, anorexia, subcutaneous edema of neck and pectoral regions, and death.

Lesions

Mammary glands are edematous and reddened, with watery, curdled milk. In animals with cardiac insufficiency, there is congestion of lungs and liver, often with dependent subcutaneous edema. There may be free fluid within the abdominal cavity, pericardial sac, and thoracic cavity; pulmonary edema may be present. The heart may contain pale streaks. Histopathologic lesions in the mammary gland include degeneration and necrosis of secretory epithelium, with interstitial edema and hemorrhage. Myocardial lesions include degeneration and necrosis of myocardial fibers, which are most pronounced in ventricular walls and septum; interstitial hemorrhage and/or edema may be present. In horses, symmetric ischemic myopathy of head muscles and tongue, as well as ischemic myelomalacia of the lumbar spinal cord, have been described.

Diagnosis

Diagnosis of avocado toxicosis relies on history of exposure and clinical signs. There are no readily available specific tests that will confirm diagnosis. Differential diagnoses include other causes of mastitis (e.g., infectious) and other myocardial disorders, including ionophore toxicosis, yew toxicosis, vitamin E/selenium deficiency, gossypol, cardiac glycoside toxicosis (e.g., oleander), cardiomyopathy, and infectious myocarditis.

Treatment

NSAID and analgesics may benefit animals with mastitis. Treatment for congestive heart failure (e.g., diuretics, antiarrhythmic drugs) may be of benefit, but may not be economically feasible in livestock.

BREAD DOUGH

Raw bread dough made with yeast poses mechanical and biochemical hazards when ingested, including gastric distention, metabolic acidosis, and CNS depression. Although any species is susceptible, dogs are most commonly involved due to their indiscriminate eating habits.

Pathogenesis

The warm, moist environment of the stomach serves as an efficient incubator for the replication of yeast within the dough. The expanding dough mass causes distention of the stomach, resulting in vascular compromise to the gastric wall similar to that seen in gastric dilatation/volvulus. With sufficient gastric distention, respiratory compromise occurs. Yeast fermentation products include ethanol, which is absorbed into the bloodstream, resulting in inebriation and metabolic acidosis.

Clinical Findings

Early clinical signs may include unproductive attempts at emesis, abdominal distention, and depression. As ethanol intoxication develops, the animal becomes ataxic and disoriented. Eventually, profound CNS depression, weakness, recumbency, coma, hypothermia, or seizures may be seen. Death is usually due to the effects of the alcohol, rather than from gastric distention; however, the potential for dough to trigger gastric dilatation/volvulus in susceptible dog breeds should not be overlooked.

Diagnosis

A presumptive diagnosis can be based on history of exposure and clinical signs. Blood ethanol levels are consistently elevated in cases of bread dough toxicosis. Differential diagnoses include gastric dilatation/volvulus, foreign body obstruction, ethylene glycol toxicosis, and ingestion of other CNS depressants (e.g., benzodiazepines).

Treatment

With recent ingestions in asymptomatic animals, emesis may be attempted, although the glutinous nature of bread dough may make removal via emesis difficult. In animals where emesis (whether induced or spontaneous) has been unsuccessful, gastric lavage may be attempted. Cold water introduced into the stomach may slow the rate of yeast fermentation and aid in removal of dough. In some cases, surgical removal of the dough mass may be required. Animals presenting with signs of alcohol toxicosis should be stabilised and any life-threatening conditions corrected before attempts to remove the dough are made. Alcohol toxicosis is managed by correcting acid/base abnormalities, managing cardiac arrhythmias as needed, and maintaining normal body temperature. Providing fluid diuresis to enhance alcohol elimination may be helpful in some cases. Anecdotally, yohimbine (0.1 mg/kg, IV) has been used to stimulate severely comatose dogs with alcohol toxicosis.

CHOCOLATE

Chocolate toxicosis may result in potentially life-threatening cardiac arrhythmias and CNS dysfunction. Chocolate poisoning occurs most commonly in dogs, although many species are susceptible. Contributing factors include indiscriminate eating habits and readily available sources of chocolate. Deaths have also been reported in livestock fed cocoa byproducts and in animals consuming mulch from cocoa-bean hulls.

Etiology

Chocolate is derived from the roasted seeds of Theobroma cacao. The toxic principles in chocolate are the methylxanthines theobromine (3, 7-dimethylxanthine) and caffeine (1, 3, 7-trimethylxanthine). Although the concentration of theobromine in chocolate is 3-10 times that of caffeine, both constituents contribute to the clinical syndrome seen in chocolate toxicosis.

The exact amount of methylxanthines in chocolate varies due to natural variation of cocoa beans and variation within brands of chocolate products. However, in general, the total methylxanthine concentration of dry cocoa powder is ~800 mg/oz (28.5 mg/g), unsweetened (baker's) chocolate is ~450 mg/oz (16 mg/g), semisweet chocolate and sweet dark chocolate is ~150-160 mg/oz (5.4-5.7 mg/g), and milk chocolate is ~64 mg/oz (2.3 mg/g). White chocolate is an insignificant source of methylxanthines. Cocoa bean hulls contain ~255 mg/oz (9.1 mg/g) methylxanthines.

The LD50 of caffeine and theobromine are reportedly 100-200 mg/kg, but severe signs and deaths may occur at much lower doses and individual sensitivity to methylxanthines varies. In general, mild signs (vomiting, diarrhea, polydipsia) may be seen in dogs ingesting 20 mg/kg, cardiotoxic effects may be seen at 40-50 mg/kg, and seizures may occur at doses =60 mg/kg. One ounce of milk chocolate per pound of body weight is a potentially lethal dose in dogs.

Pathogenesis

Theobromine and caffeine are readily absorbed from the GI tract and are widely distributed throughout the body. They are metabolised in the liver and undergo enterohepatic recycling. Methylxanthines are excreted in the urine as both metabolites and unchanged parent compounds. The half-lives of theobromine and caffeine in dogs are 17.5 hr and 4.5 hr, respectively.

Theobromine and caffeine competitively inhibit cellular adenosine receptors, resulting in CNS stimulation, diuresis, and tachycardia. Methylxanthines also increase intracellular calcium levels by increasing cellular calcium entry and inhibiting intracellular sequestration of calcium by the sarcoplasmic reticulum of striated muscle. The net effect is increased strength and contractility of skeletal and cardiac muscle. Methylxanthines may also compete for benzodiazepine receptors within the CNS and inhibit phosphodiesterase, resulting in increased cyclic AMP levels. Methylxanthines may also increase circulating levels of epinephrine and norepinephrine.

Clinical Findings

Clinical signs of chocolate toxicosis usually occur within 6-12 hr of ingestion. Initial signs may include polydipsia, vomiting, diarrhea, abdominal distention, and restlessness. Signs may progress to hyperactivity, polyuria, ataxia, tremors, and seizures. Tachycardia, premature ventricular contractions, tachypnea, cyanosis, hypertension, hyperthermia, bradycardia, hypotension, or coma may occur. Hypokalemia may occur late in the course of the toxicosis, contributing to cardiac dysfunction. Death is generally due to cardiac arrhythmias, hyperthermia, or respiratory failure. The high fat content of chocolate products may trigger pancreatitis in susceptible animals.

Lesions

No specific lesions may be found in animals succumbing to chocolate toxicosis. Hyperemia, hemorrhages, or congestion of multiple organs may occur as agonal changes. Severe arrhythmias may result in pulmonary edema or congestion. Chocolate or cocoa bean hulls may be present in the alimentary tract at necropsy.

Diagnosis

Diagnosis is based on history of exposure, along with clinical signs. Amphetamine toxicosis, ma huang/guarana (ephedra/caffeine) toxicosis, pseudoephedrine toxicosis, cocaine toxicosis, and ingestion of antihistamines or other CNS stimulants should be considered in the differential diagnosis.

Treatment

Stabilisation of symptomatic animals is a priority in treating chocolate toxicosis. Methocarbamol (50-220 mg/kg, slow IV; no more than 330 mg/kg/24 hr) or diazepam (0.5-2.0 mg/kg, slow IV) may be used for tremors and/or mild seizures; barbiturates may be required for severe seizures. Arrhythmias should be treated as needed: propranolol (0.02-0.06 mg/kg, slow IV) or metoprolol (0.2-0.4 mg/kg, slow IV) for tachyarrhythmias, atropine (0.01-0.02 mg/kg) for bradyarrhythmias, and lidocaine (1-2 mg/kg, IV, followed by 25-80 mg/kg/min infusion) for refractory ventricular tachyarrhythmias. Fluid diuresis may assist in stabilizing cardiovascular function and hasten urinary excretion of methylxanthines.

Once animals have stabilised, or in animals presenting before clinical signs have developed (e.g., within 1 hr of ingestion), decontamination should be performed. Induction of emesis using apomorphine or hydrogen peroxide should be initiated; in animals that have been sedated due to seizures, gastric lavage may be considered. Activated charcoal (1-4 g/kg, PO) should be administered; because of the enterohepatic recirculation of methylxanthines, repeated doses should be administered every 8 hr in symptomatic animals (control vomiting with metoclopramide, 0.2-0.4 mg/kg, SC or IM, qid as needed).

Other treatment for symptomatic animals includes thermoregulation, correcting acid/base and electrolyte abnormalities, monitoring cardiac status via electrocardiography, and urinary catheter placement (methylxanthines and their metabolites can be reabsorbed across the bladder wall). Clinical signs may persist up to 72 hr in severe cases.

MACADAMIA NUTS

Ingestion of macadamia nuts by dogs has been associated with a nonfatal syndrome characterised by vomiting, ataxia, weakness, hyperthermia, and depression. Dogs are the only species in which signs have been reported.

Etiology

Macadamia nuts are cultivated from Macadamia integrifolia in the continental USA and

Macadamia tetraphylla in Hawaii and Australia. The mechanism of toxicity is not known. Dogs have shown signs after ingesting 2.4 g of nuts/kg body weight. Dogs experimentally dosed at 20 g/kg of commercially prepared macadamia nuts developed clinical signs within 12 hr and were clinically normal without treatment within 48 hr.

Clinical Findings

Within 12 hr of ingestion, dogs develop weakness, depression, vomiting, ataxia, tremors, and/or hyperthermia. Tremors may be secondary to muscle weakness. Macadamia nuts may be identified in vomitus or feces. Mild transient elevations in serum triglycerides, lipases, and alkaline phosphatase were reported in some dogs experimentally dosed with macadamia nuts; these values quickly returned to baseline. Signs generally resolve within 12-48 hr.

Diagnosis

Diagnosis is based on history of exposure, along with clinical signs. Differential diagnoses include ethylene glycol toxicosis, ingestion of hypotensive agents, and infectious diseases (e.g., viral enteritis).

Treatment

For asymptomatic dogs with recent ingestion of more than 1-2 g/kg, emesis should be induced; activated charcoal may be of benefit with large ingestions. Fortunately, most symptomatic dogs will recover without any specific treatment. Severely affected animals may be given supportive treatment such as fluids, analgesics, or antipyretics.

RAISINS/GRAPES

Ingestion of grapes or raisins has resulted in development of anuric renal failure in some dogs. Cases reported to date have been in dogs; an anecdotal report exists of a cat developing renal failure following ingestion of 1 cup of organic raisins. It is not known why many dogs can ingest grapes or raisins with impunity while others develop renal failure following ingestion. The condition has not been reproduced experimentally.

Pathogenesis

The mechanism of toxicity is unknown. Affected dogs develop anuric renal failure within 72 hr of ingestion of grapes or raisins. Estimated amounts of grapes associated with renal injury in dogs are ~32 g/kg; amounts of raisins associated with signs range from 11-30 g/kg.

Clinical Findings

Most affected dogs develop vomiting and/or diarrhea within 6-12 hr of ingestion of grapes or raisins. Other signs include lethargy, anorexia, abdominal pain, weakness, dehydration, polydipsia, and tremors (shivering). Oliguric or anuric renal failure develops within 24-72 hr of exposure; once anuric renal failure develops, most dogs die or are euthanised. Transient elevations in serum glucose, liver enzymes, pancreatic enzymes, serum calcium, or serum phosphorus develop in some dogs.

Diagnosis

Diagnosis is based on history of exposure, along with clinical signs. Other causes of renal failure (e.g., ethylene glycol, cholecalciferol) should be considered in the differential diagnosis.

Treatment

Prompt decontamination of significant ingestion of raisins or grapes is recommended. Emesis can be induced with 3% hydrogen peroxide (2 mL/kg; no more than 45 mL), followed by activated charcoal. With large ingestions or in cases where vomiting and/or diarrhea has spontaneously developed within 12 hr of ingestion of grapes or raisins, aggressive fluid diuresis for 48 hr is recommended. Renal function and fluid balance should be monitored during fluid administration. For oliguric dogs, urine production may be stimulated by using dopamine (0. 5-3 μg/kg/min, IV) and/or furosemide (2 mg/kg, IV). Anuric dogs are unlikely to survive unless peritoneal dialysis or hemodialysis is performed, and even then the prognosis is guarded.

ONION AND GARLIC POISONING

Onions and garlic are other dangerous food ingredients that cause sickness in dogs, cats and also livestock. Onions and garlic contain the toxic ingredient thiosulphate. Onions are more of a danger.

Pets affected by onion toxicity will develop haemolytic anaemia, where the pet's red blood cells burst while circulating in its body.

At first, pets affected by onion poisoning show gastroenteritis with vomiting and diarrhoea. They will show no interest in food and will be dull and weak. The red pigment from the burst blood cells appears in an affected animal's urine and it becomes breathless. The breathlessness occurs because the red blood cells that carry oxygen through the body are reduced in number.

The poisoning occurs a few days after the pet has eaten the onion. All forms of onion can be a problem including dehydrated onions, raw onions, cooked onions and table scraps containing cooked onions and/or garlic. Left over pizza, Chinese dishes and commercial baby food containing onion, sometimes fed as a supplement to young pets, can cause illness.

Onion poisoning can occur with a single ingestion of large quantities or with repeated meals containing small amounts of onion. A single meal of 600 to 800 grams of raw onion can be dangerous whereas a ten-kilogram dog, fed 150 grams of onion for several days, is also likely to develop anaemia. The condition improves once the dog is prevented from eating any further onion

While garlic also contains the toxic ingredient thiosulphate, it seems that garlic is less toxic and large amounts would need to be eaten to cause illness.

REFERENCES

Hocking A.D. et al. 2006. *Advances in Food Mycology* (Advances in Experimental Medicine and Biology) Springer.

Hans P. Riemann and Dean O. Cliver. 2006. *Foodborne Infections and Intoxications.* Elsevier.

Osweiler, G. D., T. L. Carson, W. B. Buck and G. A. Van Gelder (eds.) 1985. *Clinical and Diagnostic Veterinary Toxicology,* 3rd Edition, Kendall/Hunt Publishing Co., Iowa.

Pina M. Fratamico et al. 2005. *Foodborne Pathogens: Microbiology And Molecular Biology.* Caister Academic Press.

7

Poisonous Plants

Plants are responsible for keeping the animals alive in many ways. They absorb the poisonous CO_2 gas and exhales oxygen which the humans and other animals breathe. But like many contradictions observed in nature the plants can sometimes prove to be harmful. Most of the plants are beneficial but there are some poisonous plants as well.

It is imperative for one to know about these venomous plants. People who are vegetarian consume various types of plants and plants parts like stem, flower and fruits. Eating parts of a plant that has poison could prove to be detrimental for their health.

The poisonous plants can cause some serious stomach problems and diseases that affect the nervous system. Some toxic plants can also cause dermatological problems to a person who has come in contact with it.

TYPES OF POISONOUS PLANTS

The mushrooms are among the most sought after plants that people like to eat. As a matter of fact, they can be both edible and poisonous. Sometimes people confuse the poisonous as the edible ones and get into problems. The Amanita groups of mushrooms in particular have harmful consequences on human beings.

Two most problematic genres in this family are the destroying angel and death cap fungus. The major identification sign of these mushrooms are a hood or veil that wraps the top of the mushroom. The fully bloomed mushrooms have a cup surrounding the base of the stem. However, strong winds or rain can modify the appearances of the mushrooms.

There are many other genres of poisonous plants that people do not even know about. One common example is Rhubarb. It has oxalate crystals and hence can lead to poisoning if a person consumes lots of cooked or raw leaves.

The plants which have a chemical named glycoside like lily-of-the-valley and foxgloves may also have serious consequences on human beings. Apparently innocent looking plants and their fruits often turn out to be poisonous. The seeds of sweet pea are relevant in this context. People who consume the flour made of these seeds can contract a disease like paralysis.

EFFECTS OF POISONOUS PLANTS

Different type of poisonous plants leads to different types of symptoms and ailments in people. The most prevalent signs of mushroom poisoning are strong and sudden pains in the abdominal parts. A victim of mushroom poisoning can also suffer from severe stomach related ailments after eating. Such a person can suffer from diarrhea and bouts of vomiting.

This poisoning can have fatal consequences if not checked in time. The poisoning done by the Amanita species of mushrooms can eventually lead to heart and kidney failure. The mortality rate varies between 50 to 90 percent. For this type of mushroom poisoning there is no specific treatment. Some houseplants contain toxic compounds which lead to skin rashes and allergies in the children if they swallow or chew its leaves or parts by any chance.

DEALING WITH POISONOUS PLANTS

It is imperative to practice maximum caution to protect babies and adults from the Poisonous Plants. People who have pets like dogs, cat or monkey should be more careful as the pets can fall ill after chewing a poisonous plant. The garden of the house should not contain any plant that contains toxic elements. If the pets are not given immediate treatment after falling ill due to plant poisoning they might expire. The Poinsettia plants in particular are harmful for the pets.

If the pets show any signs of poisoning like salivating or rubbing their paws they should be taken to the vet immediately. It would be advisable for the parents to educate their children about the common toxic plants so that they can avoid them. Apart from that people should only buy plants for eating that they know to be safe. If anybody develops any kind of skin irritation or stomach disorder due to plant poisoning expert medical care should be sought.

POISONOUS HOUSEPLANTS AND ORNAMENTALS

Plants are an important part of the decor of homes; pets often chew on or ingest these plants, which can result in toxicoses. Inquiries to poison control centers on plants ingested by chldren <5 yr old are estimated at 5-10% of all inquiries. Similar estimates (though not documented) could be made for pets.

Little research has been done on the toxicity of houseplants. Most are hybrids, and selecting for growth outside their natural environment could affect their degree of toxicity. Age of the pet, boredom, and changes in the surroundings are factors that may affect the incidence of poisoning. Puppies and kittens are very inquisitive, and mouth or chew almost everything. Pets (especially single household pets) of all ages may become bored or restless if left alone or confined for too long at any one time, and chewing on objects for relief is common. Pets of all ages also explore changes in their environment; for example, pets commonly chew the leaves or ripe berries of potentially poisonous plants that are placed in the home during holidays.

Poisonous plants are among the important causes of economic loss to the livestock industry and should be considered when evaluating illness and decreased productivity in livestock. Poisonous plants can affect animals in many ways, including death, chronic illness and debilitation, decreased weight gain, abortion, birth defects, increased parturition interval, and photosensitization. In addition to these more obvious losses, other considerations include loss of forage, additional fencing, increased labor and management costs, and frequently interference with proper harvesting of forage.

Most poisonous range plants fall into 2 general categories: those that are indigenous to a range and increase with heavy grazing, and those that invade after overgrazing or disturbance of the land. Among those not in these categories are certain locoweeds and larkspurs, both of which form part of the normal range plant community. Poisonous plants can be found in most plant communities and should be considered in most grazing situations.

Livestock poisoning by plants often can be traced to problems of management or range condition, rather than simply to the presence of poisonous plants. Usually, animals are poisoned because hunger or other conditions cause them to graze abnormally. Overgrazing, trucking, trailing, corralling, or introducing animals onto a new range tend to induce hunger or change behavior, and poisoning may occur.

Not all poisonous plants are unpalatable, and they are not restricted to overgrazed ranges and pastures. Furthermore, poisonous plants do not always kill or otherwise harm animals when consumed. Many plants can be either useful forage or toxic. For example, plants such as lupine and greasewood may be part of an animal's diet, and the animal is poisoned only when it consumes too much of the plant too fast. To prevent poisoning, it is important to understand the factors involved when a useful forage becomes a poisonous plant.

Definitive diagnosis of suspect plant poisonings is difficult. It is important to be familiar with the poisonous plants growing in the specific area and to be acutely aware of those plants and the conditions under which livestock may be poisoned. A tentative diagnosis is possible if the following information is available:

1) any local soil deficiencies or excesses (which may complicate plant toxicities or simply confuse as to cause of a syndrome),
2) the syndromes associated with each of the poisonous plants in the area,
3) the time of year during which each is most likely to cause problems,
4) the detailed history of the animal(s) over the last 6-8 mo, and
5) any change of management or environmental condition that may cause an animal to change its diet or grazing habits.

Identification of the plant is important, whatever its stage of growth, and is especially useful if it can be identified in the stomach contents of the poisoned animal. Chemical analysis of toxicants often is not useful. Metabolic profiles are useful for some toxicities, and in some, the necropsy lesions are distinctive.

PLANT POISONING

Methods of producing plant poisoning in animals:

1. Eating plant
2. Contact
3. Photosensitization
4. Imparts off flavors and odor to by products
5. Mechanical injury

Plant and animal factors contributing to plant poisoning in animals:

A. *Plant factors*
   1. Soil
   2. Climate
   3. Stage of growth
   4. Part of plant
   5. Health of plant

B. *Animal factors:*

1. Natural resistance
2. Type of digestive system
3. Acquired resistance
4. Breed of animals
5. Age of animals
6. State of nutrition
7. Sex
8. Diet of animals
9. Addiction

Types of Toxins Present in Plants

Alkaloids

Alkaloids are most frequent in plants: E. g:

— *Legumes*—Croalaria, Senecio, Lupine, Lathyrus etc.

— *Nightshade family*—physalis, nightshade, belladonna tobacco.

— Ergot, Larkspur, Jimsonweed, poison hemlock

Most alkaloids end in "ine". eg. Strychnine, atropine, monocrotaline

Alkaloids have tart taste—Animals deficient in minerals may eat them. Very active in animals but do not produce lesions. Act on CNS—Exception is pyrrolizidine alkaloids.

Glycosides

Yield one or more sugars and one or more other compounds (aglycones, toxins) when hydrolyzed (H_2O).

Glycosides are bitter and colorless. They are more widely present in plants than alkaloids but many are non-toxic.

There are several groups of glycosidal poisons. Included are:

1. Cyanogenic
2. Goitrogenic

3. Irritant oils
4. Coumarin
5. Steroidal

Main one of concern to us is cyanogenic. Toxicity is dependent on both plant and animal factors.

Plant factors:

- Drought
- Cold
- Trampling
- HCN potential of plant
- Amount of free cyanide
- Speed of release or rate of eating

Animal factors:

- Digestive system
- Diet

Hydrogen Cyanide

Hydrogen cyanide (with the historical common name of Prussic acid) is a chemical compound with chemical formula HCN. A solution of hydrogen cyanide in water is called hydrocyanic acid. Hydrogen cyanide is a colorless, extremely poisonous, and highly volatile liquid that boils slightly above room temperature at 26 °C (78. 8 °F). HCN has a faint, bitter, almond-like odor that some people are unable to detect due to a genetic trait. Hydrogen cyanide is weakly acidic and partly ionizes in solution to give the cyanide anion, CN^-. The salts of hydrogen cyanide are known as cyanides. HCN is a highly valuable precursor to many chemical compounds ranging from polymers to pharmaceuticals.

Hydrogen cyanide is a linear molecule, with a triple bond between carbon and nitrogen. It is a weak acid with a pKa of 9. 2. A minor tautomer of HCN is HNC, hydrogen isocyanide. Hydrogen cyanide forms in at least limited amounts from many combination of hydrogen, carbon, and ammonia. Hydrogen cyanide is currently produced in large quantities by several processes, as well as being a recovered waste product from the manufacture of acrylonitrile.

Method of action of HCN

HCN of plant released by action of B-glycosidase of plant with cyanogenic glycoside of plant to free HCN. Rumen microbes and pH may also break down cyanogenic molecule—HCN combines with cytochrome oxidase in the form of trivalent iron—This combination forms a HCN cytochrome oxidase complex which is quite stable. This trivalent iron does not allow O_2 transport from blood to cellular respiration resulting in asphyxiation at the cellular level.

Treatment

Therapy is directed at splitting of the cytochrome-cyanide bond and subsequent rapid removal of a cyanide complex. The cyanide- cytochrome complex is broken by the addition of sodium nitrite with the formation of methemoglobin which competes with cytochrome oxidase for the cyanide ion and cyanmethemoglobin is formed. Thiosulfate then reacts with cyanide, under influence of the enzyme rhodanase, to form thiocyanate which is readily excreted in the urine. A recommended therapeutic regimen is the intravenous administration of a mixture of 1 ml of 20 percent sodium nitrite and 3 ml of 20 percent sodium thiosulfate, giving 4 ml of this mixture per 45 kilograms body weight. Commercial solutions for treatment of prussic acid poisoning are available.

Some beneficial effect has been shown for cobalt salts administered for cyanide poisoning. However, the nitrite and thiosulfate remains most effective.

Oxalate

Found in many plants such as Rumex genus and chenopodiaceae family. Occurs in plants in soluable (Na & K) and insoluable (Ca) forms. Most injury due to soluable form—certain fungi may form oxalates in moldy hay.

Some plants that contain soluable oxalates:

1. Pigweed
2. Beet tops
3. Lamb quarter
4. Halogeton—34% DW
5. Oxalis
6. Rumex
7. Thistle, russian

8. Greasewood
9. poke weed

Plants that contain insoluable oxalates such as Ca oxalate are:

1. jack in the pulpit
2. Caladium
3. Elephants ear
4. Dumbcane—Diffenbachia
5. Philodendron

The oxalates cause Calcium deficiency or Kidney damage. 10% + DW to cause clinical kidney disease—may be 34% in Halogeton oxalates cause interference with CHO metabolism and is probably a factor in death of animal.

Clinical signs

May be sudden onset (2-6 hrs)-over 1200 sheep overnight, colic, depression, muscular weakness, ataxia, drooping head, get up and down, lag behind flock, prostration with milk fever attitude, Dyspnea, bloody froth from nose and mouth, polyuria and bloat. Some cases show tetney.

Treatment

Oxalate poisoning can be treated with none specific Ca gluconate, fluids.

- Prevention: 5% dicalcium phosphate in pelleted feed.
- Free choice 75lb. salt and 25lb. dicalcium phosphate.

Resins or Resinoids

Based on physical characteristics Resins or Resinoids are amorphous gummy, brittle, burn, soluable in organic solvents but not water. Cause injury to nerve tissue and muscle tissue. They are very poisonous.

Plants containing resins are:

1. milkweed
2. marihuana
3. water hemlock

4. Mt. laurel and Rhododendron

5. chinaberry

Phyto Toxins or Toxalbumins

May be most toxic of poisons: much more toxic if injected. Absorbed from gut more easily than most protein toxins.

Plants containing phytotoxins:

1. Rosary pea
2. Castorbeans
3. Black locust
4. Tung tree
5. Barbadosnut

Phytotoxins:

— cause severe gastroenteritis

— cause lysis and hemolysis of RBC in vitro

— causes ammonia accumulation due to protein breakdown

— may be detoxified with heat.

— may be lag period between time consumed and onset of clinical signs.

Nitrates

Nitrates are one of the most important of toxic substances in plants. They are found in many crop plants including:

1. Oats
2. Sorghums
3. Rye
4. Corn
5. Wheat
6. Sweet potato vines

And in weeds such as :

1. Pigweed
2. Thistle
3. Jimsonweed
4. Dock
5. Nightshade
6. Johnson grass

In plants nitrate as KN03 is toxic at 1. 5% or in water at 1500+ ppm. Lower levels may cause other signs as well as abortion—Clinical signs are seen when methemoglobin levels reach 30-40% and death at 80-90%. Nitrate in serum above 25 micrograms/ml and nitrite above. 75 micrograms/ml.

Nitrate more toxic in ruminants than mono-gastric animals—10X Urea feeding does not affect nitrate poisoning.

Toxic action

- Nitrite ion oxidizes ferrous iron of hemoglobin to ferric state forming methhemoglobin.
- Methhemoglobin cannot accpet molucular oxygen.
- Veripuncture shows dark blood. Turns red on exposure to air.

Clinical Signs

- Early onset
- Irritant action of NO_3 may cause salivation, diarrhea, colic, polyurea, abortion etc.
- Mainly signs of respiratory distress due to anoxia. Same as cyanide and also marked cyanosis—Brown blood.
- Nitroso compounds—Carcinogenic—occurs in meat curing from nitrite and heat.
- Nitrogenous gases—Silo fillers disease—Atypical Int. Pneumonia and pulmonary adenomatosis of man—silo fed animals may see idiopathic interstitial pneumonia

Selenium

Selenium is an essential element that has a narrow margin of safety. Feed supplements containing 0.1-0.3 ppm selenium are added to the diet to prevent deficiency diseases such as white muscle disease in cattle and sheep, hepatosis dietetica in pigs, and exudative diathesis in chickens. The maximum tolerable level for selenium in most livestock feed is considered to be 2 ppm or as high as 5 ppm, although some believe that levels as high as 4-5 ppm can inhibit growth.

Selenium is a component of the glutathione peroxidase enzyme that acts as an antioxidant during release of energy. In excess, selenium has 2 general effects: the direct inhibition of cellular oxidation/reduction reactions, and the replacement of sulfur in the body. The inhibition of numerous cellular functions by high levels of selenium results in acute generalized cytotoxicity. The replacement of sulfur by chronic intake of selenium leads to altered structure and function of cellular components. Altered sulfur-containing amino acids (methionine, cystine) affects cell division and growth. Especially susceptible are the cells that form keratin (keratinocytes) and the sulfur-containing keratin molecule. Selenium therefore weakens the hooves and hair, which tend to fracture when subjected to mechanical stress.

All animal species are susceptible to selenium toxicosis. However, poisoning is more common in forage-eating animals such as cattle, sheep, and horses that may graze selenium-containing plants. Plants may accumulate selenium when the element is found at high levels—generally in alkaline soil with little rainfall (<50 cm). Selenium accumulating plants have been categorized. Obligate indicator plants require large amounts of selenium for growth and contain high concentrations (often >1,000 ppm). Facultative indicator plants absorb and tolerate high levels of soil selenium accumulating up to 100 ppm under these conditions, but they do not require selenium. Nonaccumulator plants passively absorb low levels of selenium (1-25 ppm) from the soil. Poisoning may also occur in swine and poultry consuming grain raised on seleniferous soils or, more commonly, due to error in feed formulation. Selenium toxicosis after ingestion of selenium-containing shampoos or excess selenium tablets is rare in pets. Several factors are known to alter selenium toxicity; however, in general, a single acute oral dose of selenium in the range of 1-5 mg/kg is lethal in most animals. Parenteral selenium products are also quite toxic, especially to young animals, and have caused deaths in baby pigs, calves, and dogs at doses as low as 1.0 mg/kg.

Diagnosis

Severity of selenium toxicosis depends on the quantity ingested and duration of exposure. Poisoning in animals is characterized as acute, subchronic, or chronic. Diagnosis is based on clinical signs; necropsy findings; and laboratory confirmation of presence of high selenium levels in an animal's diet (feed, forage, grains), blood, or tissues (kidney, liver). Selenium levels in the diet >5 ppm may produce signs after prolonged exposure. Levels of 10-25 ppm could produce severe signs. In acute toxicosis, the blood selenium concentration may reach 25 ppm, and in chronic toxicosis, it may be 1-4 ppm. Kidney or liver may contain 4-25 ppm in both acute and chronic poisoning.

Chronic Selenium Toxicosis

Chronic selenium poisoning usually develops when livestock consume seleniferous forages and grains containing 5-50 ppm of selenium for many weeks or months. Naturally occurring seleno-amino acids in plants are readily absorbed. Until recently, 2 types of chronic selenium poisoning were recognized—alkali disease and blind staggers. Blind staggers is no longer believed to be caused by selenium but by sulfate toxicity due to consumption of high-sulfate alkali water. Excess sulfate (>2% of diet) leads to polioencephalomalacia and the classical signs of blind staggers. Animals consuming milk vetch (Astragalus bisulcatus) have demonstrated clinical signs similar to blind staggers. Although milk vetch contains high levels of selenium, evidence now indicates that the alkaloid swainsonine in milk vetch, responsible for locoism, produces the signs.

Alkali disease has been reported in cattle, sheep, and horses. Affected animals are dull, emaciated, and lack vitality. The most distinctive lesions are those involving the keratin of the hair and hooves. The animal has a rough hair coat and the long hairs of the mane and tail break off at the same level giving a "bob" tail and "roached" mane appearance. Abnormal growth and structure of horns and hooves results in circular ridges and cracking of the hoof wall at the coronary band. Extremely long, deformed hooves that turn upwards at the ends may be seen. Subsequent lameness is compounded by degeneration of joint cartilage and bone. Reduced fertility and reproductive performance occurs especially in sheep. Reproductive performance may be depressed with a dietary level of selenium lower than that required to produce typical signs of alkali disease. Other lesions may include anemia, liver cirrhosis and ascites, and atrophy of the heart.

Birds also may be affected with chronic selenium toxicosis. Eggs with >2. 5 ppm selenium from birds in high selenium areas have low hatchability, and the embryos are usually deformed. Teratologic effects include underdeveloped feet and legs, malformed eyes, crooked beaks, and ropy feathers. This has been a problem with waterfowl in southern California, where selenium was leached by agricultural water and concentrated in lakes by runoff.

Blood levels of selenium in chronic cases are usually 1-4 ppm. Other changes in blood include decreased fibrinogen level and prothrombin activity; increased serum alkaline phosphatase, ALT, AST, and succinic dehydrogenase; and reduced glutathione. Hair may have >5 ppm selenium in chronic poisoning. A "garlicky" odor on the animal's breath may be noted.

There is no specific treatment for selenium toxicosis. Eliminating the source and exposure and symptomatic and supportive care of the animal should be started as soon as possible. Addition of substances that antagonize or inhibit the toxic effects of selenium in the diet may help reduce the risk of selenium toxicosis. A high protein diet, linseed oil meal, sulfur, arsenic, silver, copper, cadmium, and mercury have reduced selenium toxicity in laboratory animals, but their use under field conditions is limited. Addition of arsenic salt at 0.00375% to enhance biliary excretion of selenium or use of a high-protein diet to bind free selenium may help reduce incidence of selenium poisoning in cattle.

Subchronic Selenium Toxicosis

Pigs fed a diet supplemented with selenium >20-50 ppm for >3 days develop a subchronic selenium toxicosis characterized by neurologic abnormalities. Animals are initially ataxic and uncoordinated followed by anterior paresis, then quadriplegia. Pigs continue to eat. The hooves show breaks and impaired growth similar to those seen in cattle; alopecia is observed. In sows, conception rate decreases and number of pigs born dead increases. Lesions of subchronic toxicosis include focal symmetric poliomyelomalacia, which is most prominent in the cervical and thoracic spinal cord. Death may result from complications of permanent paralysis. Hoof and hair damage is similar to but in most cases less severe than that observed in chronic selenium toxicosis. Treatment is similar to that for chronic toxicosis, but spinal lesions are usually permanent.

Acute Selenium Toxicosis

Acute selenium poisoning due to consumption of plants with levels >50 ppm (dosages 3-20 mg/kg) is rare but has caused large losses in cattle, sheep, and pigs. Animals usually avoid these plants because of their offensive odor; however, when pasture is limited, accumulator plants may be the only food available. Young animals are most susceptible to acute parenteral selenium toxicosis with dosages of 0.2-0.5 mg/kg. Clinical signs are different from those of chronic selenosis and are characterized by abnormal behavior, respiratory difficulty, gastrointestinal upset, and sudden death. Abnormal posture and depression, anorexia, unsteady gait, diarrhea, colic, increased pulse and respiration rates, frothy nasal discharge, moist rales, and cyanosis may be noted.

Death usually follows within a few hours of consumption or injection. The major lesions are lung edema and congestion, and necrosis of multiple organs, including lung, liver, and kidney. Sheep usually do not show these signs, but instead become depressed and die suddenly.

Blood selenium concentration in acute poisoning is much higher than in chronic poisoning. In acute cases, blood selenium may reach 25 ppm. Treatment consists of symptomatic and supportive care. Acetylcysteine to boost glutathione levels is beneficial.

Molybdenum

Found in certain soils and may be taken up in plants in toxic concentrations. Found in US in Calif, Nevada, Florida and few other places. First recognized in England called "Teart".

Molybdenum and copper are antagonistic in diets—both are strongly influenced by inorganic sulfate. Normal molybdenum and low copper may see molybdenum toxicosis. Normal copper and low molybdenum may see copper poisoning.

Toxicity

Most likely seen in alkaline soils. Soils with more than 5 ppm toxic—Hi organic matter in soils may be toxic at 3 ppm. Sulfates enhance secretion of molybdenum in urine.

Legumes take up more than grass. +/- 20 ppm in forage may be toxic.

Clinical signs

Usually seen in ruminants. Main classical sign is greying of dark hair coat. Other signs are:

1. Diarrhea—more severe in calves
2. Anemia
3. Stiffness
4. Reproduction difficulties

Prevention & Treatment

- Add copper to diet—CU:MO level > 2:1 Need >7PPM in ration
- Injectible copper glycernate—good for 3-9 months -

- $CuSO_4$ in salt or water
- Acid soil reduce plant uptake
- Legumes take up more than grasses

Compounds causing photosensitization:

May occur by 2 methods.

1. Photodynamic substances in plants—e. g. Buckwheat—Hypericin (Hypericum perforatum)

   St. John's Wort—Fagopyrin (Fagopyrum sagittatum)

   Blue Green Algae—Phyocyan

   Probably others also.

2. Hepatogenic phtosentization—many plants e. g. clover, vetch, lantana, crotolaria, ceral grain, grasses and many others.

3. Contact dermatitis—unknown

   Plants causing mechanical injury—self explanatory. Examples:

   1. grain owns
   2. spear grass
   3. cockle burs
   4. squirrel tail grass

Gossypol

Gossypol poisoning, which is usually subacute to chronic, cumulative, and sometimes insidious, follows consumption of cottonseed or cottonseed products that contain excess free gossypol. It is of most concern in domestic livestock, especially immature ruminants and pigs. However, gossypol toxicosis can also affect high-producing dairy cows with high feed intake and other mature ruminants fed excess gossypol for long periods of time. It has also been reported in dogs fed cottonseed meal in diets.

Gossypol, the predominant pigment and probably the major toxic ingredient in the cotton plant (Gossypium spp), and other polyphenolic pigments are contained within small discrete structures called pigment glands found in various parts of the cotton plant. Gossypol occurs in cottonseed as both protein-bound and free forms; only the free form is toxic. Gossypol content of cottonseeds varies from a trace to >6% and is affected by plant species and variety and by environmental factors such as climate, soil type, and fertilization. Gossypol is a natural component of all but the rarely produced "glandless" variety of cotton.

Cottonseed is processed into edible oil, meal, linters (short fibers), and hulls. Cottonseed meal is marketed with 50-90% protein, depending on intended use. Cottonseed and cottonseed meal are widely used as protein supplements in animal feed. Cottonseed oil soapstock (foots) is the principal byproduct of cottonseed oil refining. Cottonseed soapstocks are being increasingly used as animal feed additives; cottonseed hulls are used as a source of additional fiber in animal feeds and usually contain much lower gossypol concentrations than do whole cottonseeds. Lipid-soluble gossypol is readily absorbed from the GI tract. It is highly protein-bound to amino acids, especially lysine, and to dietary iron. Conjugation, metabolism, and urinary excretion of gossypol is limited; most is eliminated in the feces.

All animals are susceptible, but monogastrics, immature ruminants, and poultry appear to be affected most frequently. Pigs, guinea pigs, and rabbits are reported to be sensitive. Dogs and cats appear to have intermediate sensitivity. Holstein calves seem to be the most sensitive of cattle breeds. Horses appear relatively unaffected. Toxic effects usually only occur after longterm exposure to gossypol, often after weeks to months.

Clinical Findings

Signs may relate to effects on the cardiac, hepatic, renal, reproductive, or other systems. Prolonged exposure can cause acute heart failure resulting from cardiac necrosis. Also, a form of cardiac conduction failure similar to hyperkalemic heart failure can result in sudden death with no visible cardiac lesions. Pulmonary effects and chronic dyspnea are most likely secondary to cardiotoxicity from congestive heart failure.

Hepatotoxicity can be a primary effect from direct damage to hepatocytes or metabolism of phenolic compounds to reactive intermediates, or liver necrosis may be secondary to congestive heart failure. Gossypol inhibits glutathione-S-transferase, impairing the liver's ability to metabolize xenobiotic compounds. Hematologic effects include anemia with reduced numbers of RBC and increased RBC fragility, decreased oxygen release from oxyhemoglobin, and reduced oxygen-carrying capacity of blood with lowered Hgb and PCV values due to complexing of iron by gossypol.

Reproductive effects include reduced libido with decreased spermatogenesis and sperm motility, as well as sperm abnormalities (which may be reversible) resulting from enzyme inhibition of steroid synthesis in testicular Leydig cells in males. Effects in females may include irregular cycling, luteolytic disruption of pregnancy, and direct embryotoxicity. Green discoloration of egg yolks and decreased egg hatchability have been reported in poultry.

Signs of prolonged excess gossypol exposure in many animals are weight loss, weakness, anorexia, and increased susceptibility to stress. Young lambs, goats, and calves may suffer cardiomyopathy and sudden death; if the course is more chronic, they may be depressed, anorectic, and have pronounced dyspnea. Adult dairy cattle may show weakness, depression, anorexia, edema of the brisket, and dyspnea, and also have gastroenteritis, hemoglobinuria, and reproductive problems. In monogastric animals, acute exposure may result in sudden circulatory failure, while subacute exposure may result in pulmonary edema secondary to congestive heart failure; anemia may be another common sequela. Violent dyspnea ("thumping") is the outstanding clinical sign in pigs. In dogs, gossypol poisoning is primarily reflected by cardiotoxic effects; condition deteriorates progressively, and ascites may be marked. Affected dogs may show polydipsia and have serum electrolyte imbalances, most notably hyperkalemia, with pronounced ECG abnormalities.

Some animals have no obvious gross postmortem lesions, but copious amounts of tan to red-tinged fluid with fibrin clumps are frequently found in abdominal, thoracic, and pericardial cavities. An enlarged, flabby, pale, streaked, and mottled heart with pale myocardial streaking, enlarged and dilated ventricles, and valvular edema may be evident. Skeletal muscles may also be pale. A froth-filled trachea and edematous, congested lungs are common, with interstitial pulmonary edema and markedly edematous interlobular septa. Generalized icterus and an enlarged, congested, mottled or golden, friable liver with distinct lobular patterns can be seen. The kidneys, spleen, and other splanchnic organs may be congested, possibly with petechiae; mild renal tubular nephrosis may be present. Hemoglobinuria and edema and hyperemia of the visceral mucosa may occur. Cardiomyopathy in affected dogs has been characterized as focal or general, granular myocardial degeneration with edema between and within myofibers; severe abnormalities in contractility have resulted in right-sided congestive heart failure without pronounced dilatation, and pulmonary or hepatic changes can be minimal.

Diagnosis

Diagnosis is based on the following:

1) a history of dietary exposure to cottonseed meal or cottonseed products over a relatively long period;

2) signs, especially sudden death or chronic dyspnea, affecting multiple animals within a group;

3) lesions consistent with the reported syndrome and associated cardiomyopathy and hepatopathy, with increased amounts of fluids in various body cavities;

4) no response to antibiotic therapy; and

5) the presence of significant concentrations of free gossypol in the diet.

Analyses of dietary components for free gossypol must be correlated with history, clinical signs, and postmortem findings. However, as with many feed-induced toxicoses, the responsible feed may be already completely consumed and not available for analysis. Free gossypol at >100 mg/kg (100 ppm) of feed in the diet of pigs or young ruminants <4 mo old supports a presumptive diagnosis. Adult ruminants can detoxify higher concentrations of gossypol, but intake should still be <1,000 ppm in the diet. However, dietary gossypol concentrations of 400-600 ppm in mature ruminants have caused toxicity after longterm exposure; rumen function is a variable, as is binding of gossypol to available proteins.

Adverse effects on semen quality (decreased sperm motility and morphologic abnormalities) occurred in young bulls fed a concentrate containing 1,500 ppm free gossypol (providing 8.2 g free gossypol/head/day). Cottonseed meal containing 26.6% (266,000 ppm) total gossypol and 0.175% (1,750 ppm) free gossypol was toxic when fed to adult dogs for an unspecified length of time; however, the equivalent oral dosage of free gossypol fed was <6 mg/kg/day. Gossypol can accumulate in liver and kidney, which are additional specimens for postmortem analyses. In sheep, gossypol concentrations (free or bound) >10 ppm in the kidneys and >20 ppm in the liver suggest excess gossypol exposure. However, background and significantly increased tissue gossypol concentrations have not been determined in all animal species, so tissue analyses may be of limited diagnostic value.

Differential diagnoses include poisonings by cardiotoxic ionophoric antibiotics (eg, monensin, lasalocid, salinomycin, narasin) and ammonia, nutritional or metabolic disorders (eg, selenium, vitamin E, or copper deficiency), infectious diseases, noninfectious diseases (eg, pulmonary adenomatosis, emphysema), mycotoxicoses caused by Fusarium-contaminated grain, and toxicoses caused by plants with cardiotoxic and other effects. Cardiotoxic plants, which may cause confusing or similar clinical signs and postmortem lesions, include English yew (Taxus baccata), Japanese yew (T cuspidata), laurel (Kalmia spp), azalea (Rhododendron spp), oleander (Nerium oleander), yellow oleander or yellow-be-still tree (Thevetia peruviana), purple foxglove (Digitalis purpurea), lily-of-the-valley (Convallaria majalis), dogbane (Apocynum spp), coffee senna (Cassia occidentalis), bracken fern (Pteridium aquilinum), white snakeroot (Eupatorium rugosum), death camas (Zygadenus spp), lantana (Lantana camara), monkshood (Aconitum napellum), and milkweed (Asclepias spp).

Prevention, Treatment, and Control

There is no effective treatment. Adsorbents such as activated charcoal and saline cathartics are of little value due to the chronic exposure and cumulative nature of gossypol. If gossypol toxicity is suspected, all cottonseed products should be removed from the diet immediately. However, severely affected animals may still die up to 2 wk later. Recovery depends primarily on the extent of toxic cardiopathy. Because exposure is usually chronic and life-threatening lesions may be advanced before a diagnosis is made, a favorable prognosis for complete recovery may be unrealistic. Mild to moderate myocardial lesions may be reversible with time if stress is minimized and animals are carefully handled. However, poor weight gains in affected livestock and increased susceptibility to stress may persist for several weeks after cottonseed products are removed from the diet. A high-quality diet supplemented with lysine, methionine, and fat-soluble vitamins should be included in supportive therapy.

A high intake of protein, calcium hydroxide, or iron salts appears to be protective in cattle. Cattle should also be given =40% of dry-matter intake from a forage source. Added iron of up to 400 ppm in swine diets and up to 600 ppm in poultry diets was reported to be effective in preventing signs and tissue residues of dietary gossypol exposure when used in ratios of 1:1 to 4:1 of iron to free gossypol. The best preventative approach is analysis of all dietary components containing cottonseed products prior to incorporating into animal diets as part of a managed feeding program.

Prevention of tissue residues in animal organ meats consumed by humans is an important public health consideration for those individuals already consuming cottonseed oil and cottonseed flour products in their daily diets. Until pharmacokinetic parameters of gossypol are more completely characterized in all food animal species, immediate salvage and consumption of animals surviving excess gossypol exposure is not recommended. Only those animals living for =1 mo after exposure should be considered safe for human food sources.

Strychnine

Strychnine is an indole alkaloid obtained from the seeds of the Indian tree Strychnos nux-vomica. It is mainly used as a pesticide to control rats, moles, gophers, and coyotes. Commercial baits (usually <0. 5%) are pelleted and often dyed red or green. Strychnine is highly toxic to most domestic animals. Its oral LD50 in dogs, cattle, horses, and pigs is between 0. 5-1 mg/kg, and in cats is 2 mg/kg. Malicious or accidental strychnine poisoning, although not very common in the USA, occurs mainly in small animals, especially dogs and occasionally cats, and rarely in livestock.

Pathogenesis

Strychnine is ionized in an acidic pH and then rapidly and completely absorbed in the small intestine. It is metabolized in the liver by microsomal enzymes. The highest concentrations of strychnine are found in the blood, liver, and kidneys. Strychnine and its metabolites are excreted in the urine. Depending on the quantity ingested and treatment measures taken, most of the toxic dose is eliminated within 24-48 hr.

Strychnine inhibits competitively and reversibly the inhibitory neurotransmitter glycine at postsynaptic neuronal sites in the spinal cord and medulla. This results in unchecked reflex stimulation of motor neurons affecting all the striated muscles. Because the extensor muscles are relatively more powerful than the flexor muscles, they predominate to produce generalized rigidity and tonic-clonic seizures. Death results from anoxia and exhaustion.

Clinical Findings

The onset of strychnine poisoning is fast. After oral exposure, clinical signs may appear within 30-60 min. Presence of food in the stomach can delay onset. Early signs, which may often be overlooked, consist of apprehension, nervousness, tenseness, and stiffness. Vomiting usually does not occur. Severe tetanic seizures may appear spontaneously or may be initiated by stimuli such as touch, sound, or a sudden bright light. An extreme and overpowering extensor rigidity causes the animal to assume a "sawhorse" stance. Hyperthermia (104-106°F [40-41°C]) due to stiffness and seizures is often present in dogs.

The tetanic convulsions may last from a few seconds to ~1 min. Respiration may stop momentarily. Intermittent periods of relaxation are seen during convulsions but become less frequent as the clinical course progresses. The mucous membranes become cyanotic, and the pupils dilated. Frequency of the seizures increases, and death eventually occurs from exhaustion or asphyxiation during seizures. If untreated, the entire syndrome may last only 1-2 hr. There are no characteristic necropsy lesions. Sometimes, due to prolonged convulsions before death, agonal hemorrhages of heart and lungs and cyanotic congestion from anoxia may be seen. Animals dying from strychnine poisoning have rapid rigor mortis.

Diagnosis

Tentative diagnosis of strychnine poisoning is usually based on history of exposure and clinical signs. Recovery of strychnine alkaloid from the stomach contents, vomitus, liver, kidneys, or urine should be considered diagnostic. Sometimes, urine may not have a detectable amount of strychnine present; therefore, multiple samples should be collected and analyzed. Strychnine poisoning can be confused with poisonings by several other substances such as metaldehyde; organochlorine, organophosphate, or carbamate insecticides; fluoroacetate (1080); zinc phosphide; nicotine; 4-aminopyridine; or human medications. Acute, massive hepatic necrosis (hepatic encephalopathy) can also produce clinical signs that resemble those of strychnine poisoning.

Treatment

Strychnine poisoning is an emergency, and treatment should be instituted quickly. Treatment should be aimed at decontamination, control of seizures, prevention of asphyxiation, and supportive care.

Decontamination consists of removal of gastric contents by inducing emesis or gastric lavage, and binding of remaining bait in the GI tract with activated charcoal. Due to the rapid onset of clinical signs, emesis may be of limited value in most cases. If exposure is recent and no clinical signs are present, emesis should be induced with 3% hydrogen peroxide (small animals and pigs) at 1-2 mL/kg, PO, maximum 3 tbsp, repeated once after 30 min if vomiting has not occurred; apomorphine (dogs only) at 0.03 mg/kg, IV, or 0.04 mg/kg, IM; or xylazine (dogs or cats) at 0.5-1 mg/kg, IV or IM. If emesis cannot be induced, gastric lavage should be performed with tepid water. Animals that are already seizuring should be anesthetized first (with pentobarbital) and an endotracheal tube passed before gastric lavage. After emesis or gastric lavage, activated charcoal should be administered at 2-3 g/kg in small animals and 0.5-1 g/kg in large animals with magnesium sulfate at 250 mg/kg, PO.

Seizures should be controlled in small animals with pentobarbital, IV to effect, repeated as necessary. Muscle relaxants such as methocarbamol at 100-200 mg/kg, IV, also work well; they should be repeated as needed with a maximum dose of 330 mg/kg/day. In large animals, chloral hydrate or xylazine can be used to control seizures. Other medications such as glyceryl guaiacolate (5%, 110 mg/kg), diazepam, and xylazine have been used in dogs to control seizures with variable success.

Severely affected dogs should be intubated and artificial respiration provided. Acidification of urine with ammonium chloride (100 mg/kg, bid, PO) may be useful for ion-trapping and urinary excretion of the alkaloid. Intravenous fluids should be administered to force diuresis and maintain normal kidney function. Hyperthermia treatment (fans, cool bath) should be given if necessary. Acid-base balance should be monitored and corrected as needed.

Pyrrolizidine Alkaloidosis

Typically, pyrrolizidine alkaloidosis is a chronic poisoning that results in hepatic failure. It is caused by many toxic plants, most commonly of the genera Senecio, Crotalaria, Heliotropium, Amsinckia, Echium, Cynoglossum, and Trichodesma. These plants grow mainly in temperate climates, but some (e.g., Crotalaria spp.) require tropical or subtropical climates. The plants most often implicated are ragwort (*S.jacobea*), woolly groundsel (*S.redellii, S.longilobus*), rattleweed (*Crotalaria retusa*), and seeds of yellow tarweed (*A.intermedia*).

Cattle, horses, farmed deer, and pigs are most susceptible; sheep and goats require ~20 times more plant material than cattle. Individual susceptibility varies greatly within species; young growing animals are most susceptible.

Etiology and Pathogenesis:

More than 30 toxic factors (alkaloids with a pyrrolizidine base) have been found in the plants. It is likely that their toxic effects are unique. Senecio jacobea contains jacobine; retrorsine, seneciphylline, and monocrotaline are other pyrrolizidine alkaloids frequently incriminated in toxicities.

These plants, which under normal conditions are avoided by grazing animals, may be eaten during drought conditions. Some animals may eat these plants preferentially as roughage when they are available on extremely lush pasture. Animals are also poisoned by eating the plant material in hay, silage, or pellets. Seeds from Crotalaria, Amsinckia, and Heliotropium spp, which have been harvested with grain, have caused the disease in horses, cattle, pigs, and poultry. The toxic alkaloids are metabolized to highly reactive pyrroles, which produce cytotoxic effects on target sites, most commonly the nuclei of hepatocytes. Other target sites may include the epithelial and vascular tissues of the kidneys and lungs. The pyrroles cross-link DNA strands and also unite DNA with nucleoproteins such as actin. These molecular alterations are presumed to create the antimitotic and megalocytic effects characteristic of pyrrolizidine alkalosis.

Clinical Findings

The clinical signs and hepatic pathology are similar in all animal species regardless of the species of plant involved or the toxic pyrrolizidine alkaloids it contains. Acute intoxication is characterized by sudden death from hemorrhagic liver necrosis and visceral hemorrhages. This is a rare event, as the poor palatability of these plants makes rapid ingestion of large quantities of the toxins uncommon. More chronic exposure is typical, and the liver reflects the cumulative and progressive effects of repeated ingestion of small doses of toxin.

Clinical signs may not be seen for several weeks or months after initial exposure. Consumption of the offending plant may even have ceased months earlier. The ongoing hepatic damage in these instances is suspected to be due to the recycling of toxic pyrroles as they are released from one dying cell and taken up by another. Clinical progression may also be altered by concurrent hepatic pathology; a hemolytic crisis may be precipitated in sheep with excessive hepatic copper stores.

In horses and cattle, signs include loss of condition, anorexia, dullness, and constipation or diarrhea. Tenesmus and passing of bloodstained feces may be followed by rectal prolapse, especially in cattle. Ascites and icterus may be present, and cattle and sheep sometimes show intermittent photosensitization. Some animals become progressively weaker and reluctant to move. Others exhibit signs of hepatic encephalopathy such as head-pressing, aimless wandering, ataxia, or even frenzied and aggressive behavior. Pica may be seen. Death may occur suddenly or after prolonged recumbency with hepatic coma and high levels of ammonia in the blood.

Lesions: In acute cases, the liver may be enlarged, hemorrhagic, and icteric. In chronic cases, it is atrophied, fibrous, finely nodular, and usually pale with a glistening surface due to fibrous thickening of the capsule. Other livers are markedly icteric. The gallbladder is often edematous and grossly distended with thick, mucoid bile. Edema of the abomasum and segments of the bowel, mesentery, and associated lymph nodes is common, and there may be ascites. In some cases, numerous small hemorrhages are present in the abdominal serous membranes.

Characteristic histologic changes occur in the liver. Irreversible enlargement of individual hepatocytes (megalocytosis) is often seen; it is conspicuous in horses and sheep but less pronounced in cattle. In cattle, marked perivenous fibrosis of sublobular veins is usually present, but this is not a consistent finding in horses and sheep. In all species, increases in connective tissue, both within and around the lobules, are marked. Bile duct hyperplasia is variable but may be the most striking microscopic change seen in some livers. Pigs may show pulmonary congestion, hemorrhage, septal fibrosis, alveolar epithelialization, and emphysema. Renal tubular lining cells and glomerular epithelial cells also may be individually enlarged.

Diagnosis

A diagnosis based on history, clinical signs, and gross necropsy findings can usually be confirmed by histologic examination of liver and renal tissue. Chemical analyses of the liver for toxic metabolites are available for confirmation of exposure but are seldom necessary. When hepatic cirrhosis is extensive, hypoalbuminemia and hyperglobulinemia develop. Serum levels of fibrinogen, bilirubin, glutamyltransferase, and glutamate dehydrogenase may be increased, but it should be recognized that the insidious nature of this disease can result in surprisingly mild serum biochemical changes. Other hepatotoxins, such as copper or aflatoxin, as well as infections such as chronic fascioliasis, must be considered before making the diagnosis.

Treatment and Control

Further intake of toxic plant material must be prevented. Animals showing signs rarely recover, and lesions present in asymptomatic animals may progress and result in further losses over several months. Because high protein intake may prove harmful, rations high in carbohydrates are indicated. Methionine in 10% dextrose solution, IV, may be of value in treating horses.

The diminished ability of the liver to regenerate after pyrrolizidine alkaloid poisoning suggests a guarded prognosis. Preventing further outbreaks by reducing or eliminating contributory factors should be stressed. Sheep are commonly used for grazing control of these plants, but this practice carries risks unless sheep destined for early slaughter are used. Biologic control of plants with predator moths, flea beetles, and seed flies has met with variable success. Senecio and related toxic species in pastures have been controlled satisfactorily by annual herbicide applications, preferably in spring before hay or silage conservation. Measures that enhance destruction of the alkaloids in the rumen of sheep also have shown some promise.

Quercus

Most animals are susceptible to Quercus poisoning, although cattle and sheep are affected most often. Most species of oak (Quercus spp) found in Europe and North America are considered toxic. Clinical signs occur several days after consumption of large quantities of young oak leaves in the spring or green acorns in the fall. High mortality is often observed. Malformed calves and abortions have been reported in dams consuming acorns during the second trimester of pregnancy. The toxic principle, which appears to be gallotannins, polyhydroxyphenolic compounds, or their metabolites, causes GI and renal dysfunction. Signs include anorexia, depression, emaciation, dehydration, rumen stasis, tenesmus, smell of ammonia on the breath, serous ocular or nasal discharge, polydipsia, polyuria, hematuria, icterus, and constipation followed by mucoid to hemorrhagic diarrhea. Renal insufficiency may be evidenced by increased BUN and creatinine, proteinuria, hyperphosphatemia, hypocalcemia, and urine with a low specific gravity. Pale swollen kidneys, perirenal edema, subcutaneous edema, ascites, and hydrothorax are common necropsy findings. Edema and subserosal petechial or ecchymotic hemorrhage of intestinal mucosa and ulceration of the esophagus and rumen may be seen. Diagnosis is based on clinical findings, necropsy, history, and histopathologic examination of the kidney (ie, nephrosis). Other common diseases that resemble oak poisoning include pigweed (Amaranthus spp) poisoning and aminoglycoside antibiotic poisoning.

Consumption of a pelleted ration supplement (1 kg/head/day) containing 10-15% calcium hydroxide plus access to more palatable feeds may be used as a preventive measure if exposure to acorns or oak leaves cannot be avoided. Calcium hydroxide, ruminatorics, and purgatives (such as mineral oil [1 L/500 kg], sodium sulfate [1 kg/400 kg], or magnesium sulfate [450 g/400 kg]) may be effective antidotes if administered early in the course of disease. Fluid therapy to correct dehydration and acidosis and transplantation of ruminal microflora may be beneficial. Clinical recovery usually occurs within 60 days but is rare if renal dysfunction is severe.

MAJOR TOXIC PLANTS

Algal Poisoning

Algal poisoning is often an acute, fatal condition caused by high concentrations of toxic blue-green algae (more commonly known as cyanobacteria—literally blue-green bacteria) in the drinking water. Fatalities and severe illness of livestock, pets, wildlife, birds, and fish from heavy growths of waterblooms of blue-green algae occur in almost all countries of the world. Poisoning usually occurs during warm seasons when the waterblooms are more intense and of longer duration. Most poisonings occur among animals drinking algal-infested freshwater, but marine animals, especially maricultured fish and shrimp, are also affected. The toxins of cyanobacteria comprise 5 distinct chemical classes collectively called cyanotoxins.

Etiology, Epidemiology, and Pathogenesis:

Although toxic strains within species of Anabaena, Aphanizomenon, Cylindrospermopsis, Microcystis, Nodularia, Nostoc, and Planktothrix (Oscillatoria) are responsible for most cases of toxicity, there are >30 species of cyanobacteria that can be associated with toxic waterblooms. Neurotoxic alkaloids (called anatoxins) can be produced by Anabaena, Aphanizomenon, and Planktothrix, while saxitoxins can be produced by Anabaena, Aphanizomenon, and Lyngbya. Hepatotoxic peptides (called microcystins and nodularins) can be produced by Anabaena, Microcystis, Nodularia, Nostoc, and Planktothrix. Cylindrospermopsis can produce a potent hepatotoxic alkaloid called cylindrospermopsin. Some genera, especially Anabaena, can produce both neuro- and hepatotoxins. If a toxic waterbloom contains both types of toxins, the neurotoxin signs are usually observed first because their effects occur much sooner (minutes) than the hepatotoxins (1 to a few hours).

Poisoning usually does not occur unless there is a heavy waterbloom that forms a dense surface scum. Factors that contribute to heavy waterblooms are nutrient-rich eutrophic to hypereutrophic water and warm, sunny weather. Agriculture practices (eg, runoff of fertilizers and animal wastes) that lead to nutrient enrichment often contribute to waterbloom formation. The problem is augmented by light winds or wind conditions that lead to leeward shore concentrations of cyanobacteria in areas where livestock drink. Experiments with both toxin groups have revealed a steep dose-response curve, with up to 90% of the lethal dose being ingested without measurable effect. Animal size and species sensitivity influence the degree of intoxication. Monogastric animals are less sensitive than ruminants and birds. Depending on bloom densities and toxin content, animals may need to ingest only a few ounces or up to several gallons to experience acute or lethal toxicity.

While the species sensitivity and signs of poisoning can vary depending on the type of exposure, the gross and histopathologic lesions are quite similar among species poisoned by the hepatopeptides and neurotoxic alkaloids. Death from hepatotoxicosis induced by cyclic peptides is generally accepted as being the result of intrahepatic hemorrhage and hypovolemic shock. This conclusion is based on large increases in liver weight as well as in hepatic hemoglobin and iron content that account for blood loss sufficient to induce irreversible shock. In animals that live more than a few hours, hyperkalemia or hypoglycemia, or both, may lead to death from liver failure within a few days.

Neurotoxicosis, with death occurring in minutes to a few hours from respiratory arrest, may result from ingestion of the cyanobacteria that produce neurotoxic alkaloids. Species and strains of Anabaena, Aphanizomenon, and Planktothrix can produce a potent, postsynaptic cholinergic (nicotinic) agonist called anatoxin-a that causes a depolarizing neuromuscular blockade. Strains of Anabaena can produce an irreversible organophosphate anticholinesterase called anatoxin-a(s). Anabaena, Aphanizomenon, and Lyngbya can produce the potent, presynaptic sodium channel blockers called saxitoxins.

Clinical Findings and Lesions:

One of the earliest effects (15-30 min) of microcystin poisoning is increased serum concentrations of bile acids, alkaline phosphatase, glutamyltransferase, and AST. The WBC count and clotting times increase. Death may occur within a few hours (usually within 4-24 hr), up to a few days. Death may be preceded by coma, muscle tremors, paddling, and dyspnea. Watery or bloody diarrhea may also be seen. Gross lesions include hepatomegaly due mostly to intrahepatic hemorrhage. Intact clumps of greenish algae can be found in the stomach and GI tract, and there is a greenish algal stain on the mouth, nose, legs, and feet. Hepatic necrosis begins centrilobularly and proceeds to the periportal regions. Hepatocytes are disassociated and rounded. After death, debris from disassociated hepatocytes can be found in the pulmonary vessels and kidneys. Clinical signs of neurotoxicosis progress from muscle fasciculations to decreased movement, abdominal breathing, cyanosis, convulsions, and death. Signs in birds are similar but include opisthotonos. In smaller animals, death is often preceded by leaping movements. Cattle and horses that survive acute poisoning may experience photosensitization in areas exposed to light (nose, ears, and back), followed by hair loss and sloughing of the skin.

Diagnosis

Diagnosis is based primarily on history (recent contact with an algal bloom), signs of poisoning, and necropsy findings. Samples of the waterbloom should be taken as soon as possible for microscopic examination to confirm the presence of the toxigenic cyanobacteria and for toxin analysis. Although there are nontoxic and toxic strains of all the known toxic species, it is not possible to identify a toxic strain by visual examination. Cyanobacteria are detected by light microscopy, identified using morphologic characteristics, and counted per standard volume of water. Standard protocols for sampling and monitoring cyanobacteria as well as practical keys for the identification of toxic species are available.

Some laboratories can analyze for the toxins either by chemical or biologic assay. Animal bioassays (mouse tests) have traditionally been used for detecting the presence of the entire range of cyanotoxins based on survival times and signs of poisoning. These tests provide a definitive indication of toxicity, although they cannot be used for precise quantification of compounds in water or for determining compliance with standards for environmental levels. A number of analytic techniques are available for determining microcystins in water. Analytic techniques must provide for quantitative comparison to the guideline value in terms of toxicity equivalents. The technique most suitable in this regard is high-performance liquid chromatography, although it may still involve estimation of the concentration, and therefore only an estimate of toxicity. Commercial standards for some microcystins, nodularin, and saxitoxins are available, while those for anatoxins and cylindrospermopsin should be available shortly. Newer methods of immunoassay are also available, including commercial ELISA kits in both laboratory and field formats.

Treatment

After removal from the contaminated water supply, affected animals should be placed in a protected area out of direct sunlight. Ample quantities of water and good quality feed should be made available. Because the toxins have a steep dose-response curve, surviving animals have a good chance for recovery. While therapies for cyanobacterial poisonings have not been investigated in detail, activated charcoal slurry is likely to be of benefit. In laboratory studies, an ion-exchange resin such as cholestyramine has proved useful to absorb the toxins from the GI tract, and certain bile acid transport blockers such as cyclosporin A, rifampin, and silymarin injected before dosing of microcystin have been effective in preventing hepatotoxicity. No therapeutic antagonist has been found effective against anatoxin-a, cylindrospermopsin, or the saxitoxins, but atropine and activated charcoal reduce the muscarinic effects of the anticholinesterase anatoxin-a(s).

Prevention

Removal of animals from the affected water supply is essential. If no other water supply is available, animals should be allowed to drink only from shore areas kept free (by prevailing winds) of dense surface scums of algae. Some efforts have been made to erect surface barriers (logs or floating plastic booms) to keep shore areas free of surface scum, but these are not very successful. Cyanobacteria can be controlled by adding copper sulfate ($CuSO_4$) or other algicidal treatments to the water. The usual treatment is 0.2-0.4 ppm, equivalent to 0.65-1.3 oz/10,000 gal. of water or 1.4-2.8 lb/acre-foot of water. Livestock (especially sheep) should not be watered for at least 5 days after the last visible evidence of the algal bloom. $CuSO_4$ is best used to prevent bloom formation, and care should be taken to avoid water that has dead algae cells, either from treatment with algicide or natural aging of the bloom, because most toxin is freed in the water only after breakdown of the intact algae cells.

Source water management techniques for control of cyanobacterial growth include flow maintenance in regulated rivers, water mixing techniques for both the elimination of stratification and the reduction of nutrient release from sediments in reservoirs, and the use of algicides in dedicated water supply storages. Algicides will disrupt cells and liberate intracellular toxins. Algicide use should be in accordance with local environment and chemical registration regulations. In situations where multiple offtakes are available, the selective withdrawal of water from different depths can minimize the intake of high surface accumulations of cyanobacterial cells.

Water treatment techniques can be highly effective for removal of both cyanobacterial cells and microcystins with the appropriate technology. As with other cyanotoxins, a high proportion of microcystins remain intracellular unless cells are lysed or damaged, and can therefore be removed by coagulation and filtration in a conventional treatment plant. Treatment of water containing cyanobacterial cells with oxidants such as chlorine or ozone, while killing cells, will result in the release of free toxin. Therefore, the practice of prechlorination or preozonation is not recommended without a subsequent step to remove dissolved toxins.

Microcystins are readily oxidized by a range of oxidants, including ozone and chlorine. Adequate contact time and pH control are needed to achieve optimal removal of these compounds, which will be more difficult in the presence of whole cells. Microcystins, anatoxin-a, cylindrospermopsin and some saxitoxins are also adsorbed from solution by both granular activated carbon and, less efficiently, by powdered activated carbon. The effectiveness of the process should be determined by monitoring toxin in the product water.

Bracken Fern Poisoning

Bracken fern (Pteridium aquilinum [Pteris aquilina]) is widely distributed in upland and marginal areas throughout North and South America, Europe, Australia, and Asia. Ingestion of significant quantities produces signs of acute poisoning related to thiamine deficiency in monogastric animals and bone marrow depletion (aplastic anemia) in ruminants. The toxic effects appear to be cumulative and may require 1-3 mo to develop, depending on the species of animal, quantity consumed, time of year, and other factors. Both leaves and rhizomes contain the toxic principles, which vary in concentration with the season. Most acute poisonings are seen after periods of drought when grazing is scarce; however, the plant is toxic even when present as a contaminant in hay, and cases have occurred in stabled animals.

Longterm, low-level consumption has been associated with other clinical syndromes. Enzootic hematuria with hemorrhages or tumors in the bladder is seen in cattle in many areas of the world, and similar tumors have been seen in sheep. Bright blindness with retinal degeneration and hyperreflectivity of the tapetum is found in hill sheep in parts of England, and a similar condition has been recognized in cattle grazing bracken in

Wales. Ingestion of bracken fern has been implicated in the occurrence of tumors in the upper GI tract of cattle in areas of Brazil and Scotland.

Some epidemiologic evidence suggests that regular consumption of milk from cattle with access to bracken may be associated with an increased risk of human esophageal or gastric cancer, but this is still under investigation. A greater risk to humans is direct consumption of the fern itself, a practice that continues in various countries throughout the world and is indeed promoted in some North American publications.

Bracken fern contains a number of toxic factors, some of which are not yet fully characterized. Poisoning in nonruminants is due to a thiaminase; the effects are essentially those of vitamin B1 deficiency, with myelin degeneration of the peripheral nerves. Horses seem to be particularly susceptible, while disease in pigs is rare. Thiamine deficiency is generally not a problem in ruminants because the vitamin is synthesized in the rumen, but polioencephalomalacia (Polioencephalo-malacia: Introduction) associated with impaired thiamine metabolism in sheep has been attributed to consumption of bracken fern and rock or mulga fern (Cheilanthes sieberi) in Australia.

The nature of the bone marrow toxin (aplastic anemia factor) to which cattle are particularly susceptible has not been defined, although the compound ptaquiloside has been suggested. The toxin causes death of precursor cells in the marrow so that cells with a shorter life span (the platelets) are affected first. An initial leukocytosis is followed by granulocytopenia and thrombocytopenia with resultant increased susceptibility to infection and tendency to spontaneous hemorrhage.

Bladder tumors, carcinoma of the urothelium, and hemangioendotheliomas in naturally occurring enzootic hematuria suggest that bracken fern may act as a carcinogen. This has been confirmed experimentally—inclusion of bracken fern in the diet of rats, mice, guinea pigs, quail, and Egyptian toads has resulted in tumors at various sites depending on the species and duration of feeding. Identical tumors can be produced by feeding ptaquiloside. Studies suggest that upper GI tract tumors in cattle may be due to the combined action of bracken fern and bovine papilloma virus (BPV). Bracken fern in combination with either BPV types 2 or 4 is believed to cause tumors in cattle. A flavonoid isolated from bracken fern, quercetin, is essential to fully transform bovine cells exposed to BPV type 4 in vitro.

Clinical Findings

In horses, signs of bracken-induced thiamine deficiency (bracken staggers) include anorexia, weight loss, incoordination, and a crouching stance with back and neck arched and feet placed wide apart. When forced to move, trembling muscles are noted. In severe cases, tachycardia and arrhythmias are present; death (usually 2-10 days after onset) is preceded by convulsions, clonic spasms, and opisthotonos. The rectal temperature is usually normal but may reach 104°F (40°C).

In pigs, signs of thiamine deficiency are less distinct and may resemble heart failure. Affected pigs show anorexia and weight loss. Death can occur suddenly after recumbency and dyspnea.

In cattle, acute bracken poisoning causes an acute hemorrhagic syndrome or, in some cases, sudden death. Affected cattle are weak, rapidly lose weight, and are pyrexic (106-110°F [41-43°C]); many have difficulty breathing and have icteric or pale mucosae with petechiae. Clots of blood may be passed in the feces, and there is often bleeding from body orifices. The blood frequently fails to clot normally; where tabanid flies are abundant, the skin of affected cattle is marked by streaks of blood where the insects have fed. The disease is almost always fatal; necropsy reveals multiple hemorrhages throughout the carcass. Necrotic ulcers may be present in the GI tract and bruising in the muscles. Swelling of the larynx and difficulty breathing has been reported in young cattle.

Chronic enzootic hematuria in cattle is characterized by intermittent hematuria and, ultimately, death due to anemia. The bladder contains small hemorrhages, dilated vessels, or tumors, which can be vascular, fibrous, or epithelial. In many cases, a mixture of lesions is found.

Bright blindness in sheep is a progressive retinal atrophy that derives its name from the hyperreflectivity of the tapetum. Affected sheep are permanently blind and adopt a characteristic alert attitude. The pupils respond poorly to light, and ophthalmoscopic examination of sheep with advanced disease reveals narrowing of arteries and veins and a pale tapetum nigrum with fine cracks and spots of gray.

Diagnosis

Other plants, such as horsetail (Equisetum arvense) and turnip (Beta vulgaris), can induce thiamine deficiency. In horses, the condition must be distinguished from other neurologic disorders, including rabies or poisoning due to Crotalaria sp or ragwort (Senecio jacobea). Blood thiamine levels decrease from an average normal of 80-100 mg/L to 25-30 μg/L, while blood pyruvate levels increase from a normal of ~20-30 mg/L to 60-80 μg/L; comparison with a sample from an unexposed animal of similar age and type will mitigate problems associated with correlating data from different analytic protocols. In pigs, the signs and lesions may indicate heart failure. Definitive diagnosis is established by demonstrating decreased blood thiamine levels or an increase in blood pyruvate with a decrease in RBC transketolase activity.

The acute hemorrhagic syndrome in cattle is distinctive, but signs may be confused with those of any acute septicemia (including anthrax) or other forms of poisoning such as mycotoxicosis, or poisoning by sweet clover or trichloroethylene-extracted soybean meal. Hematologic examination shows a loss of platelets from the blood, normally accompanied by loss of WBC, and pancytopenia in advanced stages.

Chronic enzootic hematuria must be distinguished from other causes of "red water," e.g., the hemoglobinemia of babesiosis. Occasionally, cases are complicated by coexisting chronic pyelonephritis.

The retinal changes of bright blindness in sheep are characteristic but subtle, so diagnosis requires the exclusion of other causes of blindness, including pregnancy toxemia, infectious keratoconjunctivitis, and cataracts.

Treatment

Treatment of thiamine deficiency in horses is highly effective if diagnosis is made early. Injection of a thiamine solution at 5 mg/kg is suggested, given initially IV every 3 hr, then IM for several days. Oral supplementation may be required for an additional 1-2 wk, although SC injection of 100-200 mg daily for 6 days has been successful in some cases. Thiamine treatment should also include animals similarly exposed but not yet showing signs, as they can develop days or weeks after removal from the source of bracken.

In acutely affected cattle, mortality is usually >90%, and the platelet count is the best prognostic indicator. Animals should be removed from contaminated pasture, but it is often difficult to convince farmers that the plant is poisonous because the disease can appear up to 2 wk after livestock are removed from the fern-infested area. Treatment with dl-batyl alcohol to stimulate the bone marrow is of doubtful value. Antibiotics may be useful to prevent secondary infections. Blood or even platelet transfusions from a donor not grazing bracken may be appropriate, but large volumes are required (minimum of 2-4 L blood). Granulocyte-macrophage colony-stimulating factor has been used to treat aplastic anemia in humans.

The other syndromes are essentially untreatable and must be controlled by preventing access to the fern.

Prevention

Bracken is usually grazed for want of more suitable food, although individual animals may develop a taste for the plant, particularly the young tender shoots and leaves. Early spring (tender bracken shoots) or late summer (poor pasture conditions) are the times when the problem is most often manifest. The disease has been prevented in ruminants and horses by improved pasture management and fertilization or by alternating bracken-contaminated and noncontaminated pasture at 3-wk intervals.

Fern growth can be retarded by close grazing or trampling in alternate grazing pasture systems. In time, a pasture can be freed of bracken using this approach or by regular cutting of the mature plant or, if the land is suitable, by deep plowing. Herbicide treatment using asulam or glyphosate can be an effective method of control, especially if combined with cutting before treatment. Biologic control by the use of microorganisms or insects has been considered, but the longterm implications are not clear.

Ryegrass

This often fatal neurotoxic disease occurs in livestock of any age that graze pastures in which annual ryegrass (Lolium rigidum) is present and in the seedhead stage of growth. It occurs in western and southern Australia and in South Africa from November to March. Hay of Festuca rubra *commutata* (Chewing's fescue) with Rathayibacter (Clavibacter) *toxicus* -infected seedhead galls has caused a similar disease in cattle and horses in Oregon. Outbreaks of ergot alkaloid toxicity in cattle on Lolium rigidum have been reported in South Africa and should not be confused with annual ryegrass staggers.

In Australia, the responsible corynetoxins (members of the tunicaminyluracil group) are produced in seedhead galls induced by the nematode Anguina funesta and colonized by Rathayibacter toxicus. These bacteria-infected galls are present in infected annual ryegrass pastures from early spring onward, but they are most toxic when the plants senesce. Hence, animals show no sign of toxicity until late spring and summer. Spread of bacteria-infested nematodes to adjacent healthy annual ryegrass pastures is slow.

The corynetoxins are highly toxic glycolipids that inhibit specific glycosylation enzymes and therefore deplete or reduce activity of essential glycoproteins. Experimentally, the corynetoxins deplete fibronectins and cause failure of the hepatic reticuloendothelial system. Cardiovascular function and vascular integrity are consequently impaired, and peripheral circulation and oxygen distribution compromised. Tunicamycin irreversibly downregulates the expression of g-aminobutyric acidA receptors and causes cell death in cultured brain neurons. Hence, the clinical expression of the disorder is nervous.

Outbreaks occur 2-6 days after animals graze a pasture that contains annual ryegrass infected at a toxic level. Deaths occur within hours, or up to 1 wk after onset of signs.

Characteristic neurologic signs are similar to those of perennial ryegrass staggers. However, mortality from annual ryegrass toxicity is commonly 40-50%, occasionally greater. The lesions include congestion, edema, hemorrhage of the brain and lungs, and degeneration of the liver and kidneys.

Diagnosis is based on the characteristic neurologic signs of tremors, incoordination, rigidity, and collapse when stressed, with animals often becoming apparently normal again when left undisturbed. When animals are severely affected, nervous spasms supervene, and convulsions could be precipitated by either forced exercise or high ambient temperatures. A thorough history and evaluation of the pastures will assist in differentiation of staggers caused by other grasses such as perennial ryegrass, phalaris, and the ergots of paspalum and other grasses. Polioencephalomalacia and enterotoxemia are other differential diagnoses.

Clinical signs identical to those of annual ryegrass toxicity have recently been described in Australia in animals grazing Agrostis avenacea (annual blown grass), Polypogon monspeliensis (annual beard grass), or Ehrharta longiflora (annual veldtgrass) infected with nematode galls containing R toxicus. These diseases have been called flood plain staggers, Stewart range syndrome, and veldtgrass staggers, respectively. Although the same bacterium is responsible for all the diseases, the Anguina nematode vectors of R toxicus for these 3 grasses are different species than the A funesta associated with annual ryegrass toxicity. Whereas the inflorescences of annual ryegrass infected with A funesta usually appear normal, nematode-infested inflorescences of these other grasses show distinctive signs.

A significant increase in survival of sheep experimentally poisoned with tunicamycin was observed following treatment with derivatives of ß-cyclodextrin. The promising result with this toxin-binding agent offers hope for treatment of animals once they have become affected with annual ryegrass staggers. Losses from the disorder can be minimized by early recognition of signs and removal to safe grazing or by reducing grazing pressure. Gall identification is difficult in annual ryegrass pastures, and in south Australia the bacterium in emerging seedheads is detected and quantified by ELISA. Early detection of toxic fields enables farmers to mow the heads off grass or to allow grazing before the grass becomes too toxic. Grazing of hay aftermath from toxic pastures should be avoided. Burning annual ryegrass pastures in the fall destroys most of the galls colonized by bacteria and minimizes the risk of toxicity in the following season.

Perennial Ryegrass Staggers

This neurotoxic condition of grazing livestock of all ages occurs only in late spring, summer, and fall and only in pastures in which perennial ryegrass (Lolium perenne) or hybrid ryegrass are the major components. Sheep, cattle, horses, farmed deer, and llamas are susceptible. In New Zealand, a high incidence most years causes considerable loss and seriously disrupts management procedures and stock movement. Perennial ryegrass staggers occurs sporadically in parts of North and South America, Europe, and Australia.

The tremorgenic neurotoxins responsible are lolitrems, mainly lolitrem B. These indole diterpene alkaloids are produced in perennial and hybrid ryegrasses infected with the endophytic fungus Neotyphodium (Acremonium) lolii. The amounts of fungal hyphae and lolitrem B in infected plants increase to toxic levels as the temperature rises in late spring and decrease again to safe levels in the cooler seasons. Mycelia of the fungus are present in all above-ground parts of infected plants but are especially concentrated in leaf sheaths, flower stalks, and seed. Infected plants exhibit no signs, and the fungus is spread only through infected seed. Viability of the endophyte gradually declines when infected seed is stored at ambient temperatures and moderate to high humidity, so that few seeds contain viable endophyte after 2 yr. Neurotoxic tremorgens are believed to cause incoordination by interference with neuronal transmission in the cerebral cortex through production of a reversible biochemical lesion; no specific histologic lesion is recognized. N lolii also produces the ergopeptine alkaloid ergovaline, which is the alkaloid responsible for fescue toxicosis. Ergovaline raises the temperature of animals in the warmer months of the year, inducing heat stress. It also depresses prolactin levels, and reduced milk yield in cows has been recorded in New Zealand and Australia.

Signs develop gradually over a few days. Fine tremors of the head and nodding movements are the first signs noted in animals approached quietly and watched carefully. Noise, sudden exercise, or fright elicits more severe signs of head nodding with jerky movements and incoordination when first moved. Running movements are stiff and bounding with marked incoordination and often result in collapse in lateral recumbency with opisthotonos, nystagmus, and flailing of stiffly extended limbs. In less severe cases, the attack soon subsides and within minutes the animal regains its feet. If again forced to run, the episode is repeated. Signs are most severe when the animal is heat stressed.

Within flocks and herds, individual susceptibility varies greatly, and this trait is heritable. In outbreaks, morbidity may reach 80-90%, but mortality is low (0-5%). Deaths are usually accidental, often by drowning when drinking from ponds or streams, or due to the inability to forage for food and water.

The strict seasonal occurrence of characteristic tremors, incoordination, and collapse in several or many animals grazing predominantly perennial ryegrass pastures strongly implicates this disease. Reference to the botanical composition of the pastures will exclude annual ryegrass toxicity and paspalum staggers, which have similar clinical signs and seasonality. Microscopic examination of the leaf sheaths of the ryegrass sward will reveal the extent of endophyte infection.

Because movement and handling of animals exacerbates signs, individual treatment is generally impractical. Recovery is spontaneous in 1-2 wk if animals are moved to nontoxic pastures or crops.

Because the endophyte and the lolitrems and ergovaline are not uniformly distributed within ryegrass plants, control by grazing management can help reduce or prevent the disease. Lolitrems and ergovaline are concentrated in the leaf sheath and inflorescences. If pastures are not overgrazed down into the leaf sheath zone or grazed when the plants are flowering, then animals should be relatively safe even when a high proportion of the ryegrass plants are infected with endophytes. Encouragement of growth of other grass species and legumes in established swards also reduces the intake of toxic grass.

Safe new pastures can be established using ryegrass seed with little or no endophyte infection. Alternatively, seed that has been stored at ambient temperatures for 18-24 mo probably contains few viable endophytes and would produce nontoxic pastures. However, the presence of endophyte in grasses makes the plants resistant to attack from many insects and so these pastures are more persistent than endophyte-free pastures. Cultivars of ryegrass artificially infected with a strain of endophyte that does not produce lolitrem B or ergovaline are now available in New Zealand. Signs of ryegrass staggers have not been seen in animals grazing these grasses.

Sorghum

Sorghum poisoning has been seen primarily in the southwestern USA and reported almost exclusively in horses, although a similar syndrome has been reported in sheep and cattle. Lathyrogenic nitriles such as ß-cyanoalanine, cyanogenic glycosides, and nitrates have been suggested as causative agents. The syndrome develops in horses after they have grazed hybrid Sudan pastures for weeks to months and produces axonal degeneration and myelomalacia in the spinal cord and cerebellum. Consumption of the seed will not produce the syndrome.

Sorghum poisoning is characterized by posterior incoordination, cystitis, urinary incontinence (which predisposes both male and female horses to cystitis), and alopecia on the hindlegs due to urine scald. The incoordination may progress to flaccid paralysis. Deformities of the fetal musculoskeletal system (arthrogryposis) and abortion during late pregnancy may occur. Consumption of sorghum hybrids with low cyanogenic potential or restriction of access to sorghum grasses may limit the incidence. Affected horses often die from pyelonephritis. Treatment with antibiotics may be helpful, but a full recovery is rare.

Sweet Clover

Sweet clover poisoning, an insidious hemorrhagic disease, is seen in animals that consume toxic quantities of spoiled sweet clover hay or silage. During the process of spoiling, the harmless natural coumarins in sweet clover are converted to toxic dicumarol. Any method of hay storage that allows molding of sweet clover promotes the likelihood of formation of dicumarol in the hay. Weathered, large round bales, particularly the outer portions, usually contain the highest levels of dicumarol. When toxic hay or silage is consumed, hypoprothro-mbinemia results, presumably because dicumarol combines with the proenzyme required for synthesis of prothrombin (by preventing formation of the active enzyme). It probably also interferes with synthesis of factor VII and other coagulation factors. Dicumarol levels of 20-30 mg/kg of hay are usually required to cause poisoning in cattle. The toxic agent crosses the placenta in pregnant animals, and newborn animals may be affected at birth. All species of animals studied are susceptible, but instances of poisoning have involved mainly cattle and, to a limited extent, sheep, pigs, and horses.

Clinical Findings and Lesions

Clinical signs are referable to hemorrhages that result from faulty blood coagulation. The time between consumption of toxic sweet clover and appearance of clinical disease varies greatly and depends on the dicumarol content of the particular sweet clover variety being fed, age of the animals, and the amount of feed consumed. If the dicumarol content of the ration is low or variable, animals may consume it for months before signs of disease appear.

The first indication of dicumarol poisoning may be the death of one or more animals. In affected animals, the first signs may be stiffness and lameness, due to bleeding into the muscles and joints. Hematomas, epistaxis, or GI bleeding may be seen. Death may occur suddenly with little preliminary evidence of disease and is caused by massive hemorrhage or bleeding after injury, surgery, or parturition. Neonatal deaths rarely occur without signs in the dam.

Hemorrhage is the characteristic necropsy finding; large extravasations of blood are common in subcutaneous and connective tissues.

Diagnosis

This is based on a history of continuous consumption of sweet clover hay or silage over relatively long periods, compatible signs and lesions, and markedly prolonged blood clotting time or demonstration of reduced prothrombin content of the plasma. The nature of the coagulopathy can be confirmed in the laboratory when the prothrombin time (PT) is prolonged. Sweet clover poisoning is normally a herd problem; signs of hemorrhage or slow blood clotting in only one animal from a group makes this diagnosis unlikely. Most diseases with hemorrhagic manifestations, such as blackleg, pasteurellosis, bracken fern poisoning, and aplastic anemia, can be readily differentiated based on clinical, pathologic, and hematologic findings. This is the only commonly acquired disease, except purpura hemorrhagica (common only in horses) and rodenticide poisoning, in which such large hemorrhages occur. Congenital or inherited diseases affecting coagulation factors or blood platelets (eg, hemophilia A) also may be characterized by large hemorrhages.

Treatment

The hypoprothrombinemia, hemorrhages, and anemia can be immediately corrected, to a degree, by IV administration of whole blood. Recommended dosages range from 2-10 L of fresh blood per 1, 000 lb (450 kg) body wt. Animals used as a source of blood must not be receiving sweet clover feed. All animals with marked signs should receive a transfusion, which can be repeated if necessary. In addition, all severely affected animals should receive parenteral administration of synthetic vitamin K1 (phytonadione).

SC or IM injection is recommended to avoid the substantial risk of anaphylaxis; SC vitamin K1 may not be as effective as IM treatment. There appears to be little advantage in outcome from IV administration. The usual dose recommended for cattle is 1 mg/kg, bid-tid for 2 days. Although it is more costly, vitamin K1 is more effective than K3 (menadione) in experimental studies and is the preferred treatment. Because reversal of the dicumarol by vitamin K1 requires synthesis of coagulation proteins, significant improvement in homeostasis requires several hours, and >24 hr is required to completely restore coagulation. Either vitamin K1 or a blood transfusion is sufficient to correct mild cases of intoxication if feeding toxic hay is stopped.

Prevention

Cultivars of sweet clover, low in coumarin and safe to feed (eg, Polara), have been developed. If one of these is not available, the only certain method of prevention is to avoid feeding sweet clover hay or silage. Although well-cured sweet clover is not dangerous, the absence of visible spoilage is insufficient evidence of safety. There is no quick chemical test for dicumarol, but suspect feed can be fed to rabbits, which develop fatal hemorrhages more rapidly than cattle. This can be combined with periodic determination of PT in the rabbits to speed up the test results. Unfortunately, some rabbits are refractory to dicumarol, which complicates negative test results.

A simple management technique involves alternating sweet clover hay suspected of containing dicumarol with other roughage such as alfalfa or a grass-legume hay mixture. A 7- to 10-day period on the sweet clover hay is followed by an equal time on the alternate hay. Alternating the forage can successfully prevent poisoning but does not completely prevent prolonged bleeding times. Some animals are at greater risk of serious hemorrhaging at calving (or lambing). They should not receive sweet clover hay for a minimum of 2-3 wk, and preferably 4 wk, prior to parturition. The goal is to allow the animal's clotting system to fully reestablish competency before a hemorrhagic stress. Dehorning and castration should also be avoided in animals consuming sweet clover hay at least until a full withdrawal period has been achieved.

Dallisgrass Poisoning

Dallisgrass poisoning (also known as Dallisgrass staggers) occurs several days after cattle ingest a significant amount of dallisgrass seedheads infected with an "ergot-like" fungus called Claviceps paspali. The seedheads typically are infected with the fungus in the fall, as the seedheads age. Rather than flat looking seeds on the heads, the infected heads have gray to black swellings that have a sticky sap material on them. Some observers say it looks like little popcorn. Usually not all the herd is affected, and it appears that it occurs when some animals develop a preference for the tips of the seedhead.

The infected seedheads contain three primary toxins, paspalinine, and paspalitrem A and B, which are tremorgenic alkaloids. The affected animals show neurological symptoms, including trembling of the major muscles and the head, jerky uncoordinated movements, and they also are spooky and sometimes aggressive. The animals will startle and run, and often will fall in unusual positions. In bad cases the animals will go down, and may stay down for several days. Convulsions and death can occur in extreme cases. The symptoms are somewhat like grass tetany, and this is often misdiagnosed, but they don't show the sudden death characteristic of grass tetany, and don't immediately respond to treatment for grass tetany.

There is no treatment for the malady, except to get the cattle off the affected grass, and provide them with high quality forage. If possible they should be put in a field with no ponds, steep slopes, etc. as they commonly stumble around and end up injuring or drowning themselves. Usually cattle can completely recover from the poisoning.

In late summer we often have reports of dallisgrass poisoning, and it seems to be getting more common now because there is more dallisgrass in pastures in North Carolina. Toxicity usually is reported on farms with rank dallisgrass seedheads and the fungus present. In many cases producers had stayed off the pastures hoping to let the grass get a little more growth on it, and as a result the seedheads got old. In other cases, there are only a few cattle in large pastures, so the Dallisgrass grew faster than the cattle could consume it. Rarely do we get a report of a case were there deaths of the affected cattle. It also seems that in many cases the younger cows are affected, which suggests that cows may learn to avoid eating too much of the seedheads after getting too much (cattle are known to learn to avoid poisonous plants in this way).

Dallisgrass is becoming a more important part of many pastures in the piedmont and coastal plain. It is a very good quality warm season perennial, and provides great benefits to pasture systems, but the one drawback is the potential for Dallisgrass staggers. By rotational grazing the grass after seedheads emerge but before the fungus grows on them the problem can be avoided, because cattle will readily eat the immature seedheads unlike some other grasses we are used to. If the seedheads do become infected, clipping them off at about 12" before grazing should help prevent the problem. Hay with high amounts of seedhead can also be a problem, so feeding Dallisgrass hay along with other hay is advised, especially if infected seedheads are present.

Bitterweed Poisoning

Bitterweed is an erect, annual, composite plant growing from 3 inches to 2 feet tall. Stems are purplish near the base. Leaves are alternate and usually woolly underneath. Bright yellow flowers bloom from April through June and occasionally in the fall. This plant has a bitter taste and a distinct odor.

Bitterweed is common in arid areas of the southern Great Plains from southwestern Kansas and central Texas to southern California and into Mexico. It is most common where soil disturbance or overgrazing has occurred. Populations can be quite variable between years.

Bitterweed is toxic to sheep and is generally unpalatable. However, starved sheep that begin eating the plant may develop a liking for it. Cases of poisoning in cattle, horses or goats are rare. The toxic agent is a sesquiterpene lactone (hymenoxon). This material appears to accumulate, with a lethal dose consisting of 1. 3 percent of an animal's weight in green plant material, whether ingested at one time or over several months. The minimum lethal dose varies considerably among individual animals, regardless of their nutritional history. From a management perspective, it is probably best to consider bitterweed toxic at all growth stages. The plant becomes much more toxic in drought, when a lethal dose is 0. 5 percent of the animal's body weight.

Chinaberry Poisoning

Chinaberry or Bead Tree, Melia azedarach(syn. M. australis, M. japonica, M. sempervivens), is a deciduous tree in the mahogany family Meliaceae, native to India, southern China and Australia. In South Africa it is commonly but erroneously called Syringa, which is in fact the lilac genus. The genus Melia includes four other species, occurring from southeast Asia to northern Australia. They are all deciduous or semi-evergreen trees.

Fruits are poisonous to humans if eaten in quantity. However, like the Yew tree, these toxins are not harmful to birds, who gorge themselves on the fruit, eventually reaching a "drunken" state. The toxins are neurotoxins and unidentified resins, found mainly in the fruits. Some birds are able to eat the fruit, spreading the seeds in their droppings. The first symptoms of poisoning appear a few hours after ingestion. They may include loss of appetite, vomiting, constipation or diarrhea, bloody faeces, stomach pain, pulmonary congestion, cardiac arrest, rigidity, lack of coordination and general weakness. Death may take place after about 24 hours. Like in relatives, tetranortriterpenoids consititute an important toxic principle. These are chemically related to Azadirachtin, the primary insecticidal compound in the commercially important Neem oil. These compounds are probably related to the wood and seed's resistance to pest infestation, and maybe to the unattractiveness of the flowers to animals.

REFERENCES

Alpin, T. E. H. *Poisonous Garden Plants and other Plants Harmful to Man in Australia.* Perth: Western Australia Dept. of Agriculture, 1976. Bot QK100 .A8 A655.

Bailey, Frederick Manson. *Plants Reputed Poisonous and Injurious to Stock.* Brisbane: J.C. Beal, 1887. Bot QK100 .A8 B35.

Buck, et. al., *Clinical and Diagnostic Veterinary Toxicology.* 2nd ed. 1976. pp. 25-37.

Casarett, L.J. and J. Doull. (eds.) *Toxicology: The Basic Science of Poisons.* 2nd Ed. Ch. 3-5, 9-12, 14-15.

Clarke, E. G. C. and M. L. Clarke. 1975. *Veterinary Toxicology,* 1st Edition. Williams and Wilkins. pp. 109-118.

de Padua, L.S. Plant Resources of South-East Asia. No. 12, *Medicinal and Poisonous Plants* 1. Leiden, The Netherlands: Backhuys, 1999. Bot SB108 .A785 P52 v.12:1.

Forsyth, A. A. *British Poisonous Plants.* London: H.M.S.O., 1968. Bot QK100 .G7 F67 1968.

Foster, Steven. *A Field Guide to Venomous Animals and Poisonous Plants,* North America North of Mexico. Boston, MA: Houghton Mifflin, 1994. MAIN QL100 .F63 1994.

Hardin, James W. *Human Poisoning from Native and Cultivated Plants.* Durham, NC: Duke University Press, 1969. Bot QK100 .N6 H37.

Kingsbury, John Merriam. *Deadly Harvest: A Guide to Common Poisonous Plants.* New York: Holt, Rinehart and Winston,1965. Bot QK100 .A1 K55.

Lampe, Kenneth F. *AMA Handbook of Poisonous and Injurious Plants.* Chicago, IL: American Medical Association, 1985. Bot REF RA1250 .L27 1985.

Murphey, Edith Van Allen. *Stock Poisoning Plants, a Stockman's Pocket Book.* Corvallis, OR: Unnamed, 1947. Bot SB617.4 .M87.

8

Industrial Poisoning

The aim of this chapter is to provide toxicologic information on industrially important toxic substances such as fluorides, certain hydrocarbons and halogenated hydrocarbons, polychlorinated biphenyls and coal tar products.

COAL-TAR POISONING

A variety of coal-tar derivatives induce acute to chronic disease in animals. Clinical effects are acute to chronic hepatic damage with signs of icterus, ascites, anemia, and death. Coal-tar pitch poisoning has been reported from Canada, Germany, Ireland, Poland, and the USA. Toxicosis in domestic food animals and pets has been reported.

Etiology

The distillation of coal tar yields a variety of compounds, 3 of which are notably toxic: cresols (phenolic compounds), crude creosote (composed of cresols, heavy oils, and anthracene), and pitch. Tars are also produced from crude petroleum or wood. Creosote contains less volatile liquid and solid aromatic hydrocarbons of coal tar and some phenols. Cresols, composed mainly of hydroxytoluenes, are used as disinfectants. Coal-tar and pine-tar pitch are the brown to black, amorphous, polynuclear hydrocarbon residues left after coal tar is redistilled. Access of animals to coal tars is often by direct chewing on or consumption of product, rather than inclusion in feed or water. Clay pigeons, tar paper, creosote-treated wood, and bitumen-based flooring are typical sources.

Phenol is the most important toxicant in coal-tar products. The approximate oral acute LD50 of phenol for most species is 0. 5 g/kg, except for cats, which are more susceptible due to their limited ability to conjugate and excrete phenols.

Cresols, which are mixtures of methylphenols, are used as disinfectants and are readily absorbed through the skin. The lethal dose is 100-200 mg/kg, except in cats, which are especially sensitive. Because creosote derived from coal tar is toxic to wood-destroying fungi and insects, it is used as a wood preserver. Sows confined to wooden farrowing crates treated with 3 brush applications of creosote were reported to have stillborn pigs, and the surviving pigs grew slowly. Some sources suggest that coal tars reduce absorption of vitamin A by sows. Other species are less susceptible (e.g., the lethal dose of creosote in calves is 4 g/kg). Pitch is used as a binder in clay pigeons, road asphalt, insulation, and tar paper and roofing compounds, and to cover iron pipes and line wooden water tanks. Pigs that consume 15 g of clay pigeons over a 5-day period will die. Floor slabs with one-third lignite pitch reduced growth rate in pigs ~25%.

Clinical Findings

The cresols are locally corrosive; they stimulate the CNS and depress the heart, which results in vascular collapse. Capillary damage and hepatic or renal damage can occur. Death can occur from 15 min to several days after exposure. The first sign of pitch poisoning often is several dead pigs. Other pigs are depressed, and signs may progress to weakness, ataxia, sternal recumbency, icterus, coma, and death. Secondary anemia may develop. Associated problems have included stillbirths in pigs and hyperkeratosis in calves. Blood glucose is reduced terminally, while thymol turbidity and serum chloride and phosphorus are increased.

Lesions

Cresols and creosote produce contact irritation and nonspecific liver and kidney lesions. In pitch poisoning, the liver is markedly swollen with a diffuse, mottled appearance. The lobules are clearly outlined by a light-colored zone, and their centers contain deep-red dots the size of a pinhead. There is centrilobular liver necrosis, with blood replacing the lost cells and filling the center of the lobule. Renal tubular degeneration and necrosis also can be present. The blood clots slowly or not at all. The carcass is icteric. Excessive fluid is found in the peritoneal cavity.

Diagnosis

Differential diagnoses include toxic plant poisonings (Crotalaria, Senecio, cocklebur), aflatoxicosis, fumonisin toxicosis, gossypol toxicosis, yellow phosphorus poisoning, and vitamin E or selenium deficiency. Fragments of clay pigeons, tar paper, or other sources of coal tars found in the GI tract, or chemical detection of coal-tar products in liver, kidney, serum, or urine, aid in confirming the diagnosis. A rapid presumptive test is to mix 1 mL of urine with 0.1 mL of 20% ferric chloride; purple color is indicative of phenol, but results should be confirmed by a laboratory.

Treatment

There is no specific antidote for animals with frank signs. For recent oral exposure, activated charcoal and saline cathartics may reduce absorption. Supportive therapy to combat shock, respiratory failure, and acidosis could be useful for valuable individual animals. Demulcents or egg whites orally may help to reduce local corrosive effects in the stomach and intestines. Oral antibiotics and high-quality-protein diets may aid recovery.

CYANIDE POISONING

Cyanide inhibits cytochrome oxidase and causes death from histotoxic anoxia.

Etiology

Cyanides are found in plants, fumigants, soil sterilizers, fertilizers, and rodenticides (e.g., calcium cyanomide). Toxicity can result from improper or malicious use, but in the case of livestock, the most frequent cause is ingestion of plants that contain cyanogenic glycosides. These include Triglochin maritima (arrow grass), Hoecus lunatus (velvet grass), Sorghum spp (Johnson grass, Sudan grass, common sorghum), Prunus spp (apricot, peach, chokecherry, pincherry, wild black cherry), Sambucus canadensis (elderberry), Pyrus malus (apple), Zea mays (corn), and Linum spp (flax). The seeds (pits) of several plants such as the peach have been the source of cyanogenic glycosides in many cases. Eucalyptus spp, kept as ornamental houseplants, have been implicated in deaths of small animals. The cyanogenic glycosides in plants yield free hydrocyanic acid (HCN), otherwise known as prussic acid, when hydrolyzed by ß-glycosidase or when other plant cell structure is disrupted or damaged, e.g., by freezing, chopping, or chewing. Microbial action in the rumen can further release free cyanide.

Apple and other fruit trees contain prussic acid glycosides in leaves and seeds but little or none in the fleshy part of the fruits. In Sorghum spp forage grasses, leaves usually produce 2-25 times more HCN than do stems; seeds contain none. New shoots from young, rapidly growing plants often contain high concentrations of prussic acid glycosides. The cyanogenic glycoside potential of plants can be increased by heavy nitrate fertilization, especially in phosphorus-deficient soils. Spraying of cyanogenic forage plants with foliar herbicides such as 2, 4-D can increase their prussic acid concentrations for several weeks after application.

The cyanogenic glycoside potential is slow to decrease in drought-stricken plants containing mostly leaves. Grazing stunted plants during drought is the most common cause of poisoning of livestock by plants that produce prussic acid.

Frozen plants may release high concentrations of prussic acid for several days. After wilting, release of prussic acid from plant tissues declines. Dead plants have less free prussic acid. When plant tops have been frosted, new shoots may regrow at the base; these can be dangerous because of glycoside content and because livestock selectively graze them.

Ruminants are more susceptible than monogastric animals, and cattle slightly more so than sheep. Hereford cattle have been reported to be less susceptible than other breeds.

Clinical Findings

Signs can occur within 15-20 min to a few hours after animals consume toxic forage. Excitement can be displayed initially, accompanied by rapid respiration rate. Dyspnea follows shortly, with tachycardia. Salivation, excess lacrimation, and voiding of urine and feces may occur. Vomiting may occur, especially in pigs. Muscle fasciculation is common and progresses to generalized spasms before death. Animals stagger and struggle before collapse. Mucous membranes are bright red but may become cyanotic terminally. Death occurs during severe asphyxial convulsions. The heart may continue to beat for several minutes after struggling and breathing stops. The whole syndrome usually does not exceed 30-45 min. Most animals that live =2 hr after onset of clinical signs recover, unless continuous absorption of cyanide from the GI tract occurs.

Lesions

In acute or peracute cyanide toxicoses, blood may be bright cherry red initially but can be dark red if necropsy is delayed; it may clot slowly or not at all. Mucous membranes may also be pink initially, then become cyanotic after respiration ceases. The rumen may be distended with gas, and the odor of "bitter almonds" may be detected after opening. Agonal hemorrhages of the heart may be seen. Liver, serosal surfaces, tracheal mucosa, and lungs may be congested or hemorrhagic; some froth may be seen in respiratory passages. Neither gross nor histologic lesions are consistently seen.

Multiple foci of degeneration or necrosis may be seen in the CNS of dogs chronically exposed to sublethal amounts of cyanide. These lesions have not been reported in livestock.

Diagnosis

Appropriate history, clinical signs, postmortem findings, and demonstration of HCN in rumen (stomach) contents or other diagnostic specimens support a diagnosis of cyanide poisoning. Specimens recommended for cyanide analyses include the suspected source (plant or otherwise), rumen or stomach contents, heparinized whole blood, liver, and muscle. Antemortem whole blood is preferred; other specimens should be collected as soon as possible after death, preferably within 4 hr. Specimens should be sealed in an airtight container, refrigerated or frozen, and submitted to the laboratory without delay. When cold storage is unavailable, immersion of specimens in 1-3% mercuric chloride has been satisfactory.

Hay, green chop, silage, or growing plants containing >220 ppm cyanide as HCN on a wet-weight (as is) basis are very dangerous as animal feed. Forage containing <100 ppm HCN, wet weight, is usually safe to pasture. Analyses performed on a dry-weight basis have the following criteria: >750 ppm HCN is hazardous, 500-750 ppm HCN is doubtful, and <500 ppm HCN is considered safe.

Normally expected cyanide concentrations in blood of most animal species are usually <0. 5 μg/mL. Minimal lethal blood concentrations are ~3. 0 μg/mL or less. Cyanide concentrations in muscle are similar to those in blood, but concentrations in liver are generally lower than those in blood.

Differential diagnoses include poisonings by nitrate or nitrite, urea, organophosphate, carbamate, chlorinated hydrocarbon pesticides, and toxic gases (carbon monoxide and hydrogen sulfide), as well as infectious or noninfectious diseases that cause sudden death.

Treatment, Control, and Prevention

Immediate treatment is necessary. Sodium nitrite (10 g/100 mL of distilled water or isotonic saline) should be given IV at 20 mg/kg body wt, followed by sodium thiosulfate (20%), IV, at =500 mg/kg; the latter may be repeated as needed with little hazard. Sodium nitrite therapy may be carefully repeated at 10 mg/kg, every 2-4 hr or as needed. In one study investigating cyanide poisoning treatment in dogs, either dimethylaminophenol (DMAP) IM at 5 mg/kg or hydroxylamine hydrochlorine IM at 50 mg/kg were as effective as nitrite and thiosulfate.

Sodium thiosulfate alone is also an effective antidotal therapy at =500 mg/kg, IV, plus 30 g/cow, PO, to detoxify any remaining HCN in the rumen. Oxygen may be helpful in supplementing nitrite or thiosulfate therapy, especially in small animals. Hyperbaric oxygen therapy (100% oxygen breathed intermittently at a pressure >1 atmosphere absolute) causes an above normal partial pressure of oxygen (PO_2) in arterial blood and markedly increases the amount of oxygen dissolved in plasma. Oxygen-dependent cellular metabolic processes benefit from heightened oxygen tension in capillaries and enhanced oxygen diffusion from capillaries to critical tissues. Activated charcoal is not efficacious in absorbing cyanide and thus is not recommended PO for antidotal therapy.

Caution is indicated in treatment. Many clinical signs of nitrate and prussic acid poisoning are similar, and injecting sodium nitrite induces methemoglobinemia identical to that produced by nitrate poisoning. If in doubt of the diagnosis, methylene blue, IV, at 4-22 mg/kg, may be used to induce methemoglobin. Because methylene blue can serve as both a donor and acceptor of electrons, it can reduce methemoglobin in the presence of excess methemoglobin or induce methemoglobin when only hemoglobin is present (but sodium nitrate is the more effective treatment for cyanide poisoning if the diagnosis is certain).

Pasture grasses (e.g., Sudan grass and sorghum-Sudan grass hybrids) should not be grazed until they are 15-18 in. tall to reduce danger from prussic acid poisoning. Forage sorghums should be several feet tall. Animals should be fed before first turning out to pasture; hungry animals may consume forage too rapidly to detoxify HCN released in the rumen. Animals should be turned out to new pasture later in the day; prussic acid release potential is reported to be highest during early morning hours. Free-choice salt and mineral with added sulfur may help protect against prussic acid toxicity. Grazing should be monitored closely during periods of environmental stress, e.g., drought or frost. Abundant regrowth of sorghum can be dangerous; these shoots should be frozen and wilted before grazing.

Green chop forces livestock to eat both stems and leaves, thereby reducing problems caused by selective grazing. Cutting height can be raised to minimize inclusion of regrowth.

Sorghum hay and silage usually lose =50% of prussic acid content during curing and ensiling processes. Free cyanide is released by enzyme activity and escapes as a gas. Although a rare occurrence, hazardous concentrations of prussic acid may still remain in the final product, especially if the forage had an extremely high cyanide content before cutting. Hay has been dried at oven temperatures for up to 4 days with no significant loss of cyanide potential. These feeds should be analyzed before use whenever high prussic acid concentrations are suspected. Potentially toxic feed should be diluted or mixed with grain or forage that is low in prussic acid content to achieve safe concentrations in the final product.

THYLENE GLYCOL TOXICITY

All animals are susceptible to ethylene glycol (EG) toxicity, but it is most common in dogs and cats. Most intoxications are associated with ingestion of radiator antifreeze, which is usually 95% EG. The widespread availability of antifreeze, its sweet taste and small minimum lethal dose, and the lack of public awareness of the toxicity (ie, improper storage and disposal) contribute to the frequency of this intoxication. In addition, antifreeze may be ingested because it is the only available liquid in cold weather or by way of intentional poisoning. Other sources of EG include some heat-exchange fluids used in solar collectors and ice-rink freezing equipment and some brake and transmission fluids. Cutaneous absorption from topical products that contain EG has been reported to cause toxicity in cats.EG intoxication occurs most commonly in temperate and cold climates because antifreeze is used both to decrease the freezing point and to increase the boiling point of radiator fluid. In colder climates, the incidence of EG intoxications is seasonal with most cases occurring in the fall, winter, and early spring.

The minimum lethal dose of undiluted EG is 1. 4 mL/kg body wt in cats, 4. 4 mL/ kg in dogs, 7-8 mL/kg in poultry, and 2-10 mL/kg in cattle (younger animals may be more susceptible).

Pathogenesis

EG is rapidly absorbed from the GI tract; in dogs, peak blood concentrations of EG occur within 3 hr of ingestion. About 50% of ingested EG is excreted unchanged by the kidneys; however, a series of oxidation reactions in the liver and kidneys metabolize the remaining EG. Toxic metabolites of EG cause severe metabolic acidosis and renal tubular epithelial damage.

The first of 2 rate-limiting biotransformation steps is the production of glycoaldehyde from EG by the enzyme alcohol dehydrogenase. Glycoaldehyde is then rapidly metabolized to glycolic acid. The oxidation of glycolic acid to glyoxylic acid is the second rate-limiting step, which allows glycolic acid to accumulate, resulting in acidosis and nephrosis. Glyoxylic acid is rapidly metabolized to formic acid, carbon dioxide, glycine, serine, and oxalate. Oxalate is not further metabolized and is cytotoxic to the renal tubular epithelium and exacerbates the metabolic acidosis. Glycolic acid and oxalate are the metabolites thought to be most responsible for acute tubular necrosis associated with EG ingestion. Oxalate also combines with calcium to form a soluble complex that is excreted via glomerular filtration. Calcium oxalate crystals form within the lumina of tubules as the concentration of the glomerular filtrate increases and the pH decreases (smaller numbers of calcium oxalate crystals may also be observed in the adventitia of blood vessel walls throughout the body).

Clinical Findings

Clinical signs are dose- and time-dependent and can be divided into those caused by unmetabolized EG and those caused by its toxic metabolites. The onset of clinical signs is almost immediate and resembles alcohol (ethanol) intoxication. Dogs and cats exhibit vomiting due to GI irritation, polydipsia and polyuria, and neurologic signs (CNS depression, stupor, ataxia, knuckling, decreased withdrawal and righting reflexes). Polydipsia occurs due to osmotic stimulation of the thirst center, and polyuria occurs due to an osmotic diuresis. As CNS depression increases in severity, dogs and cats drink less; however, the osmotic diuresis continues and results in dehydration. Dogs may appear to transiently recover from these CNS signs ~12 hr after ingestion.

Oliguric acute renal failure usually develops between 12 and 24 hr in cats and between 36 and 72 hr in dogs. Signs include lethargy, anorexia, dehydration, vomiting, diarrhea, oral ulcers, salivation, tachypnea, and possibly seizures or coma. The kidneys are often swollen and painful on abdominal palpation.

Pigs ingesting EG are usually depressed, weak, and reluctant to move; knuckling, posterior ataxia, trembling, collapse, abdominal distention, pulmonary edema, and muffled heart sounds are common sequelae. Poultry may become drowsy, ataxic, dyspneic, and recumbent; torticollis, ruffled feathers, and watery droppings are also seen. Cattle may become depressed, tachypneic, and ataxic, and develop paraparesis or recumbency. Epistaxis and hemoglobinuria have also been seen in cattle that have ingested large doses of EG.

Lesions

Renal tubular epithelial necrosis with calcium oxalate crystals in the tubular lumina is the characteristic finding of EG intoxication. Calcium oxalate crystals appear birefringent when viewed with polarized light. Pulmonary edema and hemorrhagic gastroenteritis are common secondary findings in dogs and cats. Pigs and cattle often develop renal and perirenal edema. Pigs may also have pulmonary edema with tan fluid in the pleural and peritoneal cavities. Poultry usually do not develop gross lesions.

Diagnosis

Diagnosis is often difficult due to nonspecific multisystemic signs that may appear similar to other types of CNS disease or trauma, gastroenteritis, pancreatitis, ketoacidotic diabetes mellitus, and acute renal failure due to renal ischemia or other nephrotoxicants. If ingestion of EG is not witnessed, diagnosis is usually based on a combination of history, physical examination, and laboratory data.

Within 3 hr of ingestion of toxic doses of EG, dogs and cats develop normochloremic metabolic acidosis with an increased anion gap, minimally concentrated or isosthenuric urine with an acidic pH, and marked serum hyperosmolality with an increased osmolal gap. Serum osmolality can be increased as much as 100 mOsm/kg above normal (280-310 mOsm/kg) within 3 hr of EG ingestion. The difference between measured and calculated (1. 86 [Na+ + K+] + glucose/18 + BUN/2. 8 + 9) osmolality is referred to as the osmolal gap. The gap is caused by the presence of unmeasured osmotically active particles (e.g., ethylene glycol) in the serum.

Calcium oxalate crystalluria is commonly seen as early as 3 and 6 hr after ingestion in cats and dogs, respectively. Monohydrate calcium oxalate crystals (clear, 6-sided prisms) are more common than dihydrate calcium oxalate crystals (maltese cross or envelope-shaped). EG concentrations in serum and urine are detectable by 1-2 hr after ingestion. Commercial test kits can detect serum EG concentrations of =50 mg/dL. Some antifreeze preparations contain fluorescein, which appears bright yellow-green when viewed under a Wood's lamp.

Urine fluorescence has been used as a qualitative adjunctive test in suspected EG ingestions in humans and may be of value in veterinary medicine. Hyperphosphatemia has been seen in dogs within 3 hr of ingestion of commercial antifreeze solutions that contain phosphate rust inhibitors. This hyperphosphatemia resolves before the onset of EG-induced acute renal failure and azotemia, then recurs when the animal becomes azotemic.

Treatment

The prognosis varies inversely with the amount of time that elapses between ingestion and initiation of treatment. Treatment is aimed at decreasing absorption of ingested EG, increasing excretion of unmetabolized EG, preventing metabolism of EG, and correcting the metabolic acidosis that occurs with EG metabolism. Further absorption of EG is prevented by induction of emesis or gastric lavage (or both) followed by administration of activated charcoal and sodium sulfate within 1-2 hr of ingestion. Once absorption has occurred, excretion of EG is increased by fluid therapy designed to correct dehydration and increase urine production. To prevent metabolism of EG, the activity of alcohol dehydrogenase is decreased by direct inactivation or by competitive inhibition. 4-Methylpyrazole (4-MP, fomepizole) effectively inactivates alcohol dehydrogenase in dogs without the side effects of ethanol and is the treatment of choice. The dose of 4-MP (5% solution [50 mg/mL]) is 20 mg/kg body wt, IV, initially, followed by 15 mg/kg, IV, at 12 and 24 hr, and 5 mg/kg, IV, at 36 hr. Commercial formulations of 4-MP are available.

In cats, 4-MP is ineffective at the canine dosage, and ethanol, a competitive inhibitor of alcohol dehydrogenase, is the treatment of choice. The recommended dose is 5 mL of 20% ethanol/kg body wt diluted in IV fluids and given as a drip over 6 hr for 5 treatments, and then over 8 hr for 4 more treatments.

The metabolic acidosis associated with metabolism of EG is corrected by administration of sodium bicarbonate. The formula 0.3-(0.5 × kg body wt) × (24 - plasma bicarbonate) is used to determine the dose, in mEq of bicarbonate. One-half of this dose should be given IV slowly to prevent overdose, and plasma bicarbonate concentrations should be monitored every 4-6 hr. Additional doses of bicarbonate based on the above formula are frequently necessary. Monitoring urine pH may also be helpful with a goal of maintaining the urine pH between 7.0 and 7.5.

In dogs and cats with azotemia or in oliguric acute renal failure, inhibition of alcohol dehydrogenase is of little benefit because almost all of the EG has already been metabolized. The prognosis for these animals is guarded to poor. Treatment should include correction of fluid, electrolyte, and acid-base disorders and, if possible, establishment of diuresis.

FLUORIDE POISONING

Fluorides are widely distributed in the environment and originate naturally from rocks and soil or from industrial processes. Water supplies for human consumption have been adjusted to contain 1 ppm to prevent dental caries. Fluorine at 1-2 mg/kg in animal rations is considered adequate. The maximal tolerable level varies by species, e.g., 40-50 ppm for cattle and horses, and 200 mg/kg for chickens.

Etiology

Toxic quantities of fluorides occur naturally, e.g., certain rock phosphates and the superphosphates produced from them, partially defluorinated phosphates, and the phosphatic limestones. In certain areas, drinking water from deep wells may contain high levels of fluorides. Volcanic ash may be high in fluoride. Wastes from industrial processes, fertilizers, and mineral supplements are the most common causes of chronic fluorosis. The fluorine-containing gases and dusts from manufacturing of fertilizers, mineral supplements, metal ores (steel and aluminum), and certain enamelling processes may contaminate forage crops.

Contamination of the surrounding area, particularly in the direction of the prevailing wind, may extend 5-6 miles. Forage crops grown on high-fluorine soils have increased levels due to mechanical contamination with soil particles. Feed-grade phosphates must contain no more than 1 part of fluorine to 100 parts phosphorus. A 100-g tube of fluoride toothpaste may contain 75-500 mg of sodium fluoride, depending on the brand.

There is a general correlation between solubility of a fluoride and its toxicity. Of the common fluorides, sodium fluoride is the most toxic, and calcium fluoride the least toxic. The fluorides of rock phosphates and most cryolites are of intermediate toxicity. Soluble fluorides originating from industrial fumes or dusts are more toxic than fluoride in rock phosphate.

Fluoride binds to Ca^{2+}, Mg^{2+}, and Mn^{2+}, acting as a direct cellular poison (including bacterial cells, hence its use in dental hygiene). At high levels most fluorides are corrosive to tissue. In bone, fluoride binds calcium and replaces the hydroxyl groups in the mineral part of bone, which is mostly hydroxyapatite. In teeth developed during fluoride ingestion, the enamel is less soluble (protective) and more dense (brittle, if excessive). In addition, faulty mineralization of teeth and bones occurs when excessive fluoride interferes with intracellular calcium metabolism and damages ameloblasts and odontoblasts.

Clinical Findings

Acute poisoning from inhalation of fluorine-containing gases or from ingestion of rodenticides or ascaricides containing fluoride is rare. Oral cleaning products present a danger to pets, especially dogs. The fatal dose of sodium fluoride is 5-10 mg/kg and toxic effects occur below 1 mg/kg. Fluoride (75-90% absorbed by 90 min) lowers serum calcium and magnesium. Clinically, gastroenteritis and cardiac (ventricular tachycardia and ECG abnormalities) and nervous signs may be followed within a few hours by collapse and death.

The signs of fluorosis from chronic ingestion are the same regardless of the source of fluoride. Levels too low to produce skeletal signs can cause changes in the enamel of developing teeth, leading to chalkiness or mottling, staining, and rapid and irregular wear. When exposure occurs after dental development, the teeth remain normal even if severe skeletal fluorosis develops. Clinical signs, apart from mild tooth lesions, occur in many animals when bone fluoride reaches 4, 000 ppm.

Skeletal fluorosis results in accelerated bone resorption and remodeling with production of exostoses and sclerosis. Metabolically active bones (ribs, mandible, and long bones) and growing bones in the young are most affected. Affected animals are lame, and feed and water intake and weight gain are decreased. Severely diseased cattle may move around on their knees due to spurring and bridging of the joints in the late stages. When the skeleton becomes saturated (30-40 times normal bone content), "flooding" of the soft tissue occurs, which causes a rise in plasma fluorides and metabolic breakdown evidenced by a loss of appetite and listlessness.

Lesions

Acute ingestion of high levels of fluoride causes inflammation of the gut and degenerative changes in the lungs, liver, and kidneys. In chronic cases, mottling, staining, and excessive wearing occur in teeth that develop during the time of excessive fluoride ingestion. A more advanced stage of fluorosis is marked by skeletal abnormalities; the bones become chalky white, soft, thickened, and in the extreme, develop exostoses that may be palpated, especially along the long bones and on the mandible in animals exposed at any age.

Diagnosis

Urine fluoride levels are time dependent due to rapid elimination. In cases of known ingestion, serum calcium and magnesium levels are beneficial. Casual observation of affected animals may suggest chronic debilitating arthritis; osteoporosis; or deficiency of calcium, phosphorus, or vitamin D. Lameness in advanced cases may be wrongly attributed to an accident. Nonspecific staining seen in cattle teeth may be confused with incipient fluorosis. A developing fluoride toxicosis can be recognized by the following criteria (from most to least reliable):

1) chemical analyses to determine the amount of fluorine in the diet, urine, bones, and teeth;
2) tooth effects, in animals exposed at time of permanent teeth development;
3) lameness, as the result of fluoride accumulation in bone; and
4) systemic evidence as reflected by anorexia, inanition, and cachexia.

The normal levels of fluorine in livestock are considered to be <0.2 ppm in plasma, 1-8 in urine, 200-600 in bones, and 200-500 in teeth. Normal bovine urine contains <5 ppm fluorine; in borderline toxicity, urine contains 20-30 ppm, and in cattle with systemic signs, >35 ppm. In pigs, bones appear normal with 3,000-4,000 ppm fluorine, and levels of <4,500 ppm in compact bones from cattle are considered innocuous. In cattle, toxicosis is associated with levels of >5,500 ppm in compact bone and >7,000 ppm in cancellous bone; in sheep, levels are believed to be lower (2,000-3,000 ppm in compact bone and 4,000-6,000 ppm in cancellous bone).

Treatment and Control

Acutely exposed animals require calcium gluconate (IV) and oral magnesium hydroxide or milk to bind fluoride before absorption. In chronic exposure, control is difficult unless animals are removed from affected areas. It has been suggested that affected areas may be used for animals with a relatively short production life, e.g., pigs, poultry, or finishing cattle and sheep. Feeding calcium carbonate, aluminum oxide, aluminum sulfate, magnesium metasilicate, or boron has either decreased absorption or increased excretion of fluoride, and thus could offer some control of chronic fluorosis under some conditions. However, no treatment has been shown to cure the chronic effects of fluorine toxicity.

METALDEHYDE POISONING

Metaldehyde is the active ingredient in molluscicides used especially during the wet season for slug and snail control in domestic gardens. In certain locations, it is also used for rat control. Metaldehyde comes as a liquid or bait (3. 5%) combined with bran, either as flakes or pellets, and is palatable to pets and farm animals. Some products also contain arsenic or a cholinesterase-inhibiting insecticide, which is usually less toxic at the dosage used than the metaldehyde. All species are susceptible to metaldehyde poisoning (lethal dose 100-300 mg/kg); dogs are the species most frequently poisoned (3 oz of bait is toxic to a 30-lb dog). When ingested, a portion of the metaldehyde is partially hydrolyzed in stomach acid to acetaldehyde and absorbed, while the remaining metaldehyde is well absorbed from the intestines. The great variability in onset of clinical signs of metaldehyde poisoning appears to be dependent on gastric contents and the rate of stomach emptying. Metaldehyde and acetaldehyde contribute to a decrease in brain serotonin, and noradrenaline, which is proportional to the increase in muscle activity and CNS excitatory signs.

Clinical signs of toxicosis are similar in all mammals. Nervous signs are prominent. Initial signs may include severe muscle tremors, ataxia, hyperesthesia, tachycardia, hyperthermia, and hyperpnea, followed by nystagmus, opisthotonos, and continuous tonic convulsions. Nystagmus is most severe in cats. Nervous signs are more continuous and less exaggerated by stimulation than in strychnine poisoning, which may appear clinically similar. Emesis, diarrhea, hypersalivation, and dyspnea, in all species, and profuse sweating in horses, are also seen.

Severe acidosis develops due to acid metabolites and high muscle activity in all species. Cholinergic signs (especially pupillary constriction) and a drop in blood cholinesterase may occur if the product contains a carbamate or organophosphate. In high-level exposure, death (4-24 hr) is from respiratory failure, while survivors may develop liver failure (3-4 days). Necropsy lesions are nonspecific and include congestion and edema of the liver, kidneys, and lungs, and intestinal hemorrhage. A mild formaldehyde-like odor may be present on opening the stomach or rumen. Stomach content, rapidly frozen, is the preferred sample for analysis due to the low levels and rapid loss of acetaldehyde from tissue (liver and urine).

An emetic (e.g., apomorphine) in acute exposure may not be necessary because metaldehyde is a gastric irritant. However, gastric lavage with sodium bicarbonate is recommended. Diazepam (2-5 mg/kg, IV) to effect is preferred to reduce excitement and convulsions; acepromazine has been used successfully. Barbiturates (which compete with acetaldehyde degradation) are indicated only if the animal does not respond, and gas anesthesia is suggested to maintain severely affected animals. Horses benefit from xylazine plus acepromazine. In large animals, activated carbon (1-3 g/kg, repeated every 4-8 hr at half the original dose if necessary) reduces further absorption (metaldehyde is fat soluble). Aggressive fluid therapy with sodium lactate to reduce acidosis is essential, and dextrose or calcium borogluconate is used to prevent possible liver damage. Muscle relaxants, e.g., methocarbamol, assist in reducing muscle activity and pain. Cold water rinses are recommended when fever is severe. Prognosis is good if hyperthermia and seizures are not severe and prolonged, but longterm aggressive therapy is required (=4 days).

NITRATE AND NITRITE POISONING

Many species are susceptible to nitrate and nitrite poisoning, but cattle are affected most frequently. Ruminants are especially vulnerable because the ruminal flora reduces nitrate to ammonia, with nitrite (~10 times more toxic than nitrate) as an intermediate product. Nitrate reduction (and nitrite production) occurs in the cecum of equids but not to the same extent as in ruminants. Young pigs also have GI microflora capable of reducing nitrate to nitrite, but mature monogastric animals (except equids) are more resistant to nitrate toxicosis because this pathway is age-limited.

Acute intoxication is manifested primarily by methemoglobin formation (nitrite ion in contact with RBC oxidizes ferrous iron in Hgb to the ferric state, forming stable methemoglobin incapable of oxygen transport) and resultant anoxia. Secondary effects due to vasodilatory action of the nitrite ion on vascular smooth muscle may occur. The nitrite ion may also alter metabolic protein enzymes. Ingested nitrates may directly irritate the GI mucosa and produce abdominal pain and diarrhea.

Although usually acute, the effects of nitrite or nitrate toxicity may be subacute or chronic and are reported to include retarded growth, lowered milk production, vitamin A deficiency, minor transitory goitrogenic effects, abortions and fetotoxicity, and increased susceptibility to infection. Chronic nitrate toxicosis remains a controversial issue and is not as yet well characterized, but most current evidence does not support allegations of lowered milk production in dairy cows due to excessive dietary nitrate exposure alone.

Etiology

Nitrates and nitrites are used in pickling and curing brines for preserving meats, certain machine oils and antirust tablets, gunpowder and explosives, and fertilizers. They may also serve as therapeutic agents for certain noninfectious diseases, e.g., cyanide poisoning. Toxicoses occur in unacclimated domestic animals most commonly from ingestion of plants that contain excess nitrate, especially by hungry animals engorging themselves and taking in an enormous body burden of nitrate. Nitrate toxicosis can also result from accidental ingestion of fertilizer or other chemicals. Nitrate concentrations may be hazardous in ponds that receive extensive feedlot or fertilizer runoff; these types of nitrate sources may also contaminate shallow, poorly cased wells. Although nitrate concentrations are increasing in groundwater in the USA, well water is rarely the sole cause of excess nitrate exposure.

Water with both high nitrate content and significant coliform contamination has greater potential to affect health adversely and lower productivity than do either nitrate or bacteria alone. Livestock losses have occurred during cold weather due to the concentrating effect of freezing, which increases nitrate content of remaining water in stock tanks.

Crops that readily concentrate nitrate include cereal grasses (especially oats, millet, and rye), corn (maize), sunflower, and sorghums. Weeds that commonly have high nitrate concentrations are pigweed, lamb's quarter, thistle, Jimson weed, fireweed (Kochia), smartweed, dock, and Johnson grass. Anhydrous ammonia and nitrate fertilizers and soils naturally high in nitrogen tend to increase nitrate content in forage.

Excess nitrate in plants is generally associated with damp weather conditions and cool temperatures (55°F [13°C]), although high concentrations are also likely to develop when growth is rapid during hot, humid weather. Drought conditions, particularly if occurring when plants are immature, may leave the vegetation with high nitrate content. Decreased light, cloudy weather, and shading associated with crowding conditions can also cause increased concentrations of nitrates within plants. Well-aerated soil with a low pH, and low or deficient amounts of molybdenum, sulfur, or phosphorus in soil tend to enhance nitrate uptake, whereas soil deficiencies of copper, cobalt, or manganese tend to have opposing effects. Anything that stunts growth increases nitrate accumulation in the lower part of the plant. Phenoxy acid derivative herbicides, e.g., 2, 4-D and 2, 4, 5-T, applied to nitrate-accumulating plants during early stages, cause increased growth and a high nitrate residual (10-30%) in surviving plants, which are lush and eaten with apparent relish even though previously avoided.

Nitrate, which does not selectively accumulate in fruits or grain, is found chiefly in the lower stalk with lesser amounts in the upper stalk and leaves. Nitrate in plants can be converted to nitrite under the proper conditions of moisture, heat, and microbial activity after harvesting.

Clinical Findings

Signs of nitrite poisoning usually appear suddenly due to tissue hypoxia and low blood pressure as a consequence of vasodilation. Rapid, weak heartbeat with subnormal body temperature, muscular tremors, weakness, and ataxia are early signs of toxicosis when methemo-globinemia reaches 30-40%. Brown, cyanotic mucous membranes develop rapidly as methemoglobinemia exceeds 50%.

Dyspnea, tachypnea, anxiety, and frequent urination are common. Some monogastric animals, usually because of excess nitrate exposure from nonplant sources, exhibit salivation, vomiting, diarrhea, abdominal pain, and gastric hemorrhage. Affected animals may die suddenly without appearing ill, in terminal anoxic convulsions within 1 hr, or after a clinical course of 12-24 hr or longer. Acute lethal toxicoses almost always are due to development of ^{3}80% methemoglobinemia. Under certain conditions, adverse effects may not be apparent until animals have been eating nitrate-containing forages for days to weeks.

Some animals that develop marked dyspnea recover but then develop interstitial pulmonary emphysema and continue to suffer respiratory distress; most of these recover fully within 10-14 days. Abortion and stillbirths may be seen in some cattle 5-14 days after excessive nitrate/nitrite exposure, but likely only in cows that have survived a ^{3}50% methemo-globinemia for 6-12 hr or longer. Prolonged exposure to excess nitrate coupled with cold stress and inadequate nutrition may lead to the alert downer cow syndrome in pregnant beef cattle; sudden collapse and death can result.

Lesions

Blood that contains methemoglobin usually has a chocolate-brown color, although dark red hues may also be seen. There may be pinpoint or larger hemorrhages on serosal surfaces. Dark brown discoloration evident in moribund or recently dead animals is not pathognomonic, however, and other methemoglobin inducers must be considered. If necropsy is postponed too long, the brown discoloration may disappear with conversion of methemoglobin back to Hgb.

Diagnosis

Excess nitrate exposure can be assessed by laboratory analysis for nitrate in both pre- and postmortem specimens. High nitrate and nitrite values in postmortem specimens may be an incidental finding, indicative only of exposure and not toxicity. Plasma is the preferred premortem specimen, because some plasma-protein-bound nitrate could be lost in the clot if serum was collected. Nitrite present in whole blood also continues to react with Hgb in vitro, so these specimens must be centrifuged immediately and plasma separated to prevent erroneous values of both.

Additional postmortem specimens from either toxicoses or abortions include ocular fluids, fetal pleural or thoracic fluids, fetal stomach contents, and maternal uterine fluid. All specimens should be frozen in clean plastic or glass containers before submission, except when whole blood is collected for methemoglobin analysis. Because the amount of nitrate in rumen contents is not representative of concentrations in the diet, evaluation of rumen contents is not indicated.

Bacterial contamination of postmortem specimens, especially ocular fluid, is likely to cause conversion of nitrate to nitrite at room temperature or higher; such specimens may have abnormally high nitrite concentrations with reduced to absent nitrate concentrations. Endogenous biosynthesis of nitrate and nitrite by macrophages stimulated by lipopolysaccharide or other bacterial products may also complicate interpretation of analytical findings; this should be considered as a possible maternal or fetal response to an infectious process.

Methemoglobin analysis alone is not a reliable indicator of excess nitrate or nitrite exposure except in acute toxicosis, because 50% of methemoglobin present will be converted back to Hgb in ~2 hr, and alternate forms of nonoxygenated Hgb that may be formed by reaction with nitrite are not detected by methemoglobin analysis. Nitrate and nitrite concentrations >20 μg NO_3 /mL and >0.5 μg NO_2 /mL, respectively, in maternal and perinatal serum, plasma, ocular fluid, and other similar biologic fluids are usually indicative of excessive nitrate or nitrite exposure in most domestic animal species; nitrate concentrations of up to 40 μg NO_3/mL have been present in the plasma of healthy calves at birth, but are reduced rapidly as normal neonatal renal function eliminates nitrate in the urine.

Normally expected nitrate and nitrite concentrations in similar diagnostic specimens are usually <10 μg NO_3/mL and <0.2 μg NO_2/mL, respectively. Nitrate and nitrite concentrations >10 but <20 μg NO_3/mL and >0.2 but <0.5 μg NO_2/mL, respectively, are suspect and indicate nitrate or nitrite exposure of unknown duration, extent, or origin. The possible contribution of endogenous nitrate or nitrite synthesis by activated macrophages must also be considered. The biologic half-life of nitrate in beef cattle, sheep, and ponies was determined to be 7.7, 4.2, and 4.8 hr, respectively, so it will be at least 5 biologic half-lives (24-36 hr) before elevated nitrate concentrations from excessive nitrate exposure diminish to normally expected values, allowing additional time for valid premortem specimen collection.

A latent period may exist between excessive maternal dietary nitrate exposure and equilibrium in perinatal ocular fluids. Aqueous humor is actively secreted into the anterior chamber at a rate of ~0. 1/mL/hr, and nitrate and nitrite are thought to enter the globe of the eye by this mechanism. Equilibrium between aqueous and vitreous humor is by passive diffusion rather than by active secretion, so nitrate or nitrite may be present in comparatively lesser concentrations in vitreous humor after acute exposure.

Field tests for nitrate are presumptive and should be confirmed by standard analytical methods at a qualified laboratory. The diphenylamine blue test (1% in concentrated sulfuric acid) is more suitable to determine the presence or absence of nitrate in suspected forages. Nitrate test strips (dipsticks) are effective in determining nitrate values in water supplies and can be used to evaluate nitrate and nitrite content in serum, plasma, ocular fluid, and urine.

Differential diagnoses include poisonings by cyanide, urea, pesticides, toxic gases (e.g., carbon monoxide, hydrogen sulfide), chlorates, aniline dyes, aminophenols, or drugs (e.g., sulfonamides, phenacetin, and acetaminophen), as well as infectious or noninfectious diseases (e.g., grain overload, hypocalcemia, hypomagnesemia, pulmonary adenomatosis, or emphysema) and any sudden unexplained deaths.

Treatment

Slow IV injection of 1% methylene blue in distilled water or isotonic saline should be given at 4-22 mg/kg body wt, or more, depending on severity of exposure. Lower dosages may be repeated in 20-30 min if the initial response is not satisfactory. Lower dosages of methylene blue can be used in all species, but only ruminants can safely tolerate higher dosages. If additional exposure or absorption occurs during therapy, retreating with methylene blue every 6-8 hr should be considered. Rumen lavage with cold water and antibiotics may stop the continuing microbial production of nitrite.

Control

Animals may adapt to higher nitrate content in feeds, especially when grazing summer annuals such as sorghum-Sudan hybrids. Multiple, small feedings help animals adapt. Trace mineral supplements and a balanced diet may help prevent nutritional or metabolic disorders associated with longterm excess dietary nitrate consumption. Feeding grain with high-nitrate forages may reduce nitrite production. Forage nitrate concentrations >1% nitrate dry-weight basis (10, 000 ppm NO_3) may cause acute toxicoses in unacclimated animals, and forage nitrate concentrations £5, 000 ppm NO_3 (dry-weight basis) are recommended for pregnant beef cows. However, even forage concentrations of 1, 000 ppm NO_3 dry-weight basis have been lethal to hungry cows engorging themselves in a single feeding within an hour, so the total dose of nitrate ingested is a deciding factor.

High-nitrate forages may also be harvested and stored as ensilage rather than dried hay or green chop; this may reduce the nitrate content in forages by up to 50%. Raising cutter heads of machinery during harvesting operations selectively leaves the more hazardous stalk bases in the field.

Hay appears to be more hazardous than fresh green chop or pasture with similar nitrate content. Heating may assist bacterial conversion of nitrate to nitrite; feeding high-nitrate hay, straw, or fodder that has been damp or wet for several days, or stockpiled, green-chopped forage should be avoided. Large round bales with excess nitrate are especially dangerous if stored uncovered outside; rain or snow can leach and subsequently concentrate most of the total nitrate present into the lower third of these bales. Water transported in improperly cleaned liquid fertilizer tanks may be extremely high in nitrate. Young unweaned livestock, especially neonatal pigs, can be more sensitive to nitrate in water.

NONPROTEIN NITROGEN POISONING

Poisoning by ingestion of excess urea or other sources of nonprotein nitrogen (NPN) is usually acute, rapidly progressive, and highly fatal. Sources of NPN have different toxicities in various species, but mature ruminants are affected most commonly. After ingestion, NPN undergoes hydrolysis and releases excess ammonia (NH_3) into the GI tract, which is absorbed and leads to hyperammonemia.

Etiology

The most common sources of NPN in feeds are urea, urea phosphate, ammonia (anhydrous), and salts such as monoammonium and diammonium phosphate. Because feed-grade urea is unstable, it is formulated (usually pelleted) to prevent degradation to NH_3. Biuret, a less toxic source of NPN, is used less frequently than in the past. Natural protein sources such as rice hulls, cottonseed meal, and straw or other low-quality forages may be treated with anhydrous ammonia to increase available nitrogen in supplemented livestock diets. Most sources of NPN are provided to ruminants by direct addition of dry supplement to a complete mixed or blended diet, by free-choice access to NPN-containing range blocks or cubes, or by lick tank systems combined with molasses as a supplement. Ammonia or NPN poisoning is a common sequela of abrupt change to urea or other NPN in the diet when only natural protein was previously fed; animals have to be gradually acclimated to NPN so that rumen microflora can increase in numbers to use the NH_3 produced. Also, farm animals sometimes drink liquid fertilizers or ingest dry granular fertilizers that contain ammonium salts or urea.

Ruminants are most sensitive because urease is normally present in the functional rumen after 50 days of age. Dietary exposure of unacclimated ruminants to 0.3-0.5 g of urea/kg body wt may cause adverse effects; doses of 1-1.5 g/kg are usually lethal. Urease activity in the equine cecum is ~25% that of the rumen, and horses may receive NPN as a feed additive; however, horses are more sensitive to urea than other monogastrics, and doses =4 g/kg can be lethal. Ammonium salts at 0.3-0.5 g/kg may be toxic in all species and ages of farm animals; doses =1.5 g/kg usually are fatal. Pigs and neonatal calves are generally unaffected by ingestion of urea except for a transient diuresis.

Livestock may require days or weeks for total adaptation before rumen microflora can utilize the gradually increasing amounts of urea or other NPN in the diets; however, adaptation is lost relatively quickly (1-3 days) once NPN is removed from the diet.

Diets low in energy and high in fiber are more commonly associated with NPN toxicosis, even in acclimated animals. Highly palatable supplements (such as liquid molasses or large protein blocks crumbled by precipitation) or improperly maintained lick tanks may lead to consumption of lethal amounts of NPN.

A related CNS disorder in cattle fed ammoniated high-quality hay, silage, molasses, and protein blocks is thought to be caused by the formation of 4-methylimidazole (4-MI) through the action of NH_3 on soluble carbohydrates (reducing sugars) in these feedstuffs. Cattle fed dietary components containing 4-MI develop a syndrome known as the "bovine bonkers syndrome, " named for the wildly aberrant behavior exhibited. Signs relate to CNS effects, with stampeding, ear twitching, trembling, champing, salivating, and convulsions. Because nursing calves are affected, the toxic principle apparently is excreted in milk. Ammoniated low-quality forages do not have sufficient concentrations of reducing sugars to form 4-MI, and thus serve as a relatively safe nitrogen source to acclimated animals.

A related disorder involves accidental excessive exposure of ruminants (cattle and sheep) to raw soybeans. Soybeans have high concentrations of both carbohydrates and proteins, as well as urease. Overconsumption can cause acute carbohydrate fermentation and excessive ammonia release, resulting in ammonia toxicosis and lactic acidosis. Affected animals have engorged rumens with a gray, lava-like, amorphous mass inside.

Clinical Findings

The period from urea ingestion to onset of clinical signs is 20-60 min in cattle, 30-90 min in sheep, and longer in horses. Early signs include muscle tremors (especially of face and ears), exophthalmia, abdominal pain, frothy salivation, polyuria, and bruxism. Tremors progress to incoordination and weakness. Pulmonary edema leads to marked salivation, dyspnea, and gasping.

Horses may exhibit head pressing; cattle are often agitated, hyperirritable, violent, and belligerent as toxicosis progresses; sheep usually appear depressed. An early sign in cattle is ruminal atony; as toxicosis progresses, ruminal tympany is usually evident, and violent struggling and bellowing, a marked jugular pulse, severe twitching, tetanic spasms, and convulsions may be seen. Affected cattle with violent or belligerent aberrant behavior may have produced some 4-MI in vivo through reaction of excessive NH_3, released from NPN, with carbohydrates and reducing sugars in the rumen. The PCV and serum concentrations of NH_3, glucose, lactate, potassium, phosphorus, AST, ALT, and BUN usually are significantly increased.

As death nears, animals become cyanotic, dyspneic, anuric, and hyperthermic, and blood pH decreases from 7.4 to 7.0. Regurgitation may occur, especially in sheep. Death related to excess NPN usually occurs within 2 hr in cattle, 4 hr in sheep, and 3-12 hr in horses. Survivors recover in 12-24 hr with no sequelae.

Lesions

Carcasses of animals dying of NPN poisoning appear to bloat and decompose rapidly, with no specific characteristic lesions. Frequently, pulmonary edema, congestion, and petechial hemorrhages may be seen. Mild bronchitis and catarrhal gastroenteritis are often reported. Regurgitated and inhaled rumen contents are commonly found in the trachea and bronchi, especially in sheep. The odor of NH_3 may or may not be apparent in ingesta from a freshly opened rumen or cecum. A ruminal or cecal pH =7.5 from a recently dead animal is highly suggestive of NPN poisoning. The ruminal pH remains stable for several hours after death under most circumstances but continues to rise in NPN toxicosis.

Diagnosis

Ammonia or NPN poisoning is suggested by signs, lesions, history of acute illness, and dietary exposure. Exposure to excess NPN may be evaluated through laboratory analysis for the ammonia nitrogen (NH_3-N) in both antemortem and postmortem specimens and for urea or other NPN in suspected feeds and other dietary sources. Specimens for NH_3-N analysis include ruminal-reticular fluid, serum, whole blood, and urine. All specimens should be frozen immediately after collection and thawed only for analysis; alternatively, ruminal-reticular fluid may be preserved with a few drops of saturated mercuric chloride solution added to each 100 mL of specimen.

Animals dead more than a few hours in hot ambient temperatures or 12 hr in moderate climates probably have undergone too much autolysis to be of diagnostic value. The amount of urea or the equivalent NPN in biologic specimens is meaningless; however, urea and NPN should be determined in representative feeds and other dietary sources. Values for urea and NPN in feed permit calculation of the protein equivalent (1 part protein = 0.34 parts urea; 1 part urea = 2.92 parts protein) in feed as well as the total estimated dose of NPN ingested.

Concentrations of =2 mg/100 mL NH_3-N in blood or serum indicate excess NPN exposure. The concentration of NH_3-N in ruminal-reticular fluid is >80 mg/100 mL in most cases of NPN poisoning and may be >200 mg/100 mL. Acclimated ruminants fed diets high in legume hay, soybean meal, cottonseed meal, linseed meal, fish meal, or milk byproducts may have NH_3-N concentrations in rumen fluid approaching 60 mg/100 mL with no apparent toxicity. The pH of ruminal-reticular fluid should also be determined; a pH of 7.5-8 (at time of death) is indicative of NPN toxicity.

Differential diagnoses include poisonings by nitrate/nitrite, cyanide, organophosphate/carbamate pesticides, raw soybean overload, 4-methylimidazole, lead, chlorinated hydrocarbon pesticides, and toxic gases (carbon monoxide, hydrogen sulfide, nitrogen dioxide); acute infectious diseases; and noninfectious diseases such as encephalopathies (e.g., leukoencephalomalacia, hepatic encephalopathy, polioencephalomalacia), enterotoxemia or rumen autointoxication, protein engorgement, grain engorgement, ruminal tympany, and pulmonary adenomatosis. Nutritional and metabolic disorders related to hypocalcemia, hypomagnesemia, and other elemental aberrations should also be considered.

Treatment

Examination and treatment may be difficult because of violent behavior. Animals that are recumbent and moribund usually do not respond favorably to treatment. If possible, affected animals should be treated by ruminal infusion of 5% acetic acid (0.5-2 L in sheep and goats and 2-8 L in cattle). Ruminal-reticular fluid specimens for analysis should be taken before acetic acid therapy. Concomitant infusion of iced (0-4°C) water (up to 40 L in adult cattle, proportionally less in sheep and goats) is also recommended.

Acetic acid lowers rumen pH and prevents further absorption of NH_3; administration may have to be repeated if affected animals again show clinical signs. Acetic acid also inactivates existing NH_3 in the GI tract and rapidly forms ammonium acetate, which can be used by rumen microflora but does not release NH_3. Cold water lowers the rumen temperature and dilutes the reacting media, which slows urease activity. In valuable animals, removed rumen contents should be replaced with a hay slurry, and a transfer of some rumen contents from a healthy animal may serve as an inoculum to restore normal function. Ruminal tympany should be corrected if indicated, and a trocar may be installed to prevent recurrence.

Prevention and Control

Urea should not be fed at a rate exceeding 2-3% of the concentrate or grain portion of ruminant diets and should be limited to =1% of the total diet. Additionally, NPN should constitute no more than one-third of the total nitrogen in the ruminant diet. Once the decision is made to feed NPN, animals must be slowly adapted to, and maintained on, a consistent dietary NPN content with no significant deviation. Temporary absences of NPN from the diet should be avoided at all costs. While properly adapted adult cattle can tolerate up to 1 g urea/kg body wt/day, a safer feeding rate is no more than half that amount.

PENTACHLOROPHENOL POISONING

Penta has been used as a fungicide, molluscicide, insecticide, and as a wood preservative, but registration for its use in lumber in the USA was canceled in 1986. Gradually, other registrations for this agent have been canceled and it is now only registered for industrial purposes; agricultural and domestic uses are prohibited. It is rated by the World Health Organization as highly hazardous.

It can be absorbed through intact skin and lungs and is an intense irritant to the skin and mucous membranes. When absorbed, it increases metabolism by uncoupling cellular phosphorylation. Animals fed in troughs made of lumber treated with penta may salivate and have irritated oral mucosa. Vaporization or leaching of penta in pens, enclosures, homes, and barns has caused illness and death. Signs of poisoning include nervousness, rapid pulse and respiratory rate, weakness, muscle tremors, fever, and convulsions, followed by death. Chronic poisoning results in fatty liver, nephrosis, and weight loss. Additional problems reported when penta-contaminated shavings are used as bedding include "off flavors" in broilers, impaired immune response in chickens, and possibly decreased fertility in boars.

Commercial lots of technical-grade penta contain small but biologically significant amounts of highly toxic impurities (dioxins and furans), and material available today is manufactured so that these toxic ingredients are kept at as low a concentration as possible. Penta can cause residues in animal tissues. Also, a significant amount of hexachlorobenzene is metabolized in animal tissues to penta. Pentachlorophenol is considered to be a carcinogen and a tumor promoter, although studies have shown that the pure material does not increase the incidence of tumors in rats and mice; the technical-grade material has also been shown to be immunotoxic in laboratory studies. Penta must be handled very carefully and kept away from animal contact.

Whole blood analysis for penta may aid in the diagnosis of poisoning; diagnosis is usually made on the basis of the signs and the proximity of treated lumber in the animal's environment.

Acute toxic doses of penta range from 27-350 mg/kg and the fetotoxic NOEL is 10 mg/kg in rats.

There is no known antidote. Termination of exposure, bathing dermally exposed animals, oral administration of activated charcoal, and supportive therapy may be indicated. Bathing should be done gently with cold water and detergent so as not to cause vasodilation and increased absorption. Cattle, pigs, and chickens exposed to wood treated with commercial grade penta that contained these contaminants had increased mortality, decreased productivity, and other less specific herd health problems. Antipyretics, e.g., aspirin and acetaminophen, should not be used. Treatment involves cooling the animal and removing it from the source of poison and administering fluids, electrolytes, and anticonvulsants.

PETROLEUM PRODUCT POISONING

Ingestion or inhalation of—or skin contact with—petroleum, petroleum condensate, gasoline, diesel fuel, kerosene, crude oil, or other hydrocarbon mixtures may cause illness and occasionally death in domestic and wild animals. Both dogs and cats may ingest petroleum products during grooming if their fur becomes contaminated. Dogs may ingest these products directly when they are left in open containers. Inhalation may occur when animals are confined in poorly ventilated areas where these chemicals have been used or stored. Cattle, and less frequently sheep or goats, may ingest such products because they are curious or seeking salt or other nutrients, water is not available, or food or water is contaminated. A cow may consume several gallons at one time.

Petroleum fractions have been used as insecticides and acaricides for many years, either alone or as part of formulations. Small quantities of these may be applied to the skin with few or no harmful effects, but large quantities and prolonged exposure can induce severe reactions. Pipeline breaks, accidental release from storage tanks, and tank car accidents may contaminate land and water supplies. Animals may have access to open or leaky containers of fuel or other hydrocarbon materials. The lower the molecular weight and the higher the degree of unsaturation or aromaticity, the greater the volatility. More volatile hydrocarbons are more lipid soluble and therefore more readily absorbed by inhalation or ingestion. Crude petroleum that has lost much of its lighter, more volatile components through weathering may still be hazardous.

Crude oil and gasoline contain varying amounts of aromatic hydrocarbons including benzene, toluene, ethyl-benzene, and xylene. For example, gasoline in the USA typically contains up to 2% benzene. Gasoline in some other countries may contain up to 5% benzene. These compounds, if ingested or inhaled in sufficient amounts, can have acute and chronic effects different from the other hydrocarbons that make up the majority of oil and gas products. Benzene, for example, is a known carcinogen at high levels of exposure and has a variety of hemotoxic properties. Toluene can cause profound neurologic signs and damage at sufficient doses.

Variation in composition of petroleum and petroleum-derived hydrocarbon mixtures explains some of the differences in toxic effects. Mixtures of low viscosity (e.g., gasoline, naphtha, kerosene) have a high aspiration hazard and irritant activity on pulmonary tissues. Gasoline and naphtha fractions may induce vomiting, which contributes to aspiration hazard. Fractions more viscous than kerosene are less likely to be inhaled and, even if aspirated, are somewhat less damaging to lung tissue. Older formulations of lubricating oils and greases can be particularly hazardous because of toxic additives or contaminants (e.g., lead).

Clinical Findings

Petroleum hydrocarbon toxicity may involve the respiratory, GI, or integumentary systems or the CNS. In most cases of ingestion, no clinical signs are observed. Pneumonia due to aspiration of hydrocarbons into the lungs is usually the most serious consequence of ingestion of these materials. Aspiration can occur during vomition or eructation of rumen contents. Acute bloat is not a consistent finding but has been reported to cause death very shortly after consumption of highly volatile hydrocarbons such as gasoline or naphtha.

CNS effects are usually associated with aspiration. CNS signs may be a result of the anesthetic-like action of low-molecular-weight aliphatic hydrocarbons and/or cerebral anoxia that can result from lung damage or displacement of oxygen by the more volatile hydrocarbons. Some compounds when absorbed in high doses may sensitize the myocardium to endogenous catecholamines. Anorexia, decreased rumen motility, and mild depression may begin in ~24 hr and last 3-14 days depending on dose and content. Hypoglycemia may be seen several days after ingestion. These signs and weight loss may be the only responses seen in animals that do not bloat or aspirate oil. Some animals fail to reestablish normal rumen function after ingestion and can develop a chronic wasting condition.

After ingestion of oil, the feces may not be affected until several days later, at which time they become dry and formed in the case of kerosene or lighter hydrocarbon fractions; in contrast, heavier hydrocarbon mixtures tend to be cathartic. Oil may be found in feces and rumen contents up to 2 wk following ingestion. Regurgitated or vomited oil may be seen on the muzzle and lips. Signs attributable to pulmonary adsorption of hydrocarbons or cerebral anoxia include excitability (associated with aromatic fractions—benzene, toluene, etc), depression (aliphatic or saturated low-molecular-weight hydrocarbons), shivering, head tremors, visual dysfunction (sometimes associated with lead contamination), and incoordination.

Acute pneumonia and possibly pleuritis (coughing, tachypnea, shallow respiration, reluctance to move, head held low, weakness, oily nasal discharge, dehydrated appearance) are seen in some animals that aspirate highly volatile mixtures; death usually are seen within days. Respiratory signs may be limited to dyspnea shortly before death in animals that aspirate heavier hydrocarbons. Increased PCV, Hgb, and BUN, indicating mild to moderate hemoconcentration, are associated with development of pneumonia. Neutropenia, lymphopenia, and eosinopenia occur initially and are followed by a relative increase in neutrophils.

Lesions

Aspiration pneumonia is the most consistent postmortem finding in animals that did not die of bloat. This may be accompanied by tracheitis, pleuritis, and hydrothorax if highly volatile fractions such as gasoline or naphtha are involved. Lung lesions are usually bilateral and found in the caudoventral apical, cardiac, cranioventral diaphragmatic, and intermediate lobes. Affected portions are dark red and consolidated and may contain multiple abscesses. Encapsulated pulmonary abscesses may be found in cattle surviving up to several months after aspiration. Skin lesions may be obvious after repeated topical application or severe exposure and include drying, cracking, or blistering.

Diagnosis

A hydrocarbon odor may be detected in lungs, ruminal contents, and feces. Even if ingested in large doses, hydrocarbons may not be visible in ruminal contents after ~4 days. Adding warm water to the GI contents may cause any oily contents to collect at the surface, but finding oil in the GI tract does not in itself justify a diagnosis of poisoning; most oils have low toxicity if not aspirated. Samples of GI contents, lung, liver, kidney, and the suspected source should be collected for chemical analysis to demonstrate presence of hydrocarbons in tissue (particularly lung) and GI contents and to match those found in tissues and ingesta with the suspected source. Samples must be carefully protected from cross-contamination during necropsy and transportation to the laboratory.

Check with the diagnostic laboratory to ensure collection equipment and transport containers are appropriate to prevent evaporative loss of important components and contamination. Positive chemical findings together with appropriate clinical and pathologic findings are confirmatory. Diagnosis in oil-field situations has historically been complicated by involvement of other toxicants, e.g., explosives, lead from grease and "pipe dope," arsenicals, organophosphate esters, caustics (acids or alkalis), and saltwater.

Treatment

Bloat pressure should be released by passing a stomach tube if absolutely necessary to save the life of the animal; using a trocar risks forcing oil into the peritoneal cavity, which results in peritonitis. Passing a stomach tube dramatically increases the risk of aspiration and extreme caution is necessary. In the absence of bloat, the prime objectives are to prevent aspiration and to mitigate GI dysfunction.

Rumenotomy to remove ruminal contents and replace them with healthy ruminal material is safer. More chronic cases involving primarily hypofunction of the rumen may also respond to this procedure. Cathartics, if used, should be of the saline type; however, there is no evidence that they improve prognosis. Activated charcoal has occasionally been suggested for use in small animals. Although it does not effectively adsorb petroleum distillates, it may be given if necessary to adsorb additives and other contaminants. Care should be taken to avoid inducing vomiting and aspiration.

Animals with evidence of respiratory involvement may require broad-spectrum antibiotic treatment. Pathogens can be introduced into the lungs from aspirated rumen contents mixed with the hydrocarbons. The use of steroids in hydrocarbon aspiration may further reduce the chance for recovery. Treatment of aspiration pneumonia is rarely effective, and the prognosis is poor. However, because signs of aspiration may not appear for several days, prognosis based on initial clinical findings may be misleading.

Most high-molecular-weight compounds pass through the digestive tract unchanged. Most of the petroleum hydrocarbons are highly lipophilic and will be stored for varying times in tissues with high lipid content including fat, nervous tissue, and the liver. Some of the absorbed compounds are metabolized into more toxic byproducts (e.g., benzene, toluene, n-hexane). Although most of these compounds do not remain in the body for prolonged periods, little is known about exactly how long tissue levels persist in highly exposed animals. The potential for tissue residues must be considered prior to the slaughter of animals intended for human consumption.

In poisoning or damage due to cutaneous exposure, the material should be removed from the skin with the aid of soap or mild detergents and copious amounts of cool water. The skin should not be brushed or abraded. Further treatment depends on the clinical signs and is largely restricted to supportive therapy. Petroleum hydrocarbon poisoning can be avoided only by preventing access to these materials through proper storage of home and farm chemicals and well maintained fencing around high-risk petroleum facilities.

AIR POLLUTANTS

Animals may be exposed to a large number of toxic gases under various conditions. Such situations might involve leakage in storage areas, industrial accidents and air pollution resulting from industrialization. A newer source of toxic gases is the slurry tanks that are used to store animal wastes. The four major gases released are carbon dioxide, methane, ammonia and hydrogen sulfide. Other harmful gases that may be present in the environment include carbon dioxide, sulfur oxides and nitrogen oxides.

Dust Particles

Silicosis is an example of pneumoconioses. Dust containing silicon is produced during rock cutting, drilling, grinding, mining, abrasive manufacture, pottery making and processing of diatomaceous earth. It is possible that animals living in the vicinity of such industrial operation may get exposed to silica particles and develope pneumoconioses. However, the condition is more common in workers. Many substances containing silica are capable of causing silicosis. Particles less than 5 μ in diameter appear to be the most important in causing silicosis. Threshold limit for silica dust, including natural diatomaceous earth should not exceed 20 ppm per cu. ft. of air.

Toxic Action

Silica particles smaller than 5 μ in diameter are taken up from alveoli by phagocytic cells which then travel along the lymph channels toward the lymph nodes. Some of these phagocytes do not reach the lymph nodes but collect in nodules along the lymph channels. These nodules then gradually increase in size through proliferation of fibrous tissue to form the nodule. Pathologic examination reveals nodular fibrosis of the lungs. Progression of tuberculosis is greatly increased in silicosis, but susceptibility is not increased.

Symptoms and Lesions

Acute pneumoconiosis does not occur from silica. In case of chronic pneumoconiosis, breathing silica dust for six months to 25 years causes progressive dry cough. As the disease progresses stringy mucous is produced, a shortness of breath becomes more severe. If the patient gets tuberculosis, there is increased cough, dyspnea and weight loss. Pathological changes include first diffuse granular appearance then fibrosis and later nodules are seen in the lungs. If tuberculosis is super imposed on the original disease, large nodules, cavities and pneumonic changes are found.

Treatment

Discontinue the exposure. One to two months of positive pressure breathing therapy is recommended. Administration of bronchodilators such as epinephrine isoproterenol or phenylephrine by aerosol may improve effectiveness of the breathing therapy.

CARBON MONOXIDE (CO)

Carbon monoxide is produced by incomplete combustion of carbon or carbonaceous materials. Any flame or combustion device is likely to emit carbon monoxide. The exhaust from incomplete combustion of natural gas or petroleum fuels may contain as much as 5% carbon monoxide. The exhaust from internal combustion engines contains from 3 to 7% carbon monoxide. At 20 m. p. h. an automobile produces about 200 cu. ft. of carbon monoxide per hour.

Poisoning from carbon monoxide in animals is almost always due to coal gas which contains from 5 percent upwards. The gas owes its intensely poisonous effects to its rapid absorption into the blood stream, where it reacts with hemoglobin to form carboxy hemoglobin, a form which is incapable of combining with oxygen. Exposure to air containing 0. 4% CO for 20-30 minutes results in the conversion to carboxyhemoglobin of approximately 70% of the hemoglobin in the blood; this in turn, leads to death from tissue anoxia.

Symptoms

When the CO content of the air is above 3%, death occurs almost at once from asphyxia. When present in smaller amounts, there is vertigo, muscular weakness, increased respiration, intermittent heart beat, chest pain, confusion, and death ensues in coma. Paralysis was seen as the main symptom in pigs. Tissues and blood become cherry-red.

Diagnosis

A diagnosis can usually be arrived at from the bright pink color of the visible mucous membranes and from cherry-red color of a blood sample. The characteristic feature of carboxyhemoglobin is that it is not reduced to hemoglobin by the common reducing agents such as sodiumhydrosulfite, where as oxyhemoblobin does.

Treatment

Treatment should aim at increasing the oxygen content of the blood by inhalation of oxygen containing 5 to 10% CO_2 to act as a stimulant to the respiratory center. If a deep coma persists respiratory analeptics such as nikethamide or leptazol are indicated.

Sulfur Oxides

Sulfur dioxide (SO_2) and sulfur trioxide (SO_3) are the two sulfur oxides of greatest concern in air pollutants. Sulfur dioxide poisoning in animals grazing in the vicinity of copper works has been reported. Exposure to a concentration of 500 ppm of the gas in air for one hour is considered to be dangerous. Pigs exposed to concentrations of 5-40 ppm for 8 hours showed clinical evidence of eye and respiratory tract irritation, and pulmonary hemorrhage and emphysema were found at postmortem.

Another potential hazard has arisen from the introduction of sodium bisulphite as a preservative for silage; sulfur dioxide is evolved from the bisulfite during the fermentation process. A daily dose of 80-160 gm of metabisulfite or SO_2 caused anorexia; massive doses administered through rumen fistula were fatal. The most consistent lesions were in the larynx and in the mucosa of the ventral wall of trachea. Severe intoxication from silage preserved with bisulfite is considered improbable because of the resultant anorexia. H_2SO_4 present as mist in air causes laryngeal spasm and deep lung damage which includes degeneration of respiratory tract epithelium, hyperemia, edema, emphysema and hemorrhage.

Treatment

There is no specific antidote.

Hydrogen Sulfide (H_2S)

Hydrogen sulfide is released by the decomposition of sulfur compounds and is found in petroleum refineries, tanneries, mines and rayon industries. It is intensely toxic and relatively small amount are required to cause death. The gas may be formed from sulfur within the gut or from sulfate in the rumen. Although sudden exposure to a concentration of 0.04% might be fatal to pigs, there is no permanent ill effects in animals surviving exposure to 0.1%.

Symptoms and lesions

H_2S is believed to inhibit enzyme systems concerned in cellular respiration and to paralyze the respiratory system. Symptoms are dyspnea and cyanosis together with apathy, decrease of reflex activity and convulsions. Post mortem findings include non-coagulation of the blood, endocardial and laryngeal hemorrhages, edema of lungs, toxic changes in the liver, kidney and spleen, hyperemia and edema of the digestive tract.

Treatment

Carbon dioxide may be a physiological antidote. Inhalation of a mixture of oxygen (90%) and CO_2 (10%) may increase the tolerance of animals to H_2S. Adequate ventilation is necessary.

Ammonia (NH_3)

Ammonium compounds (nitrate and sulfate) are extensively used as fertilizers. Ammonium carbonate, chloride and acetate together with dilute solution of ammonia have been used in veterinary medicine. Urea feeding has been tried for supplementing the protein requirements of ruminant animals. Toxic effects of urea are attributed to ammonia formed from it within the rumen.

Poisoning with Urea

Oral administration of urea to a ruminant produces abrupt increase in both the blood urea and ammonia levels. Urea poisoning depends on the type of mixed feed. Urea mixed with soya meal is dangerous since the urease in the latter leads to the formation of ammonia. Poisoning of cattle may be caused by urea used as fertilizer and spread unevenly on the pasture. Toxic dose of urea varies in cattle because of the development of tolerance.

Symptoms and Lesions

The characteristic feature of ammonia gas poisoning is pulmonary edema. Symptoms of poisoning with ammonium sulfate are severe colic, groaning, shivering, staggering, forced rapid breathing, a very marked jugular pulse and death after violent struggling. Similar symptoms are seen in urea poisoning. The symptoms can be correlated with the blood ammonia level. Post mortem examination in ammonium sulfate poisoning showed large hemorrhagic patches on the mucous membranes of the GI tract, with edema and ulcer. Liver was pale and enlarged.

Diagnosis

Stomach contents should be chemically examined for ammonium salts.

Treatment

Weak acid may be used as a chemical antidote. Demulcents and stimulants are recommended.

Nitrogen Dioxide (NO_2)

Animals are exposed to nitrogen dioxide in two ways. It is formed in fermenting silage and also is produced within the rumen from plant nitrates. It is postulated that high rates of fertilization increases the nitrate contents of plants. When the nitrate—containing forage is fermented in silo nitric acid is formed which then breaks down to release NO and NO_2. Cattle, pigs and chickens have been reported to die from exposure to this gas.

Toxic Action

It causes pulmonary lesions. The effects of NO_2 in the lung are likely to be initiated by the peroxidation of lipids at points of unsaturation. A condition in man known as "silo-fillers disease" has been shown to be due to inhalation of nitrogen dioxide formed in silos. The safety limit value for continuous exposure is only 1 ppm. Animals have survived exposure of 25 ppm.

Symptoms and Lesions

Symptoms include apnea, progressive dyspnea, lachrimation, excessive salivation, grunting, anorexia, emaciation and dehydration. The pathologic changes include methemoglobinemia, dark red kidneys and necrosis of skeletal muscles. Pulmonary lesions are hyperemia, edema, hemorrhage, bronchiolitis, infarction and emphysema.

Diagnosis

History and lung damage are important. KI-starch paper turns dark when exposed to NO_2.

Treatment

No specific treatment is available. Death may occur even after giving fresh air.

Carbon Dioxide (CO_2)

Carbon dioxide results from the complete combustion of hydrocarbon fuels. CO_2 is heavier than air and can settle to low spots in a room. Dry ice is another source of exposure. CO_2 is the end product of respiration and is released from the lungs. A high alveolar CO_2 level prevents the release of CO_2 resulting in CO_2 retention and acidosis. This changes tissue pH values and if severe enough cessation of CNS function and death may occur.

Symptoms

Animals may appear anxious and high exposure staggering, incoordination, anesthesia, coma and death are observed. The blood and tissue become dark.

Diagnosis

It rests on clinical history. Blood CO_2 values may be measured.

Treatment:

It includes removal to fresh air.

REFERENCES

Aronson, A.L. 1972. *Chemical Poisonings in Small Animal Practice*. Veterinary Clinics of North America, 2:379-395.

Bailey,E.M., 1979. "Management and Treatment of Toxicoses in Cattle". *VM/SAC*., pp 1650-1657.

Buck, W. B. and Bratich,P.M.1986. "Activated charcoal: Preventing unnecessary death by poisoning". *Vet. Med.* 81:73-77.

Clarke, E. G. C. and M. L. Clarke. 1975. *Veterinary Toxicology*, 1st Edition. Williams and Wilkins. pp. 109-118.

Doull, J., Klaassen, C. D. and Amdur, M. O. 1980. *The Basic Science of Poisons*. Second edition, Macmillan Publishing Co., New York,

Simon, N.M. and Krumlovsky, F.A. 1971. "The Role of Dialysis in the Treatment of Poisoning". *Rational Drug Therapy* 5(3). 7 pages.

Szabuniewicz, M.,Bailey, E.M. and Wiersig, D.O. 1971. "Treatment of some Common Poisoning in Animals". *VM/SAC*., 66:1197-1205.

Wilkinson,G.R. 1970. "Treatment of Drug Intoxication: A review of some Scientific Principles". *Clinical Toxicology*, 3:249-265.

9

Biotoxins

A toxin is a poisonous substance produced by living cells or organisms. For a toxic substance not produced by living organisms, "toxicant" is the more appropriate term, and "toxics" is an acceptable plural. Toxins can be small molecules, peptides, or proteins and are capable of causing disease on contact with or absorption by body tissues by interacting with biological macromolecules such as enzymes or cellular receptors. Toxins vary greatly in their severity, ranging from usually minor and acute (as in a bee sting) to almost immediately deadly (as in botulinum toxin).

The term "biotoxin" is sometimes used to explicitly confirm the biological origin. Toxins produced by microorganisms are important virulence determinants responsible for microbial pathogenicity and/or evasion of the host immune response. Biotoxins vary greatly in purpose and mechanism, and can be highly complex (the venom of the cone snail contains dozens of small proteins, each targeting a specific nerve channel or receptor), or relatively small protein. Biotoxins in nature have two primary functions: predation and defence.

BACTERIAL TOXINS

Adverse reactions seen in animals (primarily dogs) ingesting foods containing preformed toxins and/or grossly contaminated with bacteria.

Bacteria of Concern

Salmonella spp.; *Clostridium* spp.; *Escherichia coli*: and *Staphylococcus* spp.

- Protein decomposition products: polypeptides and amines.

Salmonella Spp.

Primary reservoir: Intestines

Excreted by carrier animals

Toxigenic spp:. *S. typhimurium. S. anatum, S. cholerasuis, S. newport. S. enteriditis.*

Endotoxic reaction: due to Salmonella proliferation and not ingested endotoxin (s)

Vomiting, diarrhea, and increased temperature 12-24 hours post ingestion.

Hyperemic gastritis, hemorrhagic to fibrinonecrotic enteritis, hemorrhagic viscera, with leukocytosis and neutrophilia.

Clostridium Spp.

Clostridium perfringens: Spore-forming anaerobic bacillus. Heat resistant strains B, C, and D are associated with acute enterotoxemia. Lectin in foods is hydrolyzed by bacterial enzyme Phospholipase C, producing phosphorylcholine which causes diarrhea. Rapid drop in blood pressure, intravascular stasis and thrombosis, elevated PCV, congested liver and kidneys, and hemorrhagic necrosis of the intestines

C. botulinum: Found in any food source with a pH>4.5 Produces a neurotoxin, which causes flaccid motor paralysis (respiratory difficulty, excess salivation, and death). Neurotoxin adsorbs to nervous tissues, thereby preventing acetylcholine release and/ or its inactivation at the synaptic sites. Variable sensitivity among species:

- Guinea pigs Extremely sensitive
- Turkey buzzard Resistant
- Dogs, Cats, and Pigs Relatively resistant
- Horses, Minks, and Poultry Most commonly affected

Escherichia coli

Normal inhabitant of the lower gastrointestinal tract and colon of all warm blooded animals. Strains having K-antigen are associated with toxicity(release of endotoxins) on Iysis and/or death of cells. Syndromes (irreversible shock and infection).

Staphylococcus aureus

Mainly associated with dairy products. The most frequently implicated species. Several toxins are involved—Hemolytic, Leukocytic, Dermonecrotic, and lethal Enterotoxin—A product of strains A, B, and C.

Unknown mechanism (s) of action. Clinical signs are observed 1-6 hours post ingestion; with marked dehydration and electrolyte disturbance; and rear cases of death.

Postmortem observations: Serosanguineous exudate in body cavities; petechial hemorrhages in the viscera; hyperemic, empty stomach and intestines; watery feces.

Polypeptides and Amines: Formed during putrefaction and decomposition of proteinaceous foods.

Structural and biologic properties similar to substances known to affect the central nervous system, cardiovascular system and/or have histamine activity. Urine pH. is generally alkaline in these conditions

Clinical Signs

Gastrointestinal and Shock: History of ingesting spoiled foods, excessive protein rich and exotic foods, and the ingestion of dead animals. Vomiting, colic, mucoid to watery diarrhea, weakness, stiffness, ataxia, nervousness, prostration, dehydration, and occasional deaths. In less severe cases—Anorexia, dull hair coat, drowsiness, and abnormal feces.

Endotoxic Shock: Dyspnia, depression, weakness, rapid pulse, prostration, cold extremities, hemorrhagic diarrhea, and death without other signs.

Factors associated with enterotoximia—like conditions: Ingestion of garbage, spoil foods and/or feces; bones and other foreign material(pica); poor quality foods; internal parasites; intestinal stasis, and achlorhydria.

Diagnosis

History, clinical signs, confirmation of specific agents, culture of suspected foods, gastrointestinal tract and other organs. and serologic identification of toxins.

Treatment

Alleviation of shock and electrolyte imbalance, elimination of toxins or other agents, and promoting normal gastrointestinal functions. Broad spectrum antibiotics and enteric sulfonamides. Kaolin Bacteria removal, acidification of fecal flora, and eliminate gas forming bacilli. Intravenous fluid and electrolyte to correct dehydration, acid-base balance, and shock. Glutamic acid hydrochloride(300mg) before meals to correct gastric hypochlorhydrin and to acidify urine.

ANIMAL TOXINS

Venomous Animals—Secrete, store, inject or deliver via specialized structures (sting, spine. tooth, fang, etc.) venomous substances

Poisonous Animals—Cause poisoning in man and animals through their ingestion In general, all venomous animals are poisonous but not all poisonous animals are venomous.

Composition of Venoms

Proteins, polypeptides, enzymes, amines, lipids, steroids, amino polysaccharides, quinones, 5-HT, glycosides, some protease's (metalloproteins), carbohydrates (glycoproteins), and free amino acids.

Reptiles

Snakes

Venomous snakes fall into 2 classes: 1) the elapines, which include the cobra, mamba, and coral snakes; and 2) the 2 families of viperines, the true vipers (eg, puff adder, Russell's viper, and common European adder) and the pit vipers (eg, rattlesnakes, cottonmouth moccasin, copperhead, and fer-de-lance). Poisonous North American snakes include pit vipers and coral snakes.

Elapine snakes have short fangs and tend to hang on and "chew" venom into their victims. Their venom is neurotoxic and paralyzes the respiratory center. Animals that survive these bites seldom have any sequelae. Viperine snakes have long, hinged, hollow fangs; they strike, inject venom (a voluntary action), and withdraw. Many bites by vipers reportedly do not result in injection of substantial quantities of venom. Viperine venom is typically hemotoxic, necrotizing, and anticoagulant, although a neurotoxic component is present in the venom of some species, eg, the Mojave rattlesnake.

Fatal snakebites are more common in dogs than in any other domestic animal. Due to the relatively small size of some dogs in proportion to the amount of venom injected, the bite of even a small snake may be fatal. Because of their size, horses and cattle seldom die as a direct result of snakebite, but deaths may follow bites on the muzzle, head, or neck when dyspnea results from excessive swelling. Serious secondary damage sometimes occurs; livestock bitten near the coronary band may slough a hoof.

Snakebite, with envenomation, is a true emergency. Rapid examination and appropriate treatment are paramount. Owners should not spend time on first aid other than to keep the animal quiet and limit its activity.

Diagnosis

In many instances, the bite has been witnessed, and diagnosis is not a problem.

However, many conditions thought by the owner to be snakebites are actually fractures, abscesses, spider envenomations, or allergic reactions to insect bites or stings. When possible, owners should be instructed to bring the *dead* snake along with the bitten animal; they should be warned not to mutilate the snake's head because identification may depend on the morphology of the head. Many bites do not result in envenomation, or are made by nonpoisonous snakes.

Typical pit viper bites are characterized by severe local tissue damage that spreads from the bite site. The tissue becomes markedly discolored within a few minutes, and dark, bloody fluid may ooze from the fang wounds if not prevented by swelling. Frequently, the epidermis sloughs when the overlying hair is clipped or merely parted. Hair may hide the typical fang marks. Sometimes, only one fang mark or multiple punctures are present. In elapine snakebites, pain and swelling are minimal; systemic neurologic signs predominate.

Treatment

Intensive therapy should be instituted as soon as possible because irreversible effects of venom begin immediately after envenomation.

Animals bitten by an elapine may be treated with antivenin (which may be available on an as-needed basis through larger human hospital emergency rooms) and supportive care, including anticonvulsants if necessary. A polyvalent antivenin (horse-serum origin) against North American pit vipers is readily available and should be used in all cases of substantial pit viper envenomation.

The progression of events after pit viper envenomation can be divided into 3 phases: the first 2 hr, the ensuing 24 hr, and a variable period (usually ~10 days) afterward. The first 2 hr is the acute stage in which untreated, severely envenomized animals usually die. If death does not occur during this period, and the untreated animal is not in shock or depressed, the prognosis usually is favorable. The acute phase can be prolonged for several hours by use of corticosteroids and, if they are administered, prognostication should be withheld. If the animal is active and alert after 24 hr, death due to the direct effects of the venom is unlikely. The third phase is a convalescent period in which infection (possibly anaerobic) may be of concern. If necrosis has been extensive, sloughing occurs and may be so severe as to involve an entire limb.

An attempt to estimate the severity of envenomation should be made. Although not infallible, it is prudent to consider the size of the snake both as an indicator of the quantity of venom injected, and as it relates to the size of the victim. In dogs and cats, mortality is generally higher from bites to the thorax or abdomen than from bites to the head or extremities. However, this may relate to the size and vulnerability of the victim because smaller animals are more likely to be bitten on the body. Sensitivity to the venom of pit vipers varies among domestic animals. In decreasing order, sensitivity is reportedly horse, sheep, goat, dog, rabbit, pig, and cat. If there has been a previous bite, the victim may have developed some degree of active humoral immunity and be less vulnerable to the toxic effects of the venom.

Treatment for pit viper envenomation should be directed toward preventing or controlling shock, neutralizing venom, preventing or controlling disseminated intravascular coagulation, minimizing necrosis, and preventing secondary infection. Any dog or cat presented within 24 hr of a snakebite showing signs of pit viper envenomation requires intensive treatment, starting with IV fluids to combat hypotension. The use of corticosteroids has been questioned, principally because they alone do not alter the ultimate outcome. They do, however, prolong the clinical course and therefore allow more time in which to institute curative measures. Rapid-acting corticosteroids may help to control shock, protect against tissue damage, and minimize the likelihood of allergic reactions to antivenin.

Antivenin is highly beneficial because its action is the only direct and specific mechanism for neutralizing snake venom. Smaller animals probably receive a larger dose (per unit body wt) of venom than more massive animals and, accordingly, require proportionally larger doses of antivenin. Up to 100 mL of antivenin may be necessary for small dogs bitten by a large snake; 5-10 mL may be injected into the tissues around the bite, and the remainder given IV. The efficacy of antivenin is diminished if the bite occurred >24 hr previously.

In the event of an anaphylactoid reaction to the heterologous (horse) serum components in antivenin, 0. 5-1 mL of 1:1, 000 epinephrine should be administered SC. If disseminated intravascular coagulation occurs, appropriate treatment, including blood products and heparin sodium (in mini dose at 5-10 U/kg/hr or low dose at 50-100 U/kg, tid), should be administered SC.

Broad-spectrum antibiotics should be given to prevent wound infection and other secondary infections. Several potential pathogens, including Pseudomonas aeruginosa, Clostridium spp, Corynebacterium spp, and staphylococci have been isolated from rattlesnakes' mouths. Antibiotics should be continued until all superficial lesions have healed.

Tetanus antitoxin also should be administered; other supportive treatment (eg, blood transfusion in the case of hemolytic or anticoagulant venoms) is administered as needed. In most cases, surgical excision is impractical or unwarranted. Antihistamines have been reported to be contraindicated, but diphenhydramine hydrochloride is frequently given along with antivenin to treat snakebite in humans. Other procedures to neutralize venom (high-voltage, low-amperage electric shock and trypsin) have not proved effective in controlled studies.

Venomous Lizards

The most common venomous lizards are : Heloderma suspectum (gila monster) and Heloderma horridum (beaded lizard)

Venom composition

Serotonin, amine oxidase, phospholipase—A2, proteolytic and hyaluronidase activities but lacks phosphomonoesterase and diesterase, and fibrinogeno coagulase activity. High hyaluronidase content (tissue edema); low proteolytic activity (minimal tissue breakdown). The major lethal factor is gilatoxin which is devoid of proteolytic, hemorrhagic, or hemolytic activity.

Clinical signs

Multiple puncture marks, fractured teeth may be found in wound, intense localized pain, swelling, little or no necrotoxic effect. Injection of a large dose of venom—fall in systemic arterial pressure, circulating volume (hypovolemic shock may be observed), loss of ventricular contractility. tachycardia, and, respiratory distress.

Diagnosis

Difficult without a history of exposure. Typical bite wound with edema and evidence of pain. Differential diagnosis—foreign body penetration, stings from other insects, contusion, and snakebites.

Treatment

Disengage the lizard from the pet (do not pack bitten limb with ice or apply any type of constricting band. Clean bite site with 2% lidocaine, Diazepam 0. 1-0. 5 mg / kg I. M. monitor for signs of hypotension and shock. Prepare for fluid therapy (I. V. catheter in place), determine the need for antibiotics or antitoxin / toxoid. Observe closely for 3-5 days. Death is rare.

Amphibians

Skin acts as a respiratory organ and as a protective membrane (prevents desiccation, secretions—odoriferous and /bad tasting, therefore discourages predation, etc. Two types of glands—1) Mucous gland (all over the body) 2) Granular gland—limited distribution (sides of head, shoulder, and dorsolateral edges). Toads are of more concern—toxicity. Potency of the secretion varies with regions (diet, climate, and unknown genetic factors); example mortality from Bufo marinus in Hawaii is 5%, low in Texas, but 100% in Florida.

Toad

Dogs and, less frequently, cats may be poisoned by oral exposure to many types of toads. Severity varies greatly, depending on extent of contact and type of toad. Venom is produced by all toads, but its potency varies with species and apparently between geographic locations within individual species. Toad venom, a defensive mechanism, is secreted by glands located dorsal and posterior to the eyes and by other dermal structures, including warts. The venom, a thick, creamy white, highly irritating substance, can be expelled quickly by the contraction of periglandular muscles in the skin. Its many components include bufagins, which have digitalis-like effects, catecholamines, and serotonin. The most toxic species in the USA appears to be the giant or marine toad, Bufo marinus, an introduced species that is established in Florida, Hawaii, and Texas. Mortality is 20-100% in untreated cases, depending on venom potency.

Diagnosis

Encounters with toads are most common in warm or mild weather. Signs of poisoning are variable and range from local effects to convulsions and death. Severity depends on host factors, extent of exposure, length of time since exposure, and species of toad. Local effects (profuse, sometimes frothy salivation, accompanied by vigorous head shaking, pawing at the mouth, and retching) are immediate, probably because the venom is extremely irritating. Vomiting is not unusual, especially in severe cases, and although it may persist for several hours, no further signs may develop in poisoning by common indigenous toads. With more severe intoxication, as from *B.marinus*, cardiac arrhythmias, dyspnea, cyanosis, and seizures are characteristic. Both cardiac and CNS involvement are life-threatening.

Treatment

A specific antidote for the toxins in toad venom is not available. Therapy is directed at minimising absorption of the venom and controlling the associated clinical signs. Minimal treatment may be required after exposure to venom in areas where less toxic toads are found. The mouth should be immediately and thoroughly flushed with copious amounts of water. The victim should be prevented from inhaling aerosols of saliva or water that contain toad venom. Atropine may reduce the volume of saliva and the risk of aspiration. More severely affected animals require more extensive therapy. Cardiac arrhythmias should be identified and controlled using standard treatment protocols. If bradyarrhythmias exist, atropine or dopamine should be considered; tachyarrhythmias should be treated with lidocaine, phenytoin, propranolol, or procainamide hydrochloride. CNS excitation, if present, should be controlled by pentobarbital anesthesia, diazepam, or a combination of the two. Thiamylal, halothane, and other forms of anesthesia may be contraindicated because they may predispose to ventricular fibrillation. Supplemental oxygen and mechanical ventilation may also be needed if cyanosis and dyspnea are prominent.

Frogs

Secretes—Zetekitoxins; Tetrodotoxin, Chiriquitoxin, Alkaloids, Batrachotoxin A, Homobatrachotoxin, Dihydrobatrachotoxin, 3-0-Methylbatrachotoxin. Generally classified as a neurotoxin but has marked effect on the heart. Peripheral nervous system—membrane depolarization, increased cell membrane permeability to sodium ions without change in potassium or calcium ions. Reversed by tetrodotoxin and saxitoxin

Newts (Taricha SDD.)

Contain tetrodotoxin in their skin, blood, muscle, and eggs.

Clinical signs

Profused salivation, Prostration, cardiac arrhythmia, pulmonary edema, convulsions, and death within minutes of mouthing or ingestion of a toad. Vomiting may occur in some dogs, and in less severe cases, spontaneous recovery. With tetrodotoxin (neurotoxin)—pupillary dilatation, weak respiratory efforts, cardiac arrhythmia, and paralysis.

Diagnosis

History of exposure (ingestion and / or playing with toads). Fragments of toad in gastrointestinal tract, pulmonary edema (not pathognomonic). Distinguished from acute chlorinated hydrocarbon insecticide toxicity (similar clinical signs).

Treatment

In mouthing cases—Wash mouth quickly with water (not effective if toad is ingested).

Administer emetic (not if dog starts convulsing). Pentobarbitol sodium I.V. to control convulsion; and Atropine to decrease salivation and control cardiac arrhythmias. Propanolol HCl 5 mg/kg rapid I.V.; repeat in 20 minutes. Slow I.V. potassium may be indicated (persistent abnormal cardiac function). Monitor vital functions every 10 minutes.

Arthropods

Ants

Poaonomvrmex Spp. (toxic venom) and *Solenopsis* spp. (toxic venom and aggressive behavior). Minimal effects on healthy moving adult animals, Not the same for neonates, juveniles, and nesting bird chicks.

Venoms

Offensive (predation); Defensive (primary function); and as Chemical communication (alarm pheromones—attack enemy as a group). Contains complex substances and species specific. Venom with high Fonnic acid content—venom sprayed on wounds (strong mandibles) causing immediate pain, and corrosive (cellular necrosis). Venom with high proteinaceous substances (enzymes and peptides):—Phospholipase and hyaluronidase predominate, other enzymes, a protein hemolysin, histamine, 5 hydroxytryptamine, acetylcholine, norepinephrine, and dopamine. Venom of the Fire ant Contain the alkaloids methyl-n-alkylpiperidine, other nonproteinceous, and biologically active compounds

Clinical signs

Pain on initial sting, urticarial weal which transforms to a vesicle and then a pustule within a short time. Focal necrotic ulcers of cornea and conjunctiva of newborn calves (fire ants).

Diagnosis

History of ant colonies in the area, observation of sting wounds and / or the presence of ants on the animal.

Treatment

Single ant bite—no treatment required. Multiple envenomation—depending on presenting signs; Prednisolone Na succinate (5-10 mg / kg I.V.) or Dexamethazone (0.2 mg / kg -anti inflammatory effect; Z.0-4.0 mg / kg—counteract shock). Epinephrine for anaphylaxis: 0. 01 mg/ kg (3. 0-5. 0 ml. of a 1:1000 (1. 0 mg / ml.) solution / 450 kg animal. 0. 01—0. 02 mg / kg of a 1:10, 000 dilution (0. 1 mg / ml)—1. 0 ml / 1 O kg dog.

Hymenoptera

Bees: (Apis spp.); Wasp (Polistes SpD.) and Hornet—Yellow jacket (VesDula SDp.)

Envenomation by bees and wasps—potentially, all animals. Effects vary depending on species, season nutritional status, and age of bee. Dog's frequently snaps at insects, therefore swelling of the tongue or in the oral cavity is frequently observed with insect stings.

Envenomation by Yellow jacket—Dogs and people. Yellow jackets are attracted to food.

Bee Venom

Contains allegens (Phospholipase A2, acid phosphatase, hyaluronidase, melittin, and an unidentified allergen Ag-l) and non-allergens (histamine, dopamine, nor adrenaline, amino acids, and volatile substances).

Clinical Signs

Syndromes—Immediate hypersensitivity; Local inflammatory response at sting site; Systemic toxicity fro non-allergen (Human). Local swelling, edema, and erythematous plaque. Classical anaphylactic reaction reported in human is not documented in livestock. Deaths have been reported in pigs envenomated by yellow jacket, and numerous other livestock by swarms of Africanized honey bees. Multiple stings—pain. excitement, followed by tachycardia, diarrhea, hemoglobinuria, icterus, and prostration. Head sting near nostrils or mouth—dyspnea from swelling which accludes air passage(livestock). Animal presented with facial, aural, or periorbital edema. Severe dyspnea when animal is stung in oral cavity and the swelling accludes the air passage. Multiple stings—Prostration, convulsion, bloody diarrhea, vomiting of bloody fluid, leukocytosis with left shift, and elevated serum urea nitrogen, and alanine transaminase indicating renal and hepatic involvement.

Treatment

I. V. electrolyte fluid (100 ml/kg/day—dog; 50-75 ml/kg/day—horse); Corticosteroids, antihistamines, diazepam to control convulsions; careful monitoring hepatic and renal functions; oxygen supplementation may be necessary for some animals.

Cantharidin

In nature, cantharidin is found in beetles belonging to the Meloidae family. Over 200 species of these beetles occur throughout the continental USA, but members of the genus Epicauta are most frequently associated with toxicosis in horses. The striped blister beetles are particularly troublesome in the southwestern USA. The black blister beetle, E pennsylvanica, has caused toxicosis in horses in Illinois. Cantharidin is the sole toxin, but its concentration in beetles varies widely.

Blister beetles usually feed on various weeds and occasionally move into alfalfa fields in large swarms. These insects are gregarious and may be found in hay in large numbers when it is baled. One flake of alfalfa may contain several hundred beetles, but a flake from the other end of the same bale may have none. Animals are usually exposed by eating alfalfa hay or alfalfa products that have been contaminated with blister beetles.

Pathogenesis

Cantharidin is an odorless, colorless compound that is soluble in various organic solvents but only slightly soluble in water. It is highly irritating and causes acantholysis and vesicle formation when in contact with skin or mucous membranes. After ingestion, it is absorbed from the GI tract and rapidly excreted by the kidneys. The minimum lethal oral dose in horses has not been established, but it appears to be <1 mg/kg body wt. As little as 4-6 g of dried beetles may be fatal to a horse. The toxicity of cantharidin does not decrease in stored hay, and cantharidin is also toxic to people, cattle, sheep, goats, dogs, cats, rabbits, and rats.

Clinical Findings

The severity of clinical signs associated with cantharidin toxicosis vary according to dose. Signs may range from mild depression or discomfort to severe pain, shock, and death. Typical signs are related to GI and urinary tract irritation, endotoxemia and shock, hypocalcemia, and myocardial dysfunction. The onset and duration of signs can vary from hours to days. The signs seen most frequently include varying degrees of abdominal pain, depression, anorexia, and frequent attempts to drink small amounts of water or submerge the muzzle in water. Some horses show only signs of depression or make frequent attempts to urinate. Urine may be blood-tinged or contain blood clots but frequently appears normal. A striking clinical feature is that affected horses invariably have dark, congested mucous membranes, even if other systemic signs of toxicosis are minimal. Sweating, delayed capillary refill time, increased heart and respiratory rates, and increased rectal temperature are other common signs. Less frequent signs include oral erosions; salivation; synchronous diaphragmatic flutter; a stiff, short-strided gait; and diarrhea that may contain blood. Horses that ingest a massive amount of toxin may show signs of severe shock and die within hours.

Diagnosis

Both high-performance liquid chromatography and gas chromatography or mass spectrometry analyses are sensitive, reliable methods of detecting cantharidin in gastric contents or in urine. The concentration of cantharidin in urine becomes negligible in 3-4 days, so urine should be collected early in the course of disease if it is to be analysed. Microscopic evaluation of stomach contents (and often cecal contents) of fatally poisoned horses may reveal fragments of the insect, which can be positively identified if from one of the 3-striped species.

Certain laboratory findings are particularly helpful in differentiating cantharidin toxicosis from other causes of acute abdominal crisis. Serum calcium concentration is usually markedly decreased and may remain low for a prolonged time. Serum magnesium concentration is also typically low, and concentration of serum creatine kinase usually increases markedly within 24 hr of onset. In acutely affected horses, urinalysis typically reveals markedly decreased specific gravity (usually <1. 010) and varying degrees of hematuria. Peritoneal fluid usually contains increased protein (>4 g/dL) but normal numbers of WBC and normal fibrinogen concentration. Other laboratory abnormalities may include mild increases of serum urea nitrogen and creatinine and development of hypoproteinemia. Acutely affected horses are almost always hyperglycemic.

Treatment

There is no specific antidote for cantharidin, but prompt, vigorous symptomatic therapy is necessary for successful treatment. Oral administration of mineral oil aids in evacuation of the GI tract, and repeated dosing may be indicated. Activated charcoal PO may be helpful if given early. Calcium and magnesium supplementation for prolonged periods is almost always indicated. Other symptomatic therapy includes administration of fluids, analgesics, and diuretics and maintenance of normal blood pH and serum electrolyte concentrations. The prognosis for affected horses improves daily if no complications occur.

Prevention

Prevention is aimed at feeding beetle-free hay. The hay field must be scouted before it is cut and during baling, because the insects can be crushed in the cutting and crimping process as well as during baling. Areas of the field that contain swarms of beetles must be avoided for a few days because most of the insects will leave. Once the beetles have left, these areas can be harvested.

First-cutting hay is almost always free of blister beetles, because the insects overwinter as subadults and usually do not emerge until late May or June in the southwestern USA. Likewise, the last cutting of hay is often safe, because it is usually harvested after the adult insects are no longer active.

Spider Bites

Brown Spiders

Envenomation of animals by spiders is relatively uncommon and difficult to recognize. It may be suspected on clinical signs, but confirmatory evidence is rare. Spiders of medical importance in the USA do not inflict particularly painful bites, so it is unusual for a spider bite to be suspected until clinical signs appear. It is also unlikely that the offending spider will remain in close proximity to the victim for the time (30 min to 6 hr) required for signs to develop. Almost all spiders are venomous, but few possess the attributes necessary to cause clinical envenomation in mammals—mouth parts of sufficient size to allow penetration of the skin and toxin of sufficient quantity or potency to result in morbidity.

The spiders in the USA that are capable of causing clinical envenomation belong to 2 groups—widow spiders (*Latrodectus* spp.) and brown spiders (mostly *Loxosceles* spp).

Widow Spiders

Widow spiders usually bite only when accidental skin contact occurs. The most common species is the black widow, *Latrodectus mactans,* characterized by a red hourglass shape on the ventral abdomen. In the western states, the western black widow, *L.hesperus,* predominates, while the brown widow, *L.bishopi,* is found in the south, and the red widow, *L.geometricus,* is found in Florida.

Latrodectus venom is one of the most potent biologic toxins. The most important of its 5 or 6 components is a neurotoxin that causes release of the neurotransmitters norepinephrine and acetylcholine at synaptic junctions, which continues until the neurotransmitters are depleted. The resulting severe, painful cramping of all large muscle groups accounts for most of the clinical signs.

Unless there is a history of a widow spider bite, diagnosis must be based on clinical signs, which include restlessness with apparent anxiety or apprehension; rapid, shallow, irregular respiration; shock; abdominal rigidity or tenderness; and painful muscle rigidity, sometimes accompanied by intermittent relaxation (which may progress to clonus and eventually to respiratory paralysis). Partial paresis also has been described.

An antivenin (equine origin) is commercially available but is usually reserved for confirmed bites of high-risk individuals. Symptomatic treatment is usually sufficient but may require a combination of therapeutic agents. Calcium gluconate IV is reportedly helpful. Meperidine hydrochloride or morphine, also given IV, provides relief from pain and produces muscle relaxation. Muscle relaxants and diazepam are also beneficial. Tetanus antitoxin also should be administered. Recovery may be prolonged; weakness and even partial paralysis may persist for several days.

Brown Spiders

There are at least 10 species of Loxosceles spiders in the USA, but the brown recluse spider, L reclusa, is the most common, and envenomation by it is typical. These spiders have a violin-shaped marking on the cephalothorax, although it may be indistinct or absent in some species. In the northwestern USA, the unrelated spider Tegenaria agrestis reportedly causes a clinically indistinguishable dermonecrosis in humans and presumably in other animals. Brown recluse spider venom has vasoconstrictive, thrombotic, hemolytic, and necrotizing properties. It contains several enzymes, including a phospholipase (sphingomylinase D) that attacks cell membranes. Pathogenetic mechanisms of the characteristic dermal necrosis are poorly understood, but activation of complement, chemotaxis, and accumulations of neutrophils affect (or amplify) the process.

A history of a bite by a "fiddleback" brown spider is useful but rare. A presumptive diagnosis may be based on the presence of a discrete, erythematous, intensely pruritic skin lesion that may have irregular ecchymoses. Within 4-8 hr, a vesicle develops at the bite wound, and sometimes a blanched zone circumscribes the erythematous area, imparting a "bull's-eye" appearance to the lesion. The central area sometimes appears pale or cyanotic. The vesicle may degenerate to an ulcer that, unless treated in a timely manner, may enlarge and extend to underlying tissues, including muscle. Sometimes, a pustule follows the vesicle and, on its breakdown, a black eschar remains. The final tissue defect may be extensive and indolent and require months to heal. However, medical authorities claim that not all brown recluse spider bites result in severe, localized dermal necrosis.

Systemic signs sometimes accompany brown recluse spider envenomation and may not appear for 3-4 days after the bite. Hemolysis, thrombocytopenia, and disseminated intravascular coagulation are more likely to occur in cases with severe dermal necrosis.

Fever, vomiting, edema, hemoglobinuria, hemolytic anemia, renal failure, and shock may result from systemic loxoscelism.

Scorpions

Centruroides spp. They may inhabit arid deserts. The bark scorpion *C.sculpturatus* is the most dangerous U.S. species (Arizona, Texas, New Mexico, and some areas in California). Cases are possible outside these areas (Tourism). They are nocturnal, and lives where moisture is available. Pet exposure is purely accidental. Movement may initiate a stinging response.

Venom

Complex mixture of neurotoxic proteins (enzymes and others). Phospholipase A2 is common, hyaluronidase, phosphomonoesterase, acetylcholinesterase, and others are only found in venoms of some species. Other compounds are—amino acids, histamine, 5 hydroxytryptamine, and serotonin. Scorpion venoms are antigenic.

Clinical signs

Local swelling with ecchymosis but no tissue necrosis. Systemic signs—Salivation, muscle fasciculation, generalized weakness, and paralysis including respiratory paralysis (parasympathomimetic). Hypertension, respiratory failure, and skeletal muscle stimulation have been reported in dogs and cats experimentally administered *C.sculpturatus* venom.

Treatment

Antivenin though available, its usefulness is questionable due to time delay before treatment. Atropine (0. 04 mg/kg) or to effect to counter parasympathomimetic effects. Corticosteroids for Shock and edema. Parenteral fluids must be carefully monitored pulmonary edema. Positive pressure respiration assistance—Respiratory failure. Meperidine hydrochloride (Demerol) and other narcotics are contraindicated—acts synergistically to increase toxicity of venom.

MARINE TOXINS

Natural toxins represent an increasing hazard to the seafood consuming public. Toxins are produced by marine algae and are accumulated through the food chain and are ultimately deposited in higher predator fish or filter-feeding bivalves. Toxins may also affect people through the air and drinking water.

Marine and freshwater toxin diseases in human populations are due to the contamination of seafood with a myriad of natural toxins created by minute marine and freshwater organisms such as dinoflagellates found throughout the marine and freshwater world, especially in coral reefs and their surroundings.

In general, the natural marine and freshwater toxins are tasteless, odorless, and heat and acid stable. Therefore, normal screening and food preparation procedures do not prevent intoxication if the fish or shellfish is contaminated.

The marine and freshwater toxin diseases are divided into two groups by their primary transvectors, i.e. those associated with the ingestion of shellfish, and those with fish consumption. In addition, there is a group of marine and freshwater diseases associated with water exposure. The shellfish-associated diseases and those associated with water exposure generally occur with algal blooms or "red tides" while fish-associated diseases are more localized to specific reef areas and/or types of fish.

Paralytic Shellfish Poisoning (PSP), Red Tide/Neurotoxic Shellfish Poisoning (NSP), Diarrheic Shellfish Poisoning (DSP), and Amnesic Shellfish Poisoning (ASP) are primarily associated with the ingestion of contaminated shellfish.

Ciguatera Poisoning and Tetrodotoxin Poisoning (Fugu or Pufferfish Poisoning) occur with the ingestion of contaminated fish.

Aerosolized Florida Red Tide/Brevetoxins, the Blue Green Algae (Cyanobacteria), and Pfiesteria and the Pfiesteria-like Organisms (PLOs) can affect humans through exposure to water droplets or even drinking water contaminated with the organisms and/or their toxins.

The primary toxic effect of the marine and freshwater toxins is to the neurologic system, however, affected individuals usually present a wide range of symptoms resulting in a confusing clinical picture. The acute onset of severe gastro-intestinal distress after eating the contaminated fish occurs within minutes to hours. In the case of PSP, Fugu, and Ciguatera, this gastro-intestinal picture can be accompanied by acute respiratory distress which may be fatal within hours (up to 50% of cases of Fugu and 10% of PSP).

In the case of Ciguatera and ASP, debilitating chronic neurologic symptoms lasting months to years have been reported. The majority of people with Ciguatera, especially in the Caribbean, suffer for weeks to months with debilitating neurologic symptoms, including profound weakness, temperature sensation changes, pain, and numbness in the extremities. ASP has left people with permanent and severe memory loss, even years after their initial illness.

In addition to increasing worldwide seafood consumption, anthropogenic causes may have furthered the spread of the dinoflagellates and their toxins. There is a body of evidence to indicate that man-induced transportation of the cysts or "seeds" of the toxic marine and freshwater organisms such as dinoflagellates, or of the dinoflagellates themselves located inside the 'spat' (young bivalve shellfish sold commercially to global markets for aquaculture) and ship ballast water (international regulations are now changing to require ship ballast water purging in the open ocean prior to docking).

Paralytic Shellfish Poisoning

A seasonal (summer) allergic, digestive and/or paralytic syndrome observed in man and other animals ingesting toxic shellfish (clams, oysters, mussels). Shellfish become toxic following the filtration of toxic dinoflagellates through their digestive and respiratory systems. Species of dinoflagellates of the genus Gonyaulaux produces the water soluble, heat stable toxin saxitoxin, which becomes localized in the digestive organs, gills, and siphon of the shellfish.

Clinical signs

Allergic—previous sensitization necessary (anaphylactic reaction). Digestive—Seen in 10-12 hours post ingestion of toxic shellfish (vomiting, abdominal pain, nausea, recovery). Paralytic—Tingling and burning sensation (lips, gums, and tongue) rapidly spreading to all parts of the body. Numbness, difficulty moving, joint pain, weakness, increased salivation, intense thirst. Generalized paralysis with death (20%). Syndromes observed commonly together in varying degrees.

Mechanism of action

Membrane permeability to sodium ion is altered; action potential is blocked thus preventing nerve conductance. Negligible effects on potassium and chloride ions to permeability. Minimal effects on neuromuscular snapsis and cardiovascular system.

Diagnosis

Difficult without a history of shellfish consumption and the observed clinical signs. No postmortem lesion. Digestive disturbances could be attributed to endotoxins, histadine and/or thiaminase exposure.

Treatment

With no specific antidote available supportive care becomes essential

Ciguatera Poisoning

A sporadic, complex syndrome (digestive, cardiovascular, and nervous systems) in man and other animals within 30 hours of ingesting certain food fish species (snapper, barracuda, grouper, kingfish, herring). Three water soluble, heat stable toxins (Ciguatoxin, Scaritoxin, and Maitotoxin), produced by the dinoflagillate Gambierdiscus toxicus have been implicated in this condition.

Clinical signs

Digestive—Nausea, vomiting, diarrhea, and abdominal pain. Cardiovascular-Bradycardia and hypotension, followed by tachycardia and hypertension. Nervous—Severe pruritis, temperature reversal, paresthesia, convulsions, muscle paralysis, and loss of equilibrium. Neurologic signs can persist for months, and recur when stressed, consumed alcohol and/or eating non-toxic fish. Most commonly, varying degrees of each syndrome is expressed. Death, though rare (7%), is generally due to respiratory paralysis. Cats are very sensitive to ciguatoxin.

Mechanism of action

Inhibits acetylcholiesterase, cholinergicomimetic effects. Competitively inhibits calcium regulates sodium ion channel.

Diagnosis

History of fish consumption and clinical signs. Differentiate between other conditions—Paralytic shellfish poisoning, Type E botulism, Organophosphate/Carbamate poisoning.

Treatment

No antidote available. Symptomatic and supportive therapy essential. Acetaminophen and indomethacin are recommended for chronic ciguatoxin poisoning. As a precaution, viscera of tropical marine should not be eaten. Since the toxin is water soluble, it would be advisable to soak the fish meat for days, and discard the water before cooking.

Tetrodotoxin Poisoning

Marine puffer fish (toad fish, globe fish, swell fish, porcupine fish, and balloon fish) have in their ovaries (roe), liver, intestines, and skin, the neurotoxin tetrodotoxin (basic, water soluble). Ingestion of improperly prepared fish results in toxicosis. Tetrodotoxin originated from either of four possible sources—Endogenous, Exogenous, Symbiotic microorganisms, or multiple origins.

Clinical signs

Within minutes (45 minutes) of ingesting toxic fish, there is a tingling (lips and tongue) followed by motor incoordination; excessive salivation, nausea, leading to vomiting and diarrhea. Generalized paralysis with convulsions and death (60%) from skeletal muscle paralysis (human). Dogs and cats may become poisoned from scavenging. Cats experimentally administered tetrodotoxin showed—gross mydriasis, flaccid paralysis, tachycardia, and depressed respiration.

Mechanism of action

Tetrodotoxin selectively blocks sodium ion channel along the axon.

Diagnosis

History of ingestion of the puffer fish and the rapid onset of neurologic signs are suggestive. Agonal hypoxic ecchymoses on serosal surface and pulmonary edema may be seen but are not pathognomonic. Differentiate from tick paralysis and ciguataria poisoning.

Treatment

No known treatment. Ventilatory support, atropine, dopamine, crystalloid infusion are primary modalities currently used.

REFERENCES

Aronson, A.L. 1972. *Chemical Poisonings in Small Animal Practice*. Veterinary Clinics of North America, 2:379-395.

Bailey,E.M., 1979. "Management and Treatment of Toxicoses in Cattle". *VM/SAC.*, pp 1650-1657.

Buck, W. B., G. D. Osweiler and G. A. Van Gelder. 1985. *Clinical and Diagnostic Veterinary Toxicology*, 3rd Ed. Kendall/Hunt. pp. 177-197; 391-393.

Mathew, H. and Lawson, A.A. 1980. *Treatment of Common Acute Poisoning*, 4th ed., Churchill Pub. New York.

Fane, L.R., Combs, H.F. and Decker, W.J. 1971. "Physical Parameters in Gastric Lavage". *Clinical Toxicology*, 4:389-395.

Simon, N.M. and Krumlovsky, F.A. 1971. "The Role of Dialysis in the Treatment of Poisoning". *Rational Drug Therapy* 5(3). 7 pages.

Szabuniewicz, M.,Bailey, E.M. and Wiersig, D.O. 1971. "Treatment of some Common Poisoning in Animals". *VM/SAC.*, 66:1197-1205.

Thoman, M.E. 1970. "The Use of Emetics in Poison Ingestion". *Clinical Toxicology*, 3:185-188.

Wilkinson,G.R. 1970. "Treatment of Drug Intoxication: A review of some Scientific Principles". *Clinical Toxicology*, 3:249-265.

10

Endocrine Toxicology

Endocrine systems of the body play an essential and pervasive role in both the short- and long-term regulation of metabolic processes. Nutritional, behavioral, and reproductive processes are intricately regulated by endocrine systems, as are growth (including bone growth/remodeling), gut, cardiovascular, and kidney function and responses to all forms of stress. Disorders of any of the endocrine systems, involving both overactive and underactive hormone secretion, result inevitably in disease, the effects of which may extend to many different organs and functions and are often debilitating or life-threatening. Viewed from this general perspective, the threat posed from environmental chemicals with endocrine activity (either agonist or antagonistic) is potentially serious. However, the fact that humans and wildlife are exposed to such chemicals does not necessarily mean that clinically manifest disturbance of the relevant endocrine system will result, because much depends on the level and duration of exposure and on the timing of exposure.

The endocrine system originally was considered to consist only of glands that secreted hormones into the blood that traveled to distant target tissues, bound to specific cellular receptors, and produced characteristic actions. Currently, our concept of "endocrine" has been broadened by the discovery of other chemical regulators, such as chemicals secreted into the blood by neurons, that are sometimes termed neurohormones. The term "cytocrine" has been applied to numerous local or intercellular chemical regulators, including growth factors. Intercellular cytocrines that travel through the extracellular fluids to other cells in a tissue also are known as paracrine and autocrine regulators, depending on whether they affect other cells or themselves, respectively.

The term "intracrine" has been suggested for intracellular regulators such as second messengers and transcription factors. Even before allowing for the increase in complexity of "endocrinology" that has resulted from recent recognition of the many cytocrine/paracrine systems that operate, it had been realized that there were numerous "classical" endocrine systems in the body that regulate processes as diverse as blood pressure, smooth muscle contraction, fluid balance, and bone resorption.

HOMEOSTASIS

The fundamental role of all endocrine systems is to enable a dynamic, coordinated response of a distant target tissue to signals originating from another organ and, in some instances, cues originating from outside of the body. For most endocrine systems, the primary objective is to maintain some form of "homeostasis," avoiding wild swings in hormone levels/responses that might otherwise have detrimental metabolic effects. A good example is the role of insulin in maintaining blood glucose levels within the normal range, that is, a range that does not fall so low as to result in unconsciousness and does not rise so high that wasteful excretion/spillage into urine occurs. When insulin levels do not respond to changing blood levels of glucose, diseases such as diabetes are the result.

All endocrine systems operate to a large extent on the "seesaw" principle (Figure 1), in which the target cells send feedback signals (usually negative feedback) to the regulating cells, with the result that secretion of the target cell-stimulating hormone is altered (usually reduced) by one or more of the products of the target cells. However, in reality, there are usually elaborations or refinements of this simple archetypal endocrine system that enable all of the endocrine systems of the body to be integrated via cross talk. The reasons for this are obvious. For example, reproduction needs to take account of age, nutritional status, and in most animals, season of the year. Similarly, stress responses, and to a lesser extent, endocrine systems regulating hunger, need to be able to override other endocrine systems when danger threatens.

This cross talk is vital for a healthy life and has important implications for the evaluation of endocrine disruptors. Exposure to an estrogenic chemical, for example, may affect not only the reproductive endocrine axis but also several other endocrine systems as well as bone, fat, and cardiovascular systems.

PROGRAMMING OF ENDOCRINE AXES

Although homeostasis, via seesaw-type mechanisms, is a central feature of all endocrine systems, it should be stressed that the balance between the two sides of the "seesaw" need to be set up or programmed before the system will work correctly. This programming will determine at what level the two sides of the seesaw will begin to respond to signals from the other side (Figure 1). For many of the endocrine systems, it appears that the setup program is established during fetal/ neonatal development in mammals and that an abnormal environment at this stage of life can result in permanent misprogramming. A good example of this is what happens as a result of fetal IUGR.

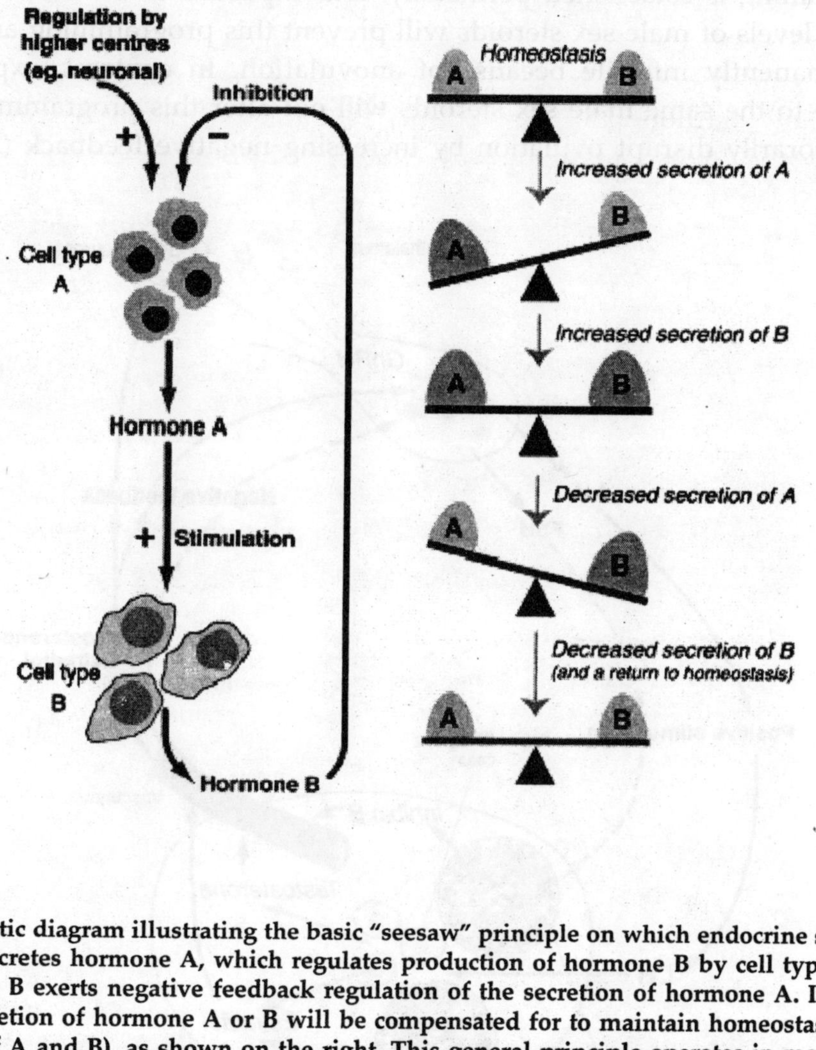

Figure 1. Schematic diagram illustrating the basic "seesaw" principle on which endocrine systems work. Cell type A secretes hormone A, which regulates production of hormone B by cell type B, and in turn, hormone B exerts negative feedback regulation of the secretion of hormone A. In this way, swings in secretion of hormone A or B will be compensated for to maintain homeostasis (i.e., the correct levels of A and B), as shown on the right. This general principle operates in most, if not all, endocrine and paracrine systems, although in reality there are usually additional factors that will interplay in the regulation of levels of A and B.

Although such offspring often reach normal growth postnatally, they show a high incidence of insulin resistance and, consequently, are at increased risk of diabetes, obesity, and cardiovascular disease in later life; they are also prone to precocious puberty. These changes are believed to represent an adaptation of the fetus to its suboptimal nutritional supply and may result from elevation of glucocorticoid levels in the fetus. A more specific example concerns programming of the hypothalamus of the female, but not of the male, to respond to gradually rising estrogen levels by triggering a positive response-the ovulatory GnRH-driven LH surge. In mammals, this programming is established perinatally, and exposure of the female at this time to moderate levels of male sex steroids will prevent this programming and render the female permanently infertile because of anovulation. In contrast, exposure of the adult female to the same male sex steroids will not alter this programming, although it may temporarily disrupt ovulation by increasing negative feedback (Figure 2).

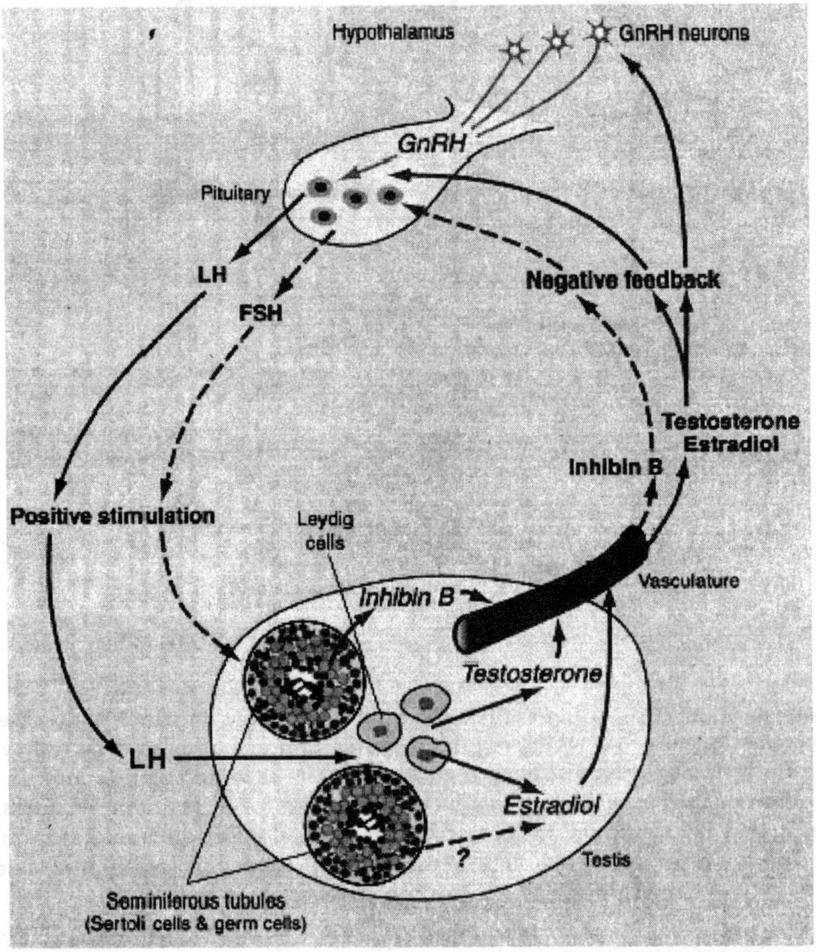

Figure 2. Diagrammatic representation of the main working components of the mammalian HPG axis.

IMPACT OF ENDOCRINE DISRUPTORS

In considering the potential impact of endocrine disruptors on bodily functions, the following points are critical:

(1) Exposure in adulthood may be compensated for by normal homeostatic mechanisms and may therefore not result in any significant or detectable effect.

(2) Exposure during the period when programming of the endocrine system is in progress may result in a permanent change of function or sensitivity to stimulatory/ inhibitory signals.

(3) Exposure to the same level of an endocrine signal at different stages in the life history or in different seasons may produce different effects.

(4) Because of cross talk between different endocrine systems, effects may occur unpredictably in endocrine systems other than the system predicted to be affected.

This is true for each of the situations in (1) through (3) above. (5) In view of (4), considerable caution should be exercised in extrapolating *in vitro* measures of hormonal activity to the situation *in vivo*.

HPG AXIS IN MAMMALS

This axis (Figure 2) involves three component parts: 1) GnRH neurons projecting from the hypothalamus of the brain; 2) gonadotropes in the anterior pituitary gland (adenohypophysis), which secrete the gonadotropins LH and FSH;, and 3) the somatic cells of the gonads (theca and granulosa cells in the ovary, Leydig and Sertoli cells in the testis). GnRH is secreted in pulses from the terminals of GnRH neurons and acts on the gonadotropes to induce secretion of both LH and FSH, which then act on their respective target cells in the gonads (LH on theca/Leydig cells; FSH on granulosa/Sertoli cells). Secretion of GnRH is modified by other neurons, and the actions of GnRH on gonadotropin release may be modified by other hypothalamic or pituitary peptides.

As a consequence, gonadal sex steroids stimulated by LH and the protein hormone inhibin (the A form in females, the B form in males) stimulated by FSH are released into the bloodstream and provide feedback to the hypothalamus and pituitary gonadotropes to reduce the secretion of GnRH, LH, and FSH, with inhibin selectively inhibiting FSH and the sex steroids inhibiting LH secretion. This description implies that the arrangement of stimulatory and negative feedback loops complies with the simple arrangement shown in Figure 1.

In reality, the arrangement is more complex and sophisticated. For example, the effects of GnRH on LH and FSH secretion are radically different, with LH release being stimulated very acutely (in pulses) by the GnRH pulses, whereas the response of FSH is extremely sluggish and takes many hours. This stems from fundamental differences in GnRH-induced synthesis, packaging, and release of LH and FSH. Similarly, although the sex steroids (primarily testosterone in the male, E_2 in the female) negatively regulate LH secretion via effects on both GnRH secretion and gonadotrope function, they also exert some negative feedback on FSH secretion; in contrast, inhibin selectively inhibits FSH secretion.

TARGET CELL SENSITIVITY

In addition to these minor refinements of the archetypal endocrine system, there are other important factors that must be considered. One such factor is modulation of target cell sensitivity to stimulation. Gonadotropes do not exhibit a constant, unchanging response to GnRH stimulation, nor do the target cells in the gonads maintain unaltered responsiveness to LH/FSH stimulation. Sensitivity of the target cell to its stimulator is regulated both acutely and chronically.

For example, an abnormally high frequency of GnRH pulses or chronic exposure to GnRH or to agonistic analogues of GnRH (which are more resistant to degradation) results in loss or down-regulation of GnRH receptors on the gonadotropes, which serves to make them more resistant (= less sensitive) to further stimulation. This happens in a matter of hours and is followed more slowly by the gradual development of "desensitization" that involves changes to the GnRH-stimulated second messenger signaling mechanisms that reduce overall responsiveness of the gonadotropes to GnRH. Analogous mechanisms operate in gonadal cells to regulate their responsiveness to LH and, to a lesser extent, to FSH. In other words, each target cell in the endocrine axis also regulates its own responsiveness to stimulation.

There is still further refinement of this process via cross talk between neighboring cells, especially in the gonads. There is good evidence, for example, that Sertoli cells in the testis are able to modulate both the numbers of LH receptors expressed in neighboring Leydig cells and their steroidogenic responsiveness via altering expression of steroid synthetic enzymes. In return, the testosterone secreted by Leydig cells exerts important paracrine regulatory effects on Sertoli cell function.

METABOLISM OF ENDOCRINE HORMONES

A further potentially modulable element in the component loops of the HPG axis is the metabolism of the secreted hormones. Increased or decreased catabolism, with a consequent change in half-life of a hormone, will change its effectiveness without altering its level of secretion. FSH has a naturally longer half-life than LH (i.e., it is metabolized more slowly), which is one reason why changes in FSH levels are more sluggish than changes in LH. Of much more importance is the role of proteins that bind the sex steroids. These include albumin and AFP in the fetus/neonate and, most important, SHBG in humans. Approximately 97-98% of testosterone and E_2 that circulate in blood in humans is bound to SHBG, and only 2-3% is free and thus biologically active. This arrangement has two important consequences:

1) the half-life of the sex steroids is considerably prolonged and
2) a new indirect pathway for regulating sex steroid action becomes evident: modulation of SHBG secretion (by the liver) can potentially alter levels of bioactive sex steroid without affecting any of the major component parts of the HPG axis.

In practice, the main (stimulatory) regulators of SHBG production are the sex steroids themselves as well as other important regulators of SHBG production that are components of other endocrine systems. Similar arguments may apply to other binding proteins (e.g., AFP).

INTERACTION OF PARACRINE AND ENDOCRINE COMPONENTS OF THE HPG AXIS

Testosterone produced by Leydig cells acts on neighboring Sertoli cells (an example of a paracrine effect). This is arguably the most important role of testosterone in the male, as its effect on Sertoli cells is the main pathway via which spermatogenesis is supported. There are analogous effects in the ovary with androgens produced by the theca cells exerting paracrine effects on granulosa cells in the adjacent, developing follicle. The most important consequence of the exposure of granulosa cells to testosterone is that they are then able to convert this androgen to E_2, which then exerts multiple endocrine effects in the uterus and elsewhere in the body, including its role in negative feedback. This conversion of testosterone to E_2 also occurs at many other sites in the body, in both the male and the female.

The ability of cells to express aromatase and/or 5α-reductase, and thus to transform an endocrine hormone (testosterone) into a locally acting paracrine hormone, appears to be far more common (especially in the male) than was initially hypothesized. These sites of paracrine action obviously depend on the supply of substrate and thus on the main endocrine axis, and "leakage" of the paracrine-generated products into the general circulation may contribute to negative feedback, although conceptually this would not appear to be important. One or both of the component parts of the paracrine mechanisms illustrated in Figure 3 are now known to be expressed in bone, muscle, the cardiovascular system, adipose tissue, the pituitary gland, and brain as well as throughout the reproductive systems of both male and female. Paracrine systems can be considered to act as local satellites of the major endocrine axis, their role being to serve local needs.

DEVELOPMENTAL ROLE OF THE HPG AXIS

The setting up of endocrine axes takes place largely during fetal/neonatal development. During this period, feedback sensitivity of the hypothalamus and pituitary gonadotropes to steroids from the gonads is established, and this will determine at what level of sex steroid a reduction in GnRH and/or LH/FSH secretion will be triggered. The details of how this occurs are incompletely understood but clearly involve programming of neuronal pathways.

At the same time, differences between male and female feedback centers are programmed. This is necessary because female reproduction usually operates around a reproductive cycle, for example, the estrous or menstrual cycle, whereas male reproduction is usually a continuous or more protracted, noncyclic event. Production of gonadal hormones in the female is therefore cyclic whereas in the male it is relatively uniform, apart from special periods such as puberty and seasonal infertility. Appropriate changes to the "wiring" of the hypothalamus of the male and female therefore have to be induced during development to ensure that the pituitary gland of an adult female will respond as in a female rather than as in a male.

Testosterone produced during fetal/neonatal life plays a role in programming the development of a "male" hypothalamus and brain, and administration of testosterone to a female during this critical programming period will result in masculinization of hypothalamic function and consequent acyclicity and anovulation in adulthood. The relative roles of testosterone, DHT, and E_2 vary from behavior to behavior in a species-specific manner. This is true for both organizational and activational influences.

In some species, all three hormones play a role in masculinization. Importantly, there are significant species differences in the organizational and activational control of the development of sexually dimorphic behaviors. For example, in the rat, activation of malelike mounting behavior in the adult female rat does not require an organizational effect of hormones during prenatal life. In at least some strains of rats, this behavior can be activated by testosterone in adult females. In contrast to the rat, androgens play an important role in the organization of mounting behavior in the nonhuman primate. This difference must be considered when extrapolating findings from the rat to humans. Rough-and-tumble play behavior is one of the few social behaviors that appears to be regulated by androgens in both the rat and rhesus monkey.

ROLE OF HORMONES IN MAMMALIAN SEX DIFFERENTIATION

As well as leading to masculinization of the brain, perinatal testosterone secretion by the testis is also responsible for masculinization of the body in general. This involves the formation of male genitalia, but effects on the many organs throughout the body also occur at this time. The role of androgens in sex differentiation is well understood. Before sex differentiation, the mammalian embryo has the potential to develop a male or a female phenotype. Following gonadal sex differentiations, testicular sections induce differentiation of the male duct system and external genitalia. The development of phenotypic sex includes persistence of either the Wolffian (male) or Müllerian (female) duct system and differentiation of the external genitalia. Generally, masculinization of the tissue/organ in question results from local conversion of circulating testosterone to either DHT or E_2, as shown in Figure 3 but for some tissues, MIS is also involved.

The female avoids developing as a male by simply not switching on secretion of testosterone by the ovary, and it is largely the absence of this endocrine signal that results in phenotypic and endocrinotypic female development. The central role of testosterone in facilitating masculinization has two important downsides. First, if a genotypic male fails to make testosterone, it will not masculinize and will develop as a phenotypic female (but with testes). Second, and conversely, if a genotypic female is exposed to sufficient testosterone (or other androgens), she will be masculinized (but will have ovaries). There are numerous examples of both of these situations that result most commonly from inactivating mutations (e.g., in the AR, resulting in lack of masculinization in males) or from abnormal androgen production (usually by the adrenal glands) by the mother or female fetus that lead to masculinization of the developing female. It is also emphasized that these are not necessarily allor-nothing events. Partial masculinization of the female or partial failure of masculinization of the male can occur, including potentially quite subtle effects. Where these affect the genitalia or other external phenotypic feature (e.g., presence/absence of horns), they may be easily detected, but if the effects are confined to the brain or to another organ, they may not be easily deducible.

Like the brain and the genitalia, other organ systems such as the liver and muscles are also "imprinted" by the hormonal milieu during development and hence may also be targets of xenobiotics that perturb the normal endocrine profile at various stages of life. For example, the development of the levator ani-bulbocavernosus muscles and their neural regulation has been employed as a model of organizational and activational roles of testosterone on the ontogeny of sexual dimorphisms in the rat. These tissues are also sexually dimorphic in humans, an effect whose critical period lies in the first trimester of pregnancy. The levator ani muscles and spinal nuclei of the bulbocavernosus are considerably larger in males than in female rats, a response that requires testosterone exposure during both the prenatal and postpubertal stages of life. As the levator ani lacks 5α-reductase, testosterone, and not DHT, is the hormone that initiates the malelike developmental pattern.

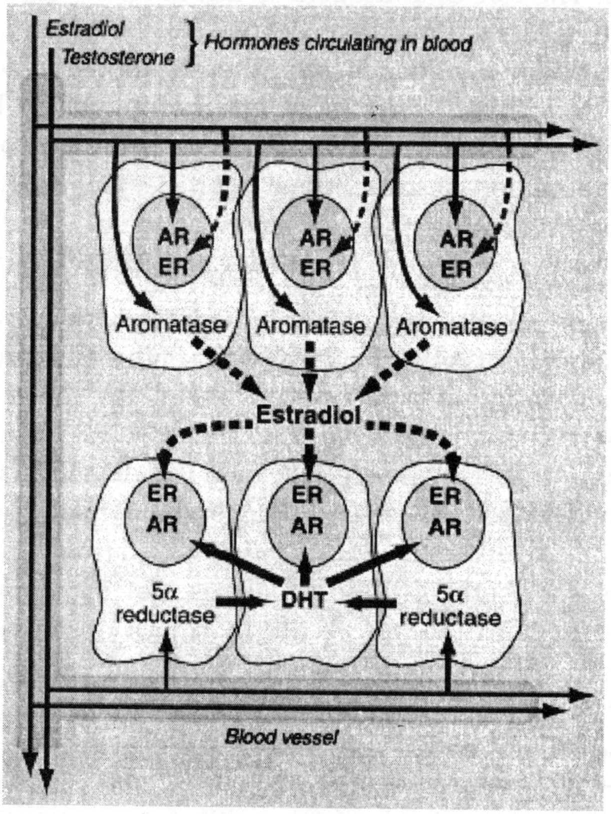

Figure 3. **Schematic illustration of the interplay between endocrine and paracrine regulatory systems as exemplified by androgens and estrogens.**

Perhaps the most important aspect of these various "programming" changes is their irreversibility. The greatest concern about environmental hormone disruptors is centered on the possibility that exposure of an animal to such an agent during perinatal life can result in a permanent adverse or abnormal change; exposure to the hormone disruptor does not need to be chronic, as transient exposure at a critical time during development is all that is required. There is added uncertainty in this regard because of emerging understanding about how different androgens and estrogens may act in different tissues-so-called SERMs and corresponding SARMs. The ability of such compounds to selectively activate or antagonize estrogen or androgen pathways in specific tissues presages the discovery of similar activities for certain environmental chemicals. Predicting the effects of such compounds in the context of programming of development of the reproductive system and its endocrine axis is extremely difficult.

THE HPG AXIS IN NONMAMMALIAN SPECIES

Nonmammalian vertebrates differ greatly from mammals and one another in their modes of reproduction, with patterns of sequential and simultaneous hermaphroditism, parthenogenesis, viviparity, and gonochorism found in many major groups. Additionally, they may be more limited in their breeding frequencies. Some species breed only once (semelparous), whereas others may breed two or more times (iteroparous). The time of gonadal activity may be very short, with the gonads remaining quiescent during most of the year. Dissociated reproduction where testicular and ovarian development actually occurs at different times of the year also is known for numerous species. However, the HPG axes of these animals are surprisingly similar in their operation, in the pattern of feedback mechanisms, and in the hormones involved to that described for mammals.

GTH release is controlled in all nonmammals by a GnRH decapeptide molecule similar to that in mammals. As in mammals, these cells develop in the nasal placodes and migrate into the preoptic area and hypothalamus during early development. Typically, at least two forms of GnRH are found, but the second form (usually chicken GnRH-II, first isolated from chickens) functions primarily as a neurotransmitter or neuromodulator and probably influences reproductive behaviors rather than the HPG axis. Furthermore, many teleosts have three forms of GnRH present in the brain. A major difference occurs in the delivery of GnRH in teleostean fishes that lack a hypothalamo-hypophysial portal system between the hypothalamus and the pituitary and exhibit direct penetration of the adenohypophysis by GnRH axons. A portal delivery system also is lacking in the jawless fishes (agnathans), in which diffusion is the mode of delivery.

There are two distinct GTHs that are not directly homologous to mammalian FSH and LH. The first GTH, called GTH-I, is responsible for gonadal growth and gamete formation. The second, GTH-II, is involved with gamete release. Administration of sufficient amounts of either GTH can produce the effects of both, but they are secreted sequentially *in vivo*. Among the tetrapods (amphibians, reptiles, birds, and mammals), only the squamate reptiles (lizards, snakes) appear to have a single, FSH-like GTH, whereas all others produce both FSH-like and LH-like GTHs.

In general, testosterone is the major androgen produced in all vertebrates, and E_2 is the major estrogen. Many male teleosts also produce 11-ketotestosterone, and it is the predominant circulating androgen in many species. Female teleosts also produce testosterone, and circulating levels of testosterone may be as great as for E_2. Teleosts also produce important progesterone-like molecules, 17α,20β-P and 17,20β,21 trihydroxy-4-pregnen-3-one that cause final oocyte maturation and ovulation. It is secreted under the influence of GTH-II. This steroid may have pheromonal roles in mating as well. In some teleosts, the corticosteroid deoxycorticosterone produced by adrenocortical cells has been shown to induce final oocyte maturation and ovulation.

Tetrapods secrete testosterone, E_2, and progesterone, which all play reproductive roles similar to those observed in mammalian development and reproduction. A secondary androgen secreted by all tetrapods is DHT. Female amphibians, like teleosts, exhibit high levels of androgens as well as estrogens during the reproductive portions of their life histories, but normally androgens are not prominent in the blood of female reptiles and birds. Knowledge of the mechanisms for steroid actions on target cells and characteristics of steroid appear to be similar to mammalian systems, although there are several differences. For example, in addition to ER-α and ER-β, a third distinct subtype, ER-γ, has been identified in teleosts.

In addition, the teleost progestin receptor differs from its mammalian counterpart in its binding affinity for steroids and does not bind many EDCs that bind to the mammalian progesterone receptor. Thus, care must be taken in extrapolating the effects of EDCs across vertebrate taxa. Complete or partial sex reversals of the gonads can be caused by early exposure of eggs, larvae, or juvenile animals to estrogens or androgens, including many paradoxical effects such as feminization by androgens. Additionally, androgens usually inhibit female duct (Müllerian) development while enhancing male duct (Wolffian) development, whereas estrogens do the reverse. Androgens may enhance degeneration of the Müllerian ducts brought about by MIH or MIS. Estrogens are thought to protect oviducts from MIH, and paradoxical actions of androgens have also been reported. Clearly, endocrine disruptors that mimic estrogens or have antiandrogenic activity could potentially have drastic effects on wildlife exposed during development or as juveniles.

Estrogens can stimulate synthesis of ovalbumin protein by cells of the avian oviduct and also the synthesis of vitellogenins by the liver. Vitellogenins are precursors used by the ovaries to synthesize yolk proteins that are incorporated into eggs. The synthesis of vitellogenin (vitellogenesis) is a dramatic biomarker for estrogenic action in adult vertebrates that produce yolky eggs (fishes, amphibians, reptiles, and birds). Estrogens produce liver hyperplasia and hypertrophy as well as elevation of plasma vitellogenins. If males or immature females are exposed to estrogens, their livers also can be induced to produce vitellogenins. Thus, plasma vitellogenin can be used as a biomarker for exposure to environmental estrogens. In teleost fishes, amphibians, and birds, vitellogenesis is enhanced by PRL or GH, whereas in elasmobranchs, lizards, and turtles, PRL seems to play an inhibitory role. PRL also stimulates parental behaviors and may enhance estrogen-dependent secondary sex characters such as the avian brood patch.

Progesterone and progesteronelike hormones regulate nongenomic- based oocyte maturation in amphibians and teleost fishes, respectively, by binding to specific receptors on the cell surface. Oviductal secretion and the sensitivity of the amphibian oviduct to contract in the presence of arginine vasotocin are dependent on progesterone. Progesterone apparently slows development of the young in the viviparous frog *Nectophrynoides ocidentalis.* In turtles, progesterone decreases contractility as it does in mammals. The fact that steroids can induce rapid, cell-surface-mediated nongenomic actions by binding to specific receptors on the cell membrane has implications for the physiological processes they help regulate as well as their disruption by environmental chemicals.

THE HPA AXIS

This axis operates in a similar way to that illustrated for the HPG axis, the major differences being in the regulatory and secretory molecules involved. CRH is secreted from the terminals of hypothalamic neurons and acts on corticotropes in the anterior pituitary gland to regulate the synthesis and secretion of ACTH, which is then transported via the bloodstream to the adrenal glands, where it stimulates the secretion of glucocorticoid hormones (cortisol and/or corticosterone). The latter have numerous effects throughout the body, including important roles in metabolism of carbohydrate, protein and fat, anti-inflammatory effects, and modulation of stress responses. As in other endocrine axes, the products of the target cell, the glucocorticoids, exert negative feedback effects at the hypothalamic and pituitary level to suppress CRH secretion.

Similar to the sex steroid hormones, much of the glucocorticoid in circulation in blood is bound to a binding protein in the human (CBG), and local release of bioactive hormone from the CBG represents one mechanism of local tissue response to pro-inflammatory changes. Increasingly, it is recognized that glucocorticoids have important "programming" effects during development and that alterations in the circulating levels of these hormones can affect the timing and set points of other endocrine axes. For example, the multiple consequences of IUGR, including the short- and long-term consequences in terms of disease risk, are believed to be triggered largely by elevation of glucocorticoid levels in the fetus. Exposure to stresses or elevated glucocorticoid levels may have profound effects on brain development, as revealed by learning and memory deficits in adults. Early effects of handling newborn rats results in better regulatory control of the stress response as well as reduced cell losses in the hippocampus and less memory loss with aging. In contrast, elevated glucocorticoids in neonatal rats result in underdeveloped axonal growth as well as a reduction in myelination, formation of dendritic spines, and synaptogenesis, resulting in learning deficits and altered motor function.

There are a number of additional refinements/complexities to the HPA axis outlined above for mammals. Initially, the adrenal glands are a source of several other important hormones, including mineralocorticoids (which act on the kidney), opioid peptides, and enkephalins, as well as catecholamines, all of which have multiple effects throughout the body. Each of these secretions is regulated by mechanisms that are not related to the HPA axis. In the context of reproduction, the most important other products of the adrenal glands are the weak androgens DHEA, DHEA sulfate, and androstenedione, the secretion of which is also stimulated by ACTH.

These adrenal androgens may be converted in target tissues to more potent androgens or to estrogens (Figure 3) and can therefore potentially affect functioning of the reproductive endocrine axis and the cell types that are responsive to androgens and estrogens. Overproduction of adrenal androgens can have major consequences, including partial sex reversal of the female fetus when this occurs *in utero* or in the pregnant mother (above). In the human, adrenal androgens also play a role in early puberty (adrenarche) and are responsible for stimulation of pubic and axillary hair growth. At the hypothalamic-pituitary level, additional control of ACTH release may be exercised via arginine vasopressin.

The HPA Axis in Nonmammals

Nonmammalian steroidogenic tissue homologous to the mammalian adrenal cortex may be termed the interrenal gland, interrenal tissue, or simply interrenal. Hence, the HPA axis often is termed the hypothalamic-pituitary-interrenal axis, especially in fishes. This steroidogenic tissue is often referred to as "adrenocortical" to emphasize its homology to the adrenal cortex of mammals. The HPA axis of nonmammals, like that of mammals, is stimulated by an initial secretion of a hypothalamic CRH-like peptide, followed in turn by release of ACTH from the pituitary and then secretion of cortisol (most fishes) or corticosterone (most amphibians, birds, and reptiles) from the adrenocortical tissue. The HPA axis is important in regulating responses to stress and appears to have anti-immune actions similar to those described in mammals. The organism may adapt to the presence of the stressor with the hormones returning to normal levels. Prolonged stress may be associated with an increase in the activity of the HPA axis, sometimes producing chronically elevated cortisol or corticosterone. In extreme cases, this may lead to exhaustion of the HPA axis and death. Chronically stressed animals may exhibit an activated HPA axis but present with normal or only slightly elevated level of glucocorticoids.

Although many nonmammals have been shown to secrete a mammalian-like CRH, other CRH-like peptides have been discovered in fishes and mammals that can increase ACTH secretion as well. Mammalian ACTH seems to be effective at stimulating adrenocortical secretion in all vertebrates, reflecting the conservation of amino acid sequence among the vertebrates in these peptides we call ACTH. A unique corticosteroid, 1-hydroxycorticosterone, is found among the elasmobranch fishes (sharks, skates, and rays), although they also produce corticosterone. In teleostean fishes, cortisol functions both as a mineralocorticoid controlling Na+ and K+ balance and as a glucocorticoid.

Small amounts of corticosterone also have been described in the plasma of teleosts. Larval and aquatic amphibians, like teleosts, produce cortisol as their major corticosteroid, but terrestrial and semiterrestrial amphibians secrete corticosterone, as do all reptiles and birds. Although all tetrapods produce aldosterone, its role in salt balance is not well studied in nonmammals. Mammals have two generalized corticosteroid receptors located in different target cells, respectively, for glucocorticoids and mineralocorticoids. The number of receptor types for corticosteroids in other vertebrates has not been examined intensively.

THE HPT AXIS

This axis operates in a very similar way to that illustrated for the HPG axis. TRH is secreted from the terminals of hypothalamic neurons and acts on thyrotropes in the anterior pituitary gland to regulate the synthesis and secretion of TSH in mammals. TSH is then transported via the bloodstream to the thyroid gland, where it acts to stimulate the synthesis of T_3 and T_4, which are released into the bloodstream and act throughout the body to stimulate general metabolic activity. In practice, the main thyroid hormone released is T_4, although T_3 is biologically much more potent. In many target tissues, T_4 is metabolized to T_3, which then exerts its effects, another example of how a simple refinement to an endocrine axis can enable greater modulation and control according to local needs. Most of the circulating T_3 results from metabolic conversion of T_4 by a liver deiodinase. Circulating T_3/T_4 feeds back to the hypothalamus and anterior pituitary gland to negatively regulate TRH and TSH release, thus completing the classical endocrine negative feedback loop.

Most of the feedback at the level of the pituitary gland is due to T_4 that is converted to T_3 in the thyrotrope. At the top end of this circuit, there is an additional controlling factor, somatostatin, which is released from hypothalamic neurons and exerts negative control of TSH release from the anterior pituitary gland. Somatostatin also plays a key role in the (negative) regulation of GH secretion from the anterior pituitary gland. However, GH stimulates cell growth whereas TSH (via T_3/T_4) stimulates cell metabolism, showing that control of these two endocrine axes is interlinked at this level.

In the present context, interest in the thyroid endocrine axis stems from a) the demonstration that certain PCBs have antithyroidal activity, that is, can antagonize the effects of T_3/T_4 levels ; and b) the important role that the thyroid axis plays in terminal differentiation of various tissues, extending from neurons to muscle and to Sertoli cells in the testis. Many of the actions of thyroid hormones are permissive in that they affect the capacity of cells to respond to other stimuli. For example, the levels of the important enzyme adenyl cyclase, responsible for generation of the second-messenger cAMP in target cells for GH, is enhanced by thyroid hormones.

The HPT Axis in Nonmammals

The structure and functions of the HPT axis of nonmammals are very similar to those of mammals. The thyroid gland has a follicular arrangement, and the mechanisms of thyroid hormone synthesis and secretion as well as peripheral deiodination of T_4 to T_3 are very similar. Patterns of metabolic degradation and excretion also are similar. One major difference in bony fishes is the diffuse nature of the thyroid follicles that are not encapsulated by a connective tissue covering, such that individual follicles are distributed among the connective tissue elements between the second and fourth aortic arches. In some cases, thyroid follicles spread to other organs, including the kidney, liver, and gonads; hence, surgical thyroidectomy is not feasible in these animals. The major differences in hypothalamic and pituitary regulation reside at the hypothalamic level. TRH is not the major stimulator of TSH release in fishes and amphibians. It appears that CRH is the principal releaser of TSH in amphibians.

However, mammalian TSH is effective at stimulating iodide accumulation by the thyroid gland and secretion of thyroid hormones in all vertebrates. Thyroid hormones play critical roles in embryonic and postembryonic development of all vertebrates, especially as related to the nervous system. They are also important for the metamorphosis of larval fishes and amphibians into the juvenile body form. These actions not only bring about dramatic morphological changes but also involve biochemical adaptations related to marked changes in habitat and diets, that is, the roles of thyroid hormones and their interactions with PRL and corticosteroids in the smoltification of salmonid fishes and in amphibian metamorphosis. The parr-to-smolt transformation (smoltification) in juvenile salmonids fishes occurs prior to their seaward migration. Studies of coho salmon smoltification have documented two- to sixfold transient increases in T_4 and cortisol, respectively, during this time as well as early surges in insulin and PRL. GH also increases and levels remain elevated in smolts.

In larval amphibians, metamorphosis to the juvenile body form involves transient increases in thyroid hormones and corticosteroids as well as a late, brief rise in PRL. In addition, specific changes in the types of deiodinase enzymes result in decreasing conversion of T_4 to the inactive metabolite reverse T_3 and increases conversion of T_4 to the more active T_3. Additionally, changes in thyroid hormone receptor types also occur during metamorphosis. Numerous gene products are up-regulated by thyroid hormones in responding tissues, and a few are down-regulated during metamorphosis.

Shedding of skin in salamanders and in reptiles is controlled by thyroid hormones. In contrast, thyroid hormones augment feather loss in birds, which is stimulated by gonadal steroids. These effects of thyroid hormones are similar to their effects on hair replacement in mammals. Thyroid hormones also work synergistically with GH to provide maximal growth rates in fishes, adult amphibians, birds, and possibly reptiles, although the latter have been less studied. Finally, thyroid hormones are important stimulators of sexual maturation and are essential for seasonal reproductive events in a wide variety of animals. The roles of thyroid hormones in controlling metabolic rates, body temperature, and thermogenesis evolved independently in accordance with homeothermy in both mammals and birds, and these hormones do not play similar roles in fishes, amphibians, and reptiles.

THE PINEAL GLAND

In mammals, the pineal gland is located above the thalamus of the brain between the cerebral cortices. Through its nocturnal secretion of the biogenic amine melatonin, the pineal has effects on the regulation of many internal physiological rhythms and may provide an important clue for translating photoperiodic stimuli into action. Furthermore, melatonin can alter coat pigmentation and hair growth; can inhibit hypothalamic regulation of the HPA, HPT, and HPG axes; and has been shown to enhance the immune response system. Photic input in birds and mammals is accomplished primarily via the optic visual system. However, the pineal of most fishes, amphibians, and reptiles also plays an important role as a direct photoreceptor, and through secretion of melatonin, it may be an important modulator of the HPA, HPT, and HPG axes as well. Any environmental factor that alters pineal function may have profound effects on the well-being of vertebrates.

Interactions of the HPG Axis with Other Endocrine Systems

The various endocrine axes of the body do not function as isolated islands, as this would clearly compromise the ability of an organism to react and adapt to changing circumstances, for example, season, food supply, and presence of predators. Various components of other endocrine axes are able to exert important modulatory effects on the HPG axis to alter the timing or efficiency of reproduction. The complexity of such interactions is illustrated in Figure 4, which highlights some of the overlapping cross talk. To give further insight into the function and complexity of these interactions, four additional points (with examples) are emphasized.

GROWTH IN UNDERSTANDING OF ENDOCRINE SYSTEMS

New pathways of communication and functional overlap between the various endocrine systems are still being discovered. One example is the relatively recent discovery of leptin following studies of the genetically obese (*ob/ob*) mouse. This hormone is produced by adipocytes and exerts important effects on feelings of satiety and hunger and on the appropriate behaviors such as feeding. As fat cell energy reserves are an important component of the insulin-glucose endocrine system, it is known that insulin can exert both direct and indirect (i.e., by altering fat deposition) effects on leptin levels (Figure 4).

There are also important interactions between leptin and the reproductive system. An animal reproduces only when the mother has appropriate energy reserves and food supply is good. Leptin provides the necessary signal that unites these various components. When food supply and maternal energy (= fat) reserves are low, elevated leptin can suppress function of the reproductive system. Such pathways play an important role in the timing/initiation of puberty, in regulation of seasonal reproduction, and in certain diseases, for example, the cessation of normal menstrual cycles in women with eating disorders such as anorexia.

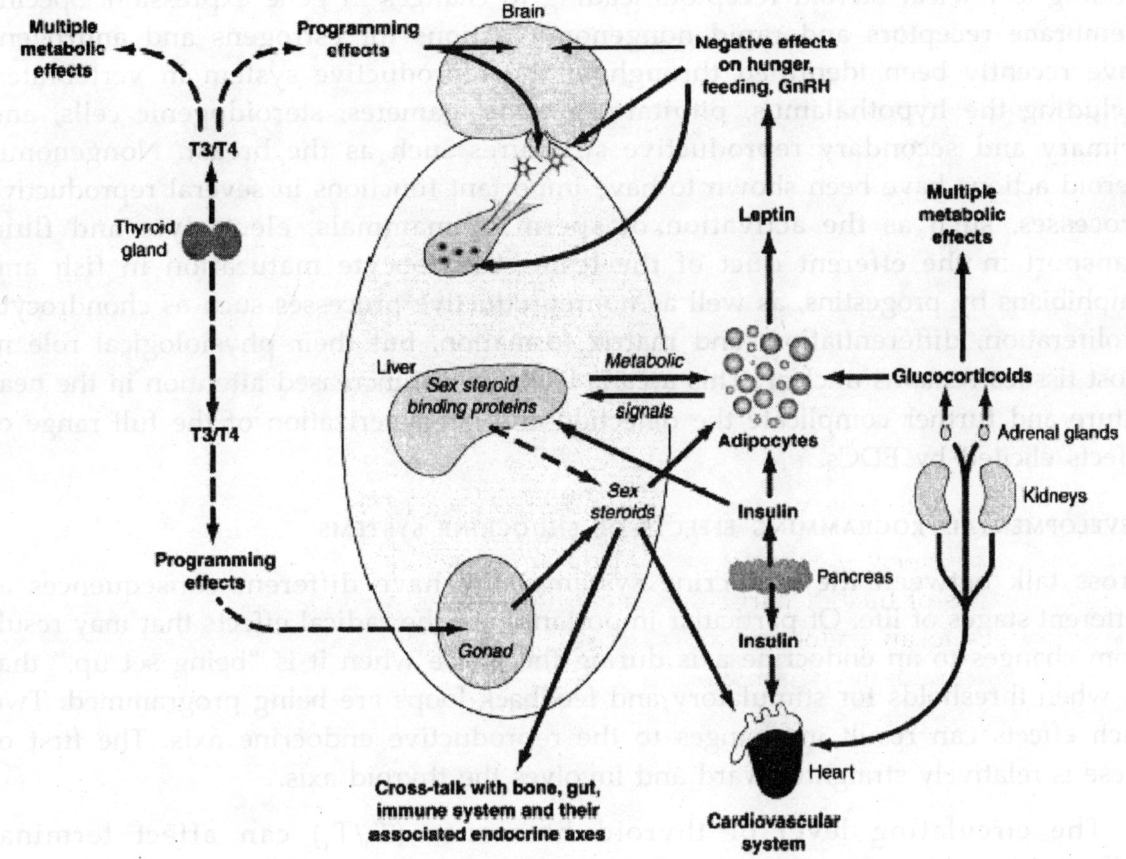

Figure 4. Schematic diagram to illustrate some of the cross talk (integration), which occurs between the mammalian HPG axis (center, shaded) and some of the other endocrine axes of the body. Note that only selective examples are shown and that, in reality, each endocrine axis interacts at multiple levels with other endocrine axes in order to integrate all bodily functions. An important consequence of this complex cross talk is that changes induced in one endocrine axis are likely to lead to changes in other endocrine axes and that such effects can be difficult to predict because of our imperfect understanding of these interactions.

Although the existence and implications for leptin in nonmammalian vertebrates remain to be explored, the importance of nutritional state to reproduction is known to be as critical as the relationship described in mammals and may exist in all vertebrates.

Another recently recognized complexity of the endocrine system involves the capability of steroids to exert rapid, nongenomic actions by binding to receptors on the cell surface of target cells and activating signal transduction pathways leading to biological responses, in addition to effects mediated by the classic mechanisms of binding to nuclear steroid receptors leading to changes in gene expression. Specific membrane receptors and rapid nongenomic actions for estrogens and androgens have recently been identified throughout the reproductive system in vertebrates, including the hypothalamus, pituitary, gonads, gametes, steroidogenic cells, and primary and secondary reproductive structures such as the breast. Nongenomic steroid actions have been shown to have important functions in several reproductive processes, such as the activation of sperm in mammals, electrolyte and fluid transport in the efferent duct of the testes, and oocyte maturation in fish and amphibians by progestins, as well as nonreproductive processes such as chondrocyte proliferation, differentiation, and matrix formation, but their physiological role in most tissues remains unclear. This area is likely to see increased attention in the near future and further complicate the detection and characterization of the full range of effects elicited by EDCs.

DEVELOPMENTAL/PROGRAMMING EFFECTS OF ENDOCRINE SYSTEMS

Cross talk between the endocrine systems may have different consequences at different stages of life. Of particular importance are the radical effects that may result from changes to an endocrine axis during the phase when it is "being set up," that is, when thresholds for stimulatory and feedback loops are being programmed. Two such effects can result in changes to the reproductive endocrine axis. The first of these is relatively straightforward and involves the thyroid axis.

The circulating level of thyroid hormones (T_3/T_4) can affect terminal differentiation of various tissues (e.g., neurons, muscle cells), and recent studies show that this extends to Sertoli cells in the male. Conversion of the Sertoli cell from an immature, proliferative cell to a mature, nonproliferating cell ready to support spermatogenesis is triggered by thyroid hormone levels in the prepubertal period. Subnormal levels of T_3/T_4 (hypothyroidism) result in prolongation of the Sertoli cell proliferative phase, whereas conversely, supranormal levels of T_3/T_4 (hyperthyroidism) attenuate the Sertoli cell proliferative phase.

The net result of such changes is to alter (up or down, respectively) final Sertoli cell number and thereby to alter final testis size and the number of sperm produced per day, because each Sertoli cell can support only a finite number of germ cells. Hypoand hyperthyroidism have many other consequences in terms of altered body growth and brain development (Figure 4), emphasizing again the pleiotropic effects that result from altered function of any individual endocrine axis. In addition to cross talk, thyroid hormones have important direct effects on differentiation of the brain as well as on its level of activity in adult animals.

In humans, thyroid deficiencies during gestation or immediately postnatally can produce irreversible mental retardation. Another, more subtle example of the dramatic consequences of "programming" cross talk between endocrine axes is that of IUGR, which has already been referred to in brief. Small-for-gestational-age offspring are "insulin resistant" as a result of their growth restriction *in utero* and have dramatically lower fat reserves and leptin levels at birth. Such offspring usually exhibit catch-up growth, presumably because of their adapted endocrine changes but remain permanently hyperinsulinemic and insulin resistant. In humans, such individuals are at increased risk of developing diabetes and becoming obese.

Such individuals are also hypertensive and are thus at increased risk of cardiovascular disease, strokes, and kidney disease unrelated to any obesity. The reproductive system is also affected in an adverse way. In the human, IUGR male offspring are at increased risk of cryptorchidism and hypospadias at birth and of developing testicular germ cell cancer and having low sperm counts in adulthood. Exactly how these changes are induced is unclear but may involve alterations in sex steroid levels. One possible pathway is illustrated in Figure 5.

It is now well established that hyperinsulinemia results in considerably reduced secretion of SHBG by the liver and a consequent rise in the circulating levels of free (biologically active) sex steroids, and because androgens bind more strongly to SHBG than do estrogens, the androgen/estrogen ratio will be altered. This is dramatically evident in one common disorder of women, polycystic ovarian disease. Such individuals are hyperinsulinemic and have supranormal blood androgen levels that lead to hirsutism as well as polycystic ovaries and anovulatory infertility. A common risk factor for developing this condition is IUGR.

NONREPRODUCTIVE EFFECTS OF SEX STEROIDS

Changes in SHBG resulting from hyperinsulinemia lead to altered androgen and estrogen bioactivity, which, predictably, can alter function of the reproductive system. However, the sex steroids (in particular, estrogens) also exert multiple other effects throughout the body. Estrogens (and, to a lesser extent, androgens) play a key role in bone formation/resorption in males and females, and estrogen action is essential for epiphyseal closure. Disorders of sex steroid production or action can lead to osteoporosis or to premature/delayed epiphyseal closure, with consequent effects on final height/body length. Additionally, the sex steroids exert pervasive effects on the cardiovascular system and, in the human, are clearly implicated in gender- and age-dependent changes in risk of developing cardiovascular disease. Multiple effects of the sex steroids on the brain, digestive system, immune system, and adipose tissue also occur and, in so doing, will interact with or modulate other endocrine axes that target these tissues. Direct or indirect effects on the HPG axis that result in changes in the absolute or relative levels of androgens and estrogens can have pervasive consequences. These effects can be acute/transient (e.g., pituitary feedback effects) or chronic (e.g., bone and cardiovascular effects) in the adult, whereas in the fetus/neonate, any effects that occur may be permanent (e.g., sexual differentiation).

ENDOCRINE CROSS TALK AND ENDOCRINE DISRUPTORS

It is emphasized that the prediction of the reproductive consequences of a given chemical from its known sex steroid hormone activity or inactivity is far from straightforward. For example, a dietary change that affects insulin levels (e.g., ingestion of a diet rich in refined sugars) has the potential to alter sex steroid hormone bioactivity via altered production of SHBG (Figure 5), but it would not be claimed that refined sugars have sex steroid hormone activity. Even when an environmental chemical is shown to have (weak) steroid hormone activity, it can possess other relevant activities.

Thus, the thyroidal activity of PCBs may be as important or even more important than the weak estrogenic/antiestrogenic effects of these compounds when considering their potential impact on the reproductive system. Other environmental chemicals may have antiandrogenic as well as estrogenic effects (e.g., DDT isomers, certain phthalates), which may confuse interpretation of potency *in vivo*. For example, administration of antiandrogens is likely to elevate endogenous estrogen levels. This occurs because antiandrogens block negative feedback loops, which leads to compensatory elevation of LH levels and thus to supranormal elevation of testosterone levels, with a consequent increase in availability of substrate for aromatization (Figure 3). If androgens positively regulate aromatase expression, as various studies suggest, further elevation of estrogen levels will occur.

Thus, the overall "estrogenic" activity of PCBs, DDT, or phthalates *in vivo* could not be predicted from measurement of their activity in any *in vitro* estrogen screening system. Some estrogens are agonists in one tissue and antagonists in another (e.g., tamoxifen, raloxifene), and emerging understanding suggests that the same will hold true for androgens. Although the basis for these differences is not understood completely, it is clear that tissuespecific expression of co-activator proteins (or adapters) is involved and, in the case of estrogens, whether ER-α and/or ER-β is expressed. As some co-activators may be shared between various members of the steroid receptor superfamily, action of one member might alter availability of co-activators to interact with androgenor estrogen-receptor complexes. Alternatively, nonreproductive hormones might regulate the expression of these co-activators. Although these possibilities are speculative, the insights afforded by tamoxifen, raloxifene, and other emerging SERMs emphasize the unpredictable pathways by which sex steroid hormone action can be altered.

Based on the considerations detailed above, it is clear that chemicals should be tested for their "reproductive" activity (i.e., the ability to alter the development or the function of the reproductive system) rather than just for their sex steroid activity in *in vitro* tests systems if the objective is to establish whether or not the compound in question is a reproductive endocrine disruptor.

EDC-RELATED TOXICITIES

As expected from the normal functioning of endocrine systems, the cellular and molecular mechanisms of endocrine disruption are not limited to receptor binding and include, for example, inhibition of hormone synthesis, metabolism, and transport. Figure 6 displays some of the mechanisms of steroid hormone action, as an example, and provides key steps in the process where EDCs have been shown to alter endocrine function. Other sites in the signal transduction process are also likely to be susceptible to disruption by anthropogenic chemicals.

Considerable homology exists in the endocrinology of vertebrates; hence, toxicants that alter endocrine function in one species are likely to produce adverse effects in another. However, there are significant differences between some species in endocrine function that warrant consideration for further interspecies extrapolations. Although the hormones, hormone synthesis, and their receptors are highly conserved, the role of specific hormones in reproductive function and development can vary greatly. Additionally, significant differences in metabolism of EDCs can result in marked species differences in responses to these chemicals.

AR-Mediated (Anti) Androgens

Vinclozolin. It is generally assumed that mammals possess a single AR, as evidenced by the complete phenotypic sex reversal displayed in humans with androgen insufficiency syndrome as a consequence of a single base substitution in the AR. Vinclozolin is a dicarboximide fungicide with AR antagonism. Of the EDCs, the cellular and molecular mechanisms of action of the antiandrogenic fungicide vinclozolin are one of the most thoroughly characterized. Vinclozolin metabolites $M_1$and M_2 competitively inhibit the binding of androgens to the mammalian AR. $M_1$and M_2 also inhibit DHT-induced transcriptional activity in cells transfected with the human AR. Kelce et al. demonstrated that vinclozolin treatment altered gene expression *in vivo* in an antiandrogenic manner. In contrast to the binding to the AR, neither vinclozolin nor its antiandrogenic metabolites display affinity for the ER, although they do have weak affinity for the progesterone receptor. Vinclozolin, M1, and M_2 do not inhibit 5α-reductase activity *in vitro*, the enzyme required for the conversion of testosterone to the more active androgen DHT. A comparison of the *in vivo* and *in vitro* dosimetry data with the biological effects of vinclozolin reveals that when $M_1$and M_2 concentrations in maternal serum approach their respective *Ki* values for AR binding, male offspring are malformed.

Change in blood levels of SHBG

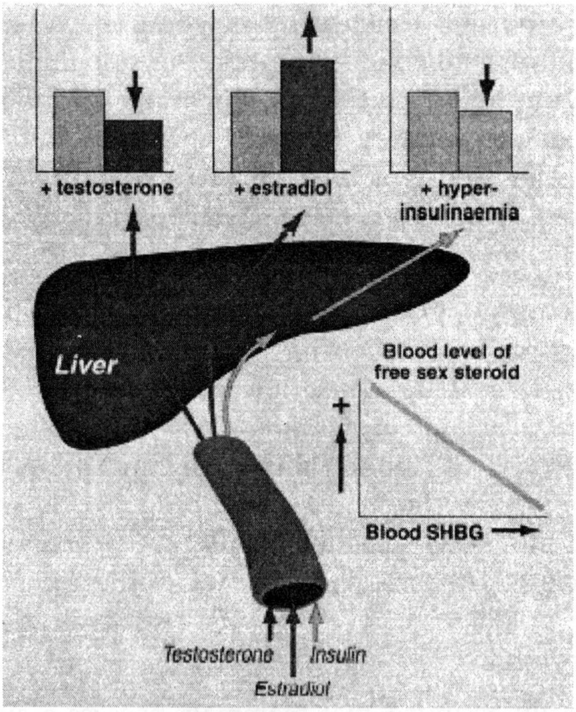

Figure 5. Diagrammatic illustration of one potentially important example of cross talk between endocrine axes in the human with particular relevance to endocrine disruption.

The ability of $M_1$and M_2 to inhibit AR-dependent gene expression has been demonstrated both *in vitro* and *in vivo*. In addition, vinclozolin inhibits growth of androgen-dependent tissues in the castrate-immature-testosterone-treated male rat, a further demonstration of its antiandrogenic action *in vivo*. The drug flutamide is metabolically activated to hydroxyflutamide, which is similar in structure to the vinclozolin metabolite M_2 and exhibits endocrine activity that is nearly identical to vinclozolin or M_2, respectively.

In addition to their antiandrogenic effects on the reproductive tract, vinclozolin and flutamide alter reproductive function at the level of the hypothalamic-pituitary axis. Oral treatment with vinclozolin or flutamide causes elevations of serum LH and testosterone levels and Leydig cell hyperplasia. In contrast to vinclozolin and flutamide, treatment with *p,p'*-DDE or MXC, which are also antiandrogenic, fails to induce any significant change in serum LH or testosterone levels. A wide variety of antiandrogenic teratogenic effects in male offspring are noted following late gestational exposure to dose levels of vinclozolin in the range of 3-200 mg/kg/day. These include a femalelike AGD, retained nipples, cleft phallus with hypospadias, suprainguinal ectopic testes, vaginal pouch, epididymal granulomas and small or absent accessory sex glands and delays in preputial separation.

In a study of the low-dose effects of vinclozolin, pregnant rats were exposed to between 3 and 100 mg/kg/day from gestation day 14 to postnatal day 3. Even the lowest dose group (3.125 mg/kg/day) produced significant effects on AGD and retention of nipples in male offspring. Malformations of the male reproductive tract were observed at 50 and 100 mg/kg/day. Even though all of these end points (reduced AGD, retained nipples, effects on accessory sex gland weight, hypospadias, epididymal agenesis) are believed to be elicited by interference at the level of the AR, they display a wide variety of effective dose levels producing statistically significant changes. Some of these changes do not exhibit an obvious threshold in the range of the experimental dose levels. Multigenerational studies are essential to detect subtle antiandrogenic effects on male reproduction, and a failure to utilize the new testing guidelines (which incorporate new antiandrogenic measures) could yield NOAELs at least an order of magnitude too high.

Dermal exposure of adolescent rabbits to 100 mg/kg of vinclozolin for 2 months resulted in reduced accessory gland weights, but sperm counts were significantly elevated. The authors suggested that the antiandrogenic effects may have blocked the negative feedback of testosterone on the hypothalamus or pituitary allowing for increased gonadotropin release.

Several other toxic substances have been shown to display AR-antagonist activity, including the DDT metabolite DDE, the MXC metabolite HPTE, the organophosphate fenitrothion, and the dicarboximide fungicide procymidone. Linuron is a urea-based herbicide that displays weak affinity for the AR, but the effects induced in male offspring indicate that it may alter mammalian sex differentiation via more than one mechanism of action. In this regard, the phytoantiandrogenic drug permixon, used clinically for prostate problems, appears to bind AR and inhibit steroid hormone synthesis as well. Tris(4-chlorophenyl)methanol is a global contaminant of unknown origin that is structurally related to DDT, has binding affinity for the AR comparable to *p,p´*-DDE. However, it has not demonstrated antiandrogenic effects *in vivo* when sexually mature rats were exposed for 28 days at doses up to 100 ppm in the diet.

Sexual dimorphisms in fish have been demonstrated to be affected by both androgens and estrogens. For example, Smith demonstrated that the formation of breeding tubercles and a mucus-secreting dorsal pad in the fathead minnow is inducible by 17α-methyltestosterone. When aromatizable (testosterone and 17α-methyltestosterone) and nonaromatizable (11-ketotestosterone and 17α-methyl-DHT) were administered to newly hatched genotypic female chinook salmon for 2 hours, dose-dependent sex reversal was observed, with the synthetic and nonaromatizable forms more potent than the natural or aromatizable forms, thus indicating a role for aromatase early in development.

Predominantly male populations of tilapia can be produced on a commercial scale by feeding androgens to fry. Administration of 25 mg of trenboline acetate for 28 days to sexually undifferentiated *Oncorhynchus aureus* resulted in 98% phenotypic males (vs. 55.7% males in the control group; higher exposures yielded lower percentages of males, presumably due to the less potent antiestrogenic activity. In similarly treated channel catfish, Davis et al. found evidence that adults were lighter and shorter and had smaller gonads and GSI and lower plasma testosterone as adults than did control males. When the reproductively mature fathead minnows were exposed to methyltestosterone for 21 days, a decrease in plasma concentrations of sex steroids and adversely affected gonadal status (as evidenced by relative weight and histopathology) was observed in both sexes. The androgenic nature of methyltestosterone was clearly evidenced by masculinization of exposed females.

Vitellogenin induction was observed in both sexes, probably as result of aromatization of the administered androgen. Although mammals are believed to possess a single AR, some piscivorous species have two ARs, termed $AR_1$and AR_2. AR_1in the brain displays binding affinities for ligands quite distinct from AR_2, which has similar ligand affinities to mammalian AR. AR_2 has been shown to bind *p,p´*-DDE and vinclozolin metabolites $M_1$and M_2, demonstrating the homology of AR function *in vitro* among diverse species of vertebrates. *In vivo*, vinclozolin treatment induces intersex in the medaka (*Oryzias latipes*), which displays a mammalian-type sex differentiation. In contrast, Makynen et al. did not obtain sex reversal in the fathead minnow with vinclozolin treatment. This may be related to several factors, including a lack of metabolic activation of vinclozolin and the undefined role for androgens in the sex differentiation process. However, in contrast to the results cited above, $M_1$and M_2 did not bind AR in this species.

Takeo and Yamashita described two distinct rainbow trout cDNA clones, which were designated rtAR-α and rtAR-β, that contain the entire AR coding region. Comparison of the predicted amino acid sequence of rtAR-α to that of rtAR-β revealed 85% identity. Despite this high homology, rtAR-α activated transcription of an androgen-responsive reporter gene in cotransfection assays, but rtAR-β did not, suggesting that rainbow trout contains two distinct isoforms of ARs whose functions differ.

Ikeuchi et al. identified 11-ketotestosterone (a potent androgen in teleosts) as the spermatogenesis-inducing hormone of the Japanese eel and cloned its receptor (eAR1) cDNA from eel testis, and also reported that they cloned a second type of AR (eAR_2) from the eel testis, encoding 797 amino acid residues. The amino acid sequence of eAR_2 shows high homology with other ARs, including eAR_1, in the DNA-binding (98-88%) and ligand-binding (59-85%) domains, whereas the other domains show low homology. In transient transfection assays of mammalian cells, the eAR_2 displayed androgen-dependent activation of transcription from the androgen-responsive murine mammary tumor virus promoter. Tissue distribution of its mRNA differed from that of eAR_1.

The degree to which the differences in amino acid sequences in the ligand binding domain between ARs of lower vertebrates and mammalian AR affect binding of natural and synthetic ligands remains to be determined. Although it is clear that differences in overall sequence homology of this region exist, it appears that the amino acids in the binding pocket of the human AR that result in loss of function when mutated are more highly conserved in the fish ARs than are other amino acids in this domain.

Other sites of action of antiandrogens: liver and adrenal. Although vinclozolin and its metabolites do not bind the glucocorticoid receptor, vinclozolin treatment has been shown to alter the pituitary-adrenal axis in several mammalian species, including rats and dogs. Indeed, the former no adverse effect level (NOAEL) was established on the effects of vinclozolin on the canine adrenal gland. The effects of vinclozolin and flutamide on liver function are also noteworthy. Although the mechanism of action for the hepatic effects of these antiandrogens has not been elucidated, androgens and antiandrogens acting via the AR are known to alter several aspects of liver growth and metabolism. In particular, cyproterone acetate, a drug that has antiandrogenic, progestational, and antiglucocorticoid activity, also acts as a liver mitogen. The mechanisms of action of vinclozolin and flutamide on the liver warrant study, as these chemicals induce adverse effects with long-term treatment (flutamide-induced morbidity due to liver failure and vinclozolin-induced liver tumors in male rats).

ER-Mediated Estrogens

The ability of pesticides to act as estrogen agonists, inducing a uterotropic response, has been known for over 30 years, and the estrogenicity of anthropogenic chemicals, for example, bisphenol A and DES, were first described in 1938. Many estrogens have been identified using *in vitro* assays (e.g., ER binding, breast cancer cell proliferation, and transcriptional activation), and several also display estrogenic activity *in vivo,* including MXC, chlordecone, octylphenol, nonylphenol, bisphenol A and B, phytoestrogens (genistein), ethynyl estradiol, and fungal mycotoxins (zearalenone). Other chemicals that have shown evidence *in vitro* of estrogenic activity have not shown similar evidence in *in vivo* systems, and caution is warranted in interpreting *in vitro* results without *in vivo* confirmation. *In vitro,* some estrogens, such as bisphenol A and E_2, have been reported to interact in an unanticipated manner, with bisphenol A antagonizing some of the effects of E_2.

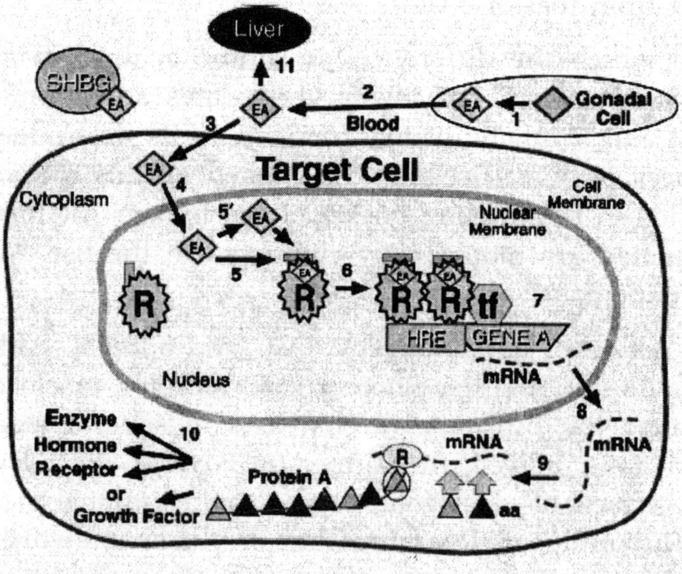

Figure 6. Schematic diagram depicting several key steps in steroid hormone action that may be sensitive to disruption by environmental chemicals

Phytoestrogens present in a variety of plants such as soy (isoflavanoids) and berries, fruits, grains, vegetables, and nuts (lignans) represent another source of exposure to estrogenic chemicals. Binding studies show that isoflavanoid phytoestrogens are high-affinity ligands for ERs, especially ER-β, but have lower potencies *in vitro* cell-based assays. *In vivo* data indicate that phytoestrogens have a wide range of biologic effects at doses and plasma concentrations seen with normal human diets. *In vivo* data effects have been reported for bone, ovary, pituitary, vasculature, prostate, and serum lipids. Effective doses in humans (0.4-10 mg/kg/day) are generally lower than those causing effects in rodents (10-100 mg/kg/day), although careful pharmacokinetic comparisons of circulating dose are not available to truly compare the species sensitivity.

MXC: An Estrogenic and Antiandrogenic Pesticide

The estrogenic pesticide MXC is still in commercial use. This DDT derivative usually does not bioaccumulate because it can be metabolized by some species more readily than the metabolites of DDT. MXC provides an example of the multiplicity of EDC action because it is an ER-α agonist, an ER-β antagonist), and an AR antagonist. *In vivo*, MXC displays estrogenic ER-α-mediated activity in many tissues, including the uterus, vagina, brain (behavior), and bone, but not in the hypothalamic-pituitary axis. MXC treatment failed to induce hyperprolactinemia, inhibit LH, or induce pituitary tumors in the rat after long-term high-dose treatment.

In the adult and pubertal male rat, MXC antagonizes the effects of androgens, which may indicate that MXC metabolites are inhibiting testosterone and DHT-induced gene expression and tissue growth and differentiation, as some of these tissues lack ER. Many natural and anthropogenic estrogens display affinity for AR, acting as AR antagonists and agonists in *in vitro* assays, albeit often at high concentrations. MXC itself is weakly active or inactive *in vitro* in ER binding and transcriptional activation assays. Purer forms of MXC (>99%) are inactive compared with less pure MXC (>95% pure).

MXC is metabolically activated to several monohydroxy and dihydroxy metabolites that display estrogenic activity. One of these, HPTE also is a relatively potent AR and ER-β antagonist as well as an ER-α agonist. Treatment of adult male rats with MXC alters fertility at very high doses by the inhibition of spermatogenesis; lower dose levels (~25-200 mg/kg/day) reduce epididymal sperm reserves and seminal vesicle weight without affecting sperm production, testicular morphology, or serum testosterone levels. If treatment is administered at weaning, MXC will induce a number of effects in male offspring, including delays in puberty and reduced accessory sex gland weights. In the adult female, MXC induces effects more typical of an estrogen, with induction of lordosis. There were no effects on circulating LH or testosterone in the presence of delayed puberty, but there was an elevation in serum PRL. The lack of an effect on LH may be suggestive that, rather than working through the pituitary, the agent may have a direct effect on the reproductive tract.

In longer term exposure, dosing of MXC for 10 months (200-400 mg/kg/day) to male rats delayed puberty by up to 10 weeks, reduced fertility, and altered reproductive behavior but did not mimic the chronic sustained effects of E_2 given via Silastic implants. In a study in which MXC was given to female rats by gavage at 0, 5, 50, or 150 mg/kg/day for the week before and the week after birth, with the pups then directly dosed with MXC from postnatal day 7, the high dose of MXC reduced litter size by approximately 17%. AGD was unchanged, although male prepuce separation was delayed at the middle and high doses by 8 and 34 days, respectively. High-dose males impregnated fewer untreated females; epididymal sperm count and testis weight were reduced at the high and top two doses, respectively. Female effects (vaginal opening, estrous cyclicity) were noted at 50 mg/kg/day and above.

Mechanisms of action of xenoestrogens in other vertebrates.

Several of the xenoestrogens bind one of the fish ERs with affinity similar to that displayed for mammalian ER. Octylphenol, nonylphenol, bisphenol A, *o,p*-DDT, ethynyl estradiol, and MXC display estrogenic activity in lower vertebrates (i.e., fish and frogs). In avian and mammalian species, *o,p′*-DDT, but not *p,p*-DDT, induced growth of the female reproductive tract.

Some of these xenoestrogens induce gonadal intersex, vitellogenin synthesis in males, and hermaphroditism and estrogen-dependent sexual dimorphisms. The toxicants that induce estrogen-dependent changes in coloration in the African reed frog are remarkably similar to those that induce a uterotropic response in the female rat, indicating a high degree of homology in ER-α function despite the differences in ER sequence.

In contrast, the estrogenicity of MXC is likely to be as widespread throughout the animal kingdom because it will not be estrogenic in those lower vertebrate species that are unable to metabolically activate it. Hydroxylation of MXC is required for estrogenicity and for excretion; hence, these species that cannot metabolically active MXC have a tendency to bioaccumulate this pesticide to the same degree as DDT. In male catfish pretreated with MXC or BNF alone or in combination, pretreatment with MXC but not BNF significantly reduced rates of MXC biotransformation, and pretreatment with MXC/BNF followed by MXC significantly induced serum vitellogenin, whereas MXC alone did not significantly elevate vitellogenin, thus demonstrating in this species that MXC can elicit estrogenic activity despite diminished capacity to form estrogenic metabolites. In a short-term reproduction test with the fathead minnow (*Pimepehales promelas*) initiated with reproductively mature animals exposed for up to 21 days, MXC decreased plasma concentrations of one or more steroids (testosterone, 11-ketotestosterone, E_2) in both sexes and caused a significant induction of plasma vitellogenin in males. A significant decrease in fecundity was also observed at the same concentration that induced vitellogenin (3.56 μg/liter).

Continuous exposure of adult male sheepshead minnow (*Cyprinodin variegates*) to *p*-nonylphenol, MXC, or endosulfan for up to 42 days was observed to induce a dose-dependent increase in hepatic vitellogenin mRNA and plasma protein within 5 days of exposure to all but endosulfan. The fact that MXC, but not its estrogenic metabolite HPTE, alters amphibian germinal vesicle breakdown, which is dependent upon cell-surface hydroxyprogesterone receptor activation, indicates that this effect is not mediated by the ER. Recent studies have shown that a variety of xenobiotic chemicals, in addition the disrupting genomic steroid actions, can also interfere with the nongenomic actions of steroids. The finding that low concentrations (100 nM, equivalent to 30-40 ppb) of the estrogenic compounds kepone and *o,p′*-DDE interfered with progestogen induction of meiotic maturation of Atlantic croaker oocytes *in vitro* provided initial evidence for this novel type of endocrine disruption.

Subsequently, disruption of oocyte maturation by estrogenic compounds was confirmed in an amphibian species, *Xenopus*, exposed to MXC. In addition, kepone was shown to partially block the stimulatory actions of progestogens on sperm motility in Atlantic croaker. Estrogenic compounds such as *o,p.*-DDT and nonylphenol have also been shown to exert rapid estrogenic (agonistic) actions on rat smooth muscle cells and on croaker testicular androgen production. Recently, direct evidence has been obtained that estrogenic compounds can disrupt nongenomic steroid actions by receptormediated mechanisms. Competition studies have shown that these compounds bind to the progestogen membrane receptors on fish oocytes and sperm and to the estrogen membrane receptor in fish testes as well as disrupting nongenomic steroid actions in these tissues.

When a genetically male population of the common carp (*Cyprinus carpio*) was exposed to 4-*tert*-pentylphenol, no effects on sexual differentiation or proliferation of primordial germ cells were evident following 3 days of exposure during the embryo-larval period. However, longer exposures, starting before and including sexual differentiation, induced the formation of an oviduct that was persistent upon returning to clean water. Exposure during these times (days 24-51 posthatch) reduced the number of primordial germ cells. Bisphenol A was observed to increase vitellogenin levels in male rainbow trout (*O. mykiss*) following 14 days of exposure to 500 μg/liter, whereas constant or decreasing levels were present at lower exposure levels. However, the ratio of responding to nonresponding animals indicated that levels as low as 70 μg/liter were effective. Average liver concentration at the 500 μg/liter exposure level was 4.36 μg/g.

INHIBITORS OF STEROID HORMONE SYNTHESIS

Several classes of fungicides have been developed to inhibit fungal membrane synthesis and growth by inhibiting specific CYP450 enzymes, especially 14α demethylation of lanosterol, in the sterol pathways. The process of steroidogenesis is sufficiently conserved that these chemicals can also inhibit mammalian steroidogenesis. There are several CYP450 enzymes in the steroid pathway, and the binding affinity for each varies from chemical to chemical. In general, however, at relatively high concentrations, these are nonspecific inhibitors of CYP450 enzymes. Hence, effects are not limited to the reproductive system and include adrenal and liver steroid metabolism in mammals and ecdysteroid synthesis in invertebrates.

Ketoconazole

The antifungal imidazole derivative ketoconazole inhibits various enzymes that belong to the CYP450-dependent mono-oxygenases in rodents and humans such as side chain cleavage of cholesterol and 11β-hydroxylase in the adrenal and 17α-hydroxylase and C17-20 lyase in rat and human testes. For example, human testicular mono-oxygenase activities *in vitro* are reduced by 50% by 3.1 μM ketoconazole. Side effects of the use of ketoconazole as a therapeutic antiandrogen include gynecomastia.

However, the effects on steroidogenesis are not selective for the testis, with ovary and adrenal effects reported. Effects on adult Leydig cell function have been noted in humans and rodents *in vitro*. When administered to adult rodents, ketoconazole can have dramatic effects on fertility even after a single dose. It is more difficult to observe effects on male reproductive development resulting from a decreased testosterone production, as other effects on ovarian and uterine steroid responses tend to interfere with pregnancy maintenance. Treatment of pregnant dams with ketoconazole is more likely to affect the ability to maintain pregnancy due to effects on ovarian progesterone synthesis resulting in abortion/litter loss that would preclude the observation of marked effects on the pups.

Aromatase inhibitors

Aromatase CYP450 converts C19 androgens to aromatic C18 estrogens. A number of pharmaceutical agents have been developed that inhibit aromatase, which have been applied as treatment for postmenopausal breast cancer. This P450 enzyme is highly conserved in a wide variety of tissues and many species, but the overall homology of the genes (as there is more than one gene) with other CYP450s is only about 30%. Hence, this enzyme is considered to be in a separate gene family within the overall superfamily. A consequence of the lack of sequence homology with other P450 enzymes in the steroid pathway, inhibitors of aromatase may display greater specificity than drugs such as ketaconazole.

A yeast-based screening assay has been proposed to test for this activity. The induction of imposex in mollusks exposed to tributyl tin has been linked to inhibition of aromatase and subsequent estrogen deficiency and enhanced androgen levels. Several fungicides inhibit aromatase activity in mammals, resulting in infertility in both sexes. Fenarimol treatment inhibits male rat mating behavior, presumably by inhibiting the conversion of androgens to estrogens in the brain, and also inhibits parturition because of the critical role of E_2 near term in the induction of labor. The effects of fenarimol in mammals differ from those seen with ketoconazole, because fenarimol does not inhibit androgen production in male rat or progesterone synthesis during pregnancy.

Fenarimol also has been shown to inhibit ecdysteroid synthesis in invertebrates, whereas in reptiles aromatase inhibitors inhibit female gonadal sex determination. Fenarimol caused a dose-related decrease in male fertility in Wistar rats, with the effect particularly evident in the anatomically normal progeny of dams treated with fenarimol throughout life, including gestation and lactation. Based on the observation that the infertility was associated with the absence of vaginal sperm at the time of mating, the effect appeared to be the result of an absence of male sexual behavior. Gray and Ostby subsequently described a dose-related decrease in male mating behavior of rats when fenarimol was administered daily from weaning through adulthood. These results suggest that fenarimol is acting centrally to decrease male sexual behavior by inhibiting the conversion of testosterone to E_2 in the brain. Consistent with a central effect, Hirsch et al. noted that fenarimol concentrations in the brain of neonates whose mothers were treated were three- to fourfold higher, and half-life was four times longer, than in other brain regions.

Exposure of genetic stocks of all female chinook salmon (*O. tshawytscha*) to fadrozole [5-(5,6,7,8-tetrahyroimidazo[1,5-α]-pyridin-5yl) benzonitrile monohyrochloride, or CGS 16949A], a nonsteroidal aromatase inhibitor, for a 2-hour period when the gonads were totipotent caused genetic females to develop as males.

Resulting males had testes that were indistinguishable in both size and function from genetic males, and were fertile. When fadrozole was given to adult female coho salmon (*O. kisutch*), a lowering in plasma E_2 was observed, associated with an increase in plasma 17α,20β-P. Ten days after injection, 67% of the fish exposed to 10 mg of fadrozole/kg body weight had ovulated, in contrast to 0% in the control group, indicating an advancement in oocyte maturation and subsequent ovulation. Administration of fadrozole to male coho salmon during sexual maturation inhibited secretion of E_2 by the brain and increased plasma 17α,20β-P, and treated males began spermiation earlier than control males. In addition, fadrozole-treated fish had higher levels of testosterone and 11-ketotestosterone than did controls within 4 days of injection.

5α-Reductase Inhibitors

5α-Reductase is the enzyme responsible for the conversion of testosterone to DHT, a more potent AR agonist. DHT acts specifically to masculinize the external genitalia of the male. Finasteride is a 5α-reductase inhibitor used clinically to combat androgen-dependent prostate cancer and more widely as a treatment for hair loss in adult men. Although this is not an environmental contaminant, it is used as an example because DHT plays such a significant role in the development of the male reproductive tract, and the impact of its inhibition on male reproductive development, especially the prostate and genitalia, is profound. Following oral exposure to rats on days 6-20 of gestation, AGD was reduced at doses as low as 0.003 mg/kg/day, hypospadias was observed beginning at 0.1 mg/kg/day, and 100% of the offspring were affected at 100 mg/kg/day. There was a significant decrease in prostate size at 25 and 50 mg/kg/day, with no further decrease at higher doses.

Unlike AR blockade with flutamide, finasteride did not totally abolish prostate differentiation or completely feminize the external genitalia, despite increasingly higher doses. These results suggest that testosterone can compensate for DHT to some degree at the level of the AR. Wolffian differentiation, however, was not affected by inhibition of DHT, demonstrating its testosterone dependency, but seminal vesicle growth was impaired. AR blockade can inhibit testicular descent more effectively than inhibition of 5α-reductase activity.

It is suggested that finasteride causes hypospadias by preventing the formation of the medial mesenchymal plate that is necessary for assisting the movement of the urogenital sinus from the base to the tip of the genital tubercle. Additionally, external genital abnormalities can be produced in male rhesus monkey fetuses when dams are exposed to an oral dose (2 mg/kg/day) of finasteride on gestation days 20-100. No external genital malformations were seen in similarly exposed female fetuses or in fetuses of either sex following daily intravenous exposure of up to 800 ng/kg/day over the same period of gestation.

Phthalates

Phthalates are a broad class of chemicals used as plasticizers in a number of manufacturing processes, and as discussed below, the developmental effects of several phthalates (e.g., the dibutyl and diethylhexyl esters) are exerted via alterations in testosterone-synthesizing ability of the fetal testes. The reproductive toxicity in adults of some phthalates has been well described. For example, DEHP has been shown to target the rat testis of adults and juveniles. The mode of action of the testicular toxicity is via a metabolite (the monoester, MEHP), with the target cell in the testis being the Sertoli cell, although the precise biochemical interaction has yet to be identified.

Attention has also been focused on the endocrine-active effects of phthalates, including interactions with both estrogen and androgen action. Zacharewski et al. reported that DBP, BBP, and DHP weakly competed with E_2 for binding to the ER in competitive ligand-binding assays. In gene expression assays using MCF-7 cells transiently transfected with Gal4-HEGO, and the Gal4-regulated luciferase reporter gene 17m5-G-Luc, 10 μM DBP, BBP, or DHP exhibited 36%, 42%, and 20% activity, respectively, when compared with the 100% response observed with 10 nM E_2. Only BBP induced luciferase activity (32%) in HeLa cells stably transfected with Gal4-HEGO and 17m5-G-Luc constructs and imparted minimal ER-mediated viability to the E_2-dependent recombinant yeast strain PL3 on selective medium.

No significant responses were observed with the five other phthalate esters in any of the *in vitro* assays. *In vivo,* none of the eight phthalate esters reproducibly induced significant increases in uterine wet weight in immature ovariectomized SD rats treated with oral doses of 20, 200, or 2,000 mg/kg of phthalate ester. Treatment with phthalate esters at the same doses did not affect the degree of vaginal epithelial cell cornification in mature ovariectomized rats. These results indicate that only selected phthalate esters (i.e., DBP, BBP, and DHP) exhibit weak ER-mediated activity in some *in vitro* assays at high concentrations, but none of the eight phthalate esters elicited *in vivo* estrogenic responses based upon results obtained from uterotrophic and vaginal cornification assays. These results serve to raise caution in assessing the potential hazard of chemicals based solely upon results of *in vitro* experiments.

More significantly, some phthalates (e.g., DEHP, DBP, BBP, di-isonyl phthalate, but not DEP, DMP or DOTP) induce antiandrogenic responses in fetal males. For example, male rat pups exposed during sexual differentiation to DBP or DEHP exhibit malformations in androgen-dependent tissues although apparently by a non-receptor-mediated mechanism. Importantly, because the critical window lies outside that of the traditionally defined "period of organogenesis," these effects have been missed in standard developmental toxicology studies.

A DBP multigenerational study showed marked effects on fertility of rats in the F_1generation compared with their parents in the F0 generation, with fewer and smaller litters and a 50% decrease in sperm count. In addition, these F_1animals showed numerous male reproductive tract malformations at the highest dose level tested (~660 mg/kg/day) that were not observed at comparable dose levels in the standard developmental toxicity studies.

Mylchreest et al. examined the critical differences in the exposure period between the F0 and F_1generations, and exposed pregnant and lactating animals and then examined their offspring. A high incidence of epididymal malformations and decreased sperm count were found, as well as delays in preputial separation and decreases in AGD of the male pups. All of the reproductive tract malformations seen in the multigeneration study could be reproduced in this shorter exposure regimen, and no effects were noted in female offspring. In another multigeneration study, however, exposure to 250 mg/kg/day DBP (the lowest dose tested) induced malformations in both male and female F_1rats.

By narrowing the exposure window to just late gestation (gestation days 12-21), Mylchreest et al. essentially reproduced their earlier findings and also reported an increased incidence of retained nipples in the male offspring. Thus, DBP had all the attributes of a classical AR antagonist in affecting reproductive tract development with a LOAEL of 100 mg/kg/day that is much lower than LOAELs and most NOAELs for other toxicities of DBP. Mylchreest et al. compared the effects of DBP to the AR antagonist flutamide and showed many similarities in the pattern of effects but also a number of differences in tissue sensitivity, with the epididymis being the prime target for DBP malformations, whereas the prostate was the major target for flutamide. Neither DBP nor monobutylphthalate interacted directly with the AR. That these effects are not mediated via AR antagonism are supported by the findings that DBP and DEHP, as well as their monoester metabolites, do not bind mammalian (rat or human) AR.

Although the precise cellular and molecular site of phthalate action in the fetal male is unknown, the testis appears to be the primary target. Maternal DEHP and DBP treatments induced dramatic reductions of fetal testosterone synthesis and fetal androgen levels, and altered Leydig cell morphology and function were evident. The fact that the selective AR for toxicity of the phthalates during development appears similar to that for testicular toxicity in pubertal males may suggest that some commonality in the initial molecular event initiates these adverse outcomes. It appears that the mechanism of action of phthalate-induced toxicity is widespread throughout vertebrates.

Developmental reproductive toxicity of the phthalates is observed in the guinea pig, ferret, rabbit, hamster (i.e., MEHP), and several strains of rats and mice, including the PPARα-knockout mouse. The fact that PPARα-knockouts display testicular and renal lesions after DEHP-treatment demonstrates that this receptor, apparently involved in the toxicity of MEHP in the liver, is not required for the expression of these other forms of toxicity. A fish multigenerational study, which exposed medaka to DBP at environmentally relevant concentrations, detected abnormal gonadal function in the F_1 by not the F0 generation, although it failed to induce estrogenlike responses in this species. DBP also has been shown to alter androgen-dependent tissues in developing anurans.

AhR Agonists: TCDD, PCBs, and PCDFs

This class of EDCs is responsible for many well-characterized reproductive and populations effects in fish and wildlife. Because these observed effects are used as support of the endocrine disruptor hypothesis and are believed to be caused by TCDD and structurally similar, synthetic halogenated hydrocarbons, it is important to understand the mechanism of action, as it relates to the endocrine disruptor hypothesis. Although the effects caused by TCDD can be classified as an effect on signal transduction, these effects are not covered by the narrow definition of receptor-mediated effects of steroid hormones. Overall, the evidence supports the hypothesis that most, if not all, TCDD effects are mediated through the AhR, a cytosolic receptor protein that was first discovered by Poland and Glover.

The AhR signaling transcription pathway is initiated by TCDD diffusion into the cell, where it binds with high affinity to the cytosolic AhR protein complex, which also includes heat-shock protein 90. The ligand binding activates AhR and stimulates the dissociation of AhR-associated proteins. The ligand-receptor complex is subsequently translocated into the nucleus, where it dimerizes with AhR nuclear translocator.

The heterodimers are capable of recognizing and binding DNA at the consensus sequence, GCGTG, of dioxinresponsive elements. This action either increases or decreases the transcription of target genes, including CYP450, NAD(P)H:quinone reductase, class 3 aldehyde dehydrogenase, and glutathione *S*-transferase. The ARNT protein also pairs with HIF-1α to regulate genes active in response to low oxygen stress.

Regulated genes include Epo for erythropoiesis, VEGF for angiogenesis, and GLUT-1 for glucose transport. AhR, ARNT, and HIF-1a belong to basic-helix-loophelix/ PAS protein family and are found in representative organisms of all five kingdoms. In addition to responding to low oxygen in the case of ARNT-HIFa heterodimers, PAS proteins are involved in development and differentiation, regulation of circadian clocks, and steroid receptor signaling. The fact that ARNT null mice are not viable beyond day 10.5 of gestation provides additional evidence of the importance of this protein. It is possible that exposure to TCDD and subsequent recruitment of ARNT through AhR may inhibit other signal transduction pathways depending on ARNT.

Thus, through its ability to interact with multiple signal transduction pathways and to induce or inhibit a variety of gene products, AhR agonists are capable of inducing a wide spectrum of biological effects at a number of different life stages and in a variety of species. Some of these responses do not easily fit the traditional definition of endocrine-mediated effects. In this assessment, biological effects that correlated with AhR occupancy were therefore not considered sufficient to invoke an endocrine-mediatedmode of action.

Male rats exposed *in utero* to a single dose of 0, 0.05, 0.20 or 0.80 μg/kg TCDD on day 15 of gestation displayed reduced fertility, as well as delayed puberty and altered reproductive organ weights. Growth and viability of the pups were reduced only at 0.80 μg/kg, eye opening was accelerated (all dosage groups), and puberty was delayed (at 0.20 and 0.80 μg/kg). Treated progeny displayed transient reductions in ventral prostate and seminal vesicle weights, and epididymal sperm reserves and glans penis size were permanently reduced. Ejaculated sperm numbers were reduced (45% in the 0.8 and by 25% in the 0.05 and 0.2 μg/kg dosage groups) to a greater degree than were cauda or caput/corpus epididymal or testicular (unaffected) sperm numbers. Female offspring from this treatment regimen showed a delay in vaginal opening at 0.80 μg/kg.

A persistent vaginal thread was present in 27% of the progeny at 0.20 and 92% at 0.80 μg TCDD/kg. These effects did not appear to result from abnormal ovarian function during prepubertal development; neither serum E_2 levels nor ovarian E_2 production was reduced in 21- or 28-day-old progeny of dams exposed to 1 μg/kg. In addition, partial to complete clefting of the phallus was displayed in TCDD-treated rats (10% at 0.20 and 60% at 0.80 μg/kg), and these dosage levels also increased the length of the urethral slit, increased distance from the urethral opening to the tip of the phallus, and decreased distance from the urethral opening to the vaginal orifice. Although fertility rates were normal, time to pregnancy was delayed by treatment with 0.80 μg/kg. When necropsied at 20 months of age, females from the TCDD-dose groups displayed histopathological alterations of the reproductive tract. Thus, TCDD affects reproductive tract development in ways both similar and different than estrogens and antiandrogens. Fetal levels of TCDD as low as 8-13 ppt are associated with these reproductive alterations.

Following exposure to a single dose of 2 μg/kg TCDD on gestation day 11.5, both control and TCDD-treated F_1females mated successfully with a control male; 20% of the F_1treated females did not become not pregnant. In addition, 38% of pregnant F_1females from the TCDD group died near-term, and there were reductions in the numbers of implants in pregnant animals and pups born live in the treated group. In the F_2, survival through weaning was drastically reduced (15% treated vs. 78% for control) by TCDD treatment of dams on postnatal day 0. F_1female hamster offspring exposed *in utero* to TCDD also displayed external urogenital malformations, with most females having complete clefting of the phallus. Thus, adverse effects of TCDD persisted through two generations ($F_1$and F_2), even though the F_1generation was only indirectly exposed during gestation and lactation. Altered neurological development is another health outcome associated with prenatal exposure to TCDD in experimental animals.

Mably et al. reported demasculinization and feminization of sexual behavior in male rats following maternal exposure. At the age when sexual behavior was tested, AhRdependent hepatic CYP450 levels and ethoxyresorutin dehydroxylase activity were not different from controls, thus demonstrating that effects on sexual behavior were due to longlasting effects of developmental exposure and disturbance of organizational effects of sex steroids. In this model, levels of ERs in different brain regions were measured.. Although the AhR receptor is present in the developing nervous system, its role, if any, in normal development is unknown, and there is as yet no direct evidence for an implication of the AhR in brain development.

3.1$_2$.6 Mechanism for *p,p´*-DDE-Induced Eggshell Thinning in Oviparous Vertebrates

During the 1960s and 1970s, when the pesticide DDT was in the North American environment at greater concentrations, populations of several sensitive bird species declined because of unsuccessful incubation of eggs due to abnormally thin egg shells. Many of these species (e.g., the double-crested cormorant) have experienced dramatic population increases since the use of DDT was banned in the United States and environmental concentrations have subsequently declined. The eggshell-thinning effect of *o,p´*-DDT and its potent, stable metabolite *p,p´*-DDE in sensitive species is well known. Species that normally produce eggs with a chalky valerite cover, including pelicans, cormorants, shags, and gannets, can produce eggs with a much reduced or completely absent cover following DDE exposure. In these species, the shell-forming process was most impacted by DDE toward its termination. Other birds such as the great blackbacked gull and the gray heron show a general reduction in all shell layers following DDE exposure. Changes in mineral composition of eggshells following DDE treatment have seldom been investigated.

Several possible mechanisms of DDE-induced eggshell thinning (which may vary among species) have been suggested. However, many of the most popular avian laboratory species, including the domestic chicken and the Japanese quail, are insensitive to DDE-induced eggshell thinning. Although the mechanism of eggshell thinning has never been completely deduced, research in this area has focused mainly on one sensitive avian species. Suggested mechanisms have included

1) limiting the supply of calcium to the shell gland from the blood by either changing uptake, excretion, or transport;
2) decreasing carbonate availability for shell formation via inhibition of carbonic anhydrase and
3) altering steroid hormone receptors or function.

Currently, the leading hypothesis regarding the mechanism of DDE-induced eggshell thinning involves an inhibition of PGs by the shell gland mucosa. PGs play an important role in the control and regulation of reproduction in birds. PG synthesis is decreased by *p,p′*-DDE in duck shell gland mucosa, both in *in vitro* experiments and following *in vivo* exposure. PG synthesis was not inhibited by *p,p′*-DDT or *o,p′*-DDE in *in vitro* experiments, in keeping with the potency of these congeners in causing egg shell thinning.

Additionally, indomethacin treatment reduced eggshell thickness. It has been hypothesized that a furosemide-insensitive, PG-stimulated HCO_3 transport could be inhibited in the shell gland mucosa of DDE-treated ducks, but further experiments have not supported that hypothesis. The mechanism of DDE-induced eggshell thinning has been suggested to be quite complex. Eggshell thinning is associated with a decreased quantity of calcium in affected eggs, and in the mallard duck the effect of DDE has been associated with a decreased transport of calcium from the eggshell gland mucosa to the lumen fluid. Treatment of birds with DDE has been associated with a variety of biochemical changes that could be related to changes in calcium transport.

Many of these biochemical end points are interrelated, and it is difficult to determine which are the direct targets of DDE and which are merely co-influenced by its action. The situation is complicated by the fact that sensitivities to DDE-induced eggshell thinning vary among avian species, and hence different mechanisms might be causing eggshell thinning in different species, as evidenced by different gross eggshell defects. Although egg shell thinning induced by DDE and related chemicals is one of the most cited examples of endocrine disruption in wildlife, given the multiple hypothesis regarding the mode of action, it cannot be stated with certainty that it is indeed an result of endocrine disruption. The strongest evidence for the linkage comes from the findings of altered PG biosynthesis in the mucosal gland.

EDC MODES OF ACTION FOR CARCINOGENESIS

Concern for the endocrine-disrupting effects of atrazine, a triazine herbicide, arose following the observation of increased incidence of mammary tumors in a chronic bioassay in female SD rats exposed to 400 ppm atrazine in the diet for 104 weeks. These tumors also appeared in control females but occurred earlier in the treated females. No other tumors were present in the treated SD female rats or in male SD rats or male and female Fischer 344 rats.

The finding of earlier-onset mammary tumors led to an investigation into the estrogenicity of atrazine, but (under equilibrium conditions) atrazine was not able to compete with E_2 for binding to rat uterine ERs. A weak competition was noted if the cytosols were preincubated at 25°C prior to incubation with the tracer. Somewhat conflicting results have been seen in other studies. Daily exposure of adult Fischer rats to 120 mg/kg for 7 days resulted in fewer treated females displaying normal estrous cycles, and the number of days in diestrous was significantly increased. Fertility was reduced in females during the first week after exposure, but pregnancy outcome was not affected in those that became inseminated.

However, treatment of adult, ovariectomized SD rats with up to 300 mg/kg atrazine by oral gavage for 3 days did not result in an increase in uterine weight, nor were there increases in uterine progesterone levels, suggesting the lack of an estrogenic potential. When E_2 (2 μg/kg s.c.) was given in conjunction with 300 mg/kg or orally administered atrazine, there was a weak inhibition (~25%) of the uterotrophic response. In a similar study, immature female SD rats were dosed with 0, 50, 150, or 300 mg/kg atrazine by gavage for 3 days. Uterine weight was not increased, but decreases in uterine progesterone receptors and peroxidase activities were noted; however, when combined with E_2, no antiestrogenic effect of atrazine was noted on the uterus, including decreases in uterine progesterone receptor binding and uterine peroxidase. In this same study, atrazine did not affect basal or

E_2-induced MCF-7 cell proliferation or display agonist or antagonist action against E_2-induced luciferase activity in MCF-7 cells transfected with Gal4-regulated human ER chimera.

To further evaluate effects on reproductive function, female LE and SD rats that had been screened for regular 4-day estrous cycles received 0, 75, 150, or 300 mg/kg/day atrazine by gavage for 2_1days. In both strains, atrazine disrupted the regular 4-day estrous cycles. For the LE rats, all dose levels were effective, whereas SD rats required a higher dose (150 mg/kg/day) for a longer time for this effect to appear. The increased time spent in vaginal diestrus was associated with elevated serum progesterone and low E_2 concentrations, indicative of a repetitive pseudopregnant condition. This hormonal condition was not considered by the authors to be conducive to the development of mammary tumors, although there was some indication of prolonged estrous at the lowest dose tested.

The strain difference noted in the premature onset of mammary tumors (insensitive Fischer 344 rats vs. sensitive SD rats) has been attributed to differences in the normal aging of the reproductive tract in these strains. Reproductive cycling in the female SD rat begins to decline in animals less than 1 year of age, presumably due to the loss of sensitivity of adrenergic neurons in the hypothalamus that control GnRH release to the pituitary. This loss of stimulation reduces FSH and LH release and ultimately delays ovulation. The delayed ovulation, in turn, allows prolonged exposure to estrogens and an effect evident as persistent vaginal cornification.

In contrast, adrenergic neurons of female Fischer 344 rats do not seem to lose their sensitivity to estrogen stimulation, and regular cycling is maintained for a much longer time period. Rather, reproductive aging in the Fischer 344 is believed due to inability to control daily PRL surges, a prolonged activity of the corpora lutea, and a higher level of progesterone release. Hence, the endocrine milieu of the aging SD rat, but not the Fischer 344 rat, favors development of mammary tumors and helps explain the difference in incidence of spontaneous tumors as females of these strains age.

Consistent with an effect on central nervous system function, atrazine exposure beginning at weaning alters the development of puberty in both the male and female rat. In the male, doses as low as 12.5 mg/kg/day beginning on postnatal day 23 delayed preputial separation. At postnatal day 53, ventral prostate weights, but not testes weights, were reduced in rats treated with 50 mg/kg/day. Female rats were somewhat less sensitive, as it required 50 mg/kg/day to delay vaginal opening, and 100 mg/kg/day altered estrous cycles in the first 15 days after vaginal opening. In addition, *in vitro* studies involving PC12 cells have suggested that atrazine inhibits the cellular synthesis of dopamine mediated by tyrosine hydroxylase, and norepinephrine mediated by dopamine β-hydroxylase and, as result, reduces the potential of the neuronlike cells to release norepinephrine. How atrazine accelerates the neuroendocrine aging of the reproductive axis in the SD rat, however, has not been determined. Atrazine may exert neuroendocrine effects in other vertebrates.

Ovulated female Atlantic salmon (*Salmo salar*) release a priming pheromone in the urine (an F-type prostagladin) that is subsequently detected by the olfactory system of the mature male salmon and results in increased levels of sex steroids and expressible milt. Short exposure of atrazine to male parr significantly reduced the olfactory response to PG F_2a. In addition, similar exposures reduced their ability to respond to the priming effect of ovulated female salmon urine. Atrazine also had an additional effect upon the testes, modifying the release of androgens and suggestive of an additional mode of action in this species.

EDC-RELATED MODES OF ACTION IN NEUROTOXICITY

There is evidence of neurotoxicity for over 850 workplace chemicals, including metals, organic solvents, agrochemicals, polyhalogenated aromatic hydrocarbons, natural neurotoxins, and pharmaceuticals/drugs of abuse. Because the reproductive endocrine system is primarily regulated by the neuroendocrine system, these chemicals are potentially EDCs. However, even with the close interactions between the nervous and endocrine systems, it has generally proven difficult to elucidate primary modes of action from secondary manifestations, even for chemicals that have known potential to influence hormone action. Although the mechanisms by which endocrine disruptors influence the nervous system are largely unknown, it is clear that two different modes of interaction of hormones with neural function must be considered:

1) effects related to activational properties of hormones in adult organisms resulting in transient changes and
2) organizational effects on hormone-dependent processes during neural development that can result in permanent changes of neurobehavioral function, particularly sex-dependent and sexual-related behaviors.

Both actions may involve specific hormone receptors, such as the estrogen or the AR, or may be due to modulations of receptors for neurotransmitters that are reported to be influenced by hormones. For instance, GABA receptors, muscarinic and nicotinic receptors, NMDA receptors, σ-receptors, and neuropeptide receptors are implicated in steroid hormone action as well as membrane receptors coupled to second messengers.

To further complicate matters, the nature of the influence on neurotransmitters and whether it is endocrine mediated may differ even with compounds that are structurally closely related. For example, prenatal/neonatal exposure to the 3,4,3′,4′-tetrachlorobiphenyl resulted in elevated concentrations of dopamine in the frontal cortex and of dopamine and its metabolites in the substantia nigra, whereas exposure to 2,4,2′,4′-tetrachlorobiphenyl resulted in significant decreases in concentrations of dopamine in the frontal cortex and caudate nucleus. In both cases, the changes persisted into adulthood.

The study suggested that the reductions in brain dopamine concentrations were a consequence of PCB congener-induced inhibition of the synthesis of dopamine in concert with changes in cholinergic receptor function, whereas the persistent elevations in brain dopamine may be mediated by alterations in steroid hormone function during key developmental periods. Coplanar congeners, in addition to their ability to interact at the AhR, also alter estrogenic function, either by enhancing the metabolism of estrogens to hydroxy- and catecholestrogens or by down-regulating ERs. Although chemicals that alter neurotransmitter concentrations, such as PCBs, are likely to influence neuroendocrine function and ultimately reproduction, there are only a few reports on this potentially important mechanism of endocrine disruption.

Reproductive impairment in Atlantic croaker exposed to Aroclor 1254 was associated with a dramatic decline in LH secretion and hypothalamic levels of 5-HT, a neurotransmitter that has a stimulatory influence on LH secretion. A subsequent study showed that that the decline in 5-HT concentrations was due to inhibition of tryptophan hydroxylase, the rate-limiting enzyme in 5-HT synthesis. The decreased 5-HT activity after PCB exposure resulted in decreased hypothalamic concentrations of LHRH and its secretion, leading to the down-regulation of LHRH receptors on gonadotropes and a decreased LH response to LHRH stimulation. Moreover, a specific inhibitor of tryptophan hydroxylase, parachlorine phenylanaline, mimicked these neuroendocrine effects of the PCB mixture as well as the subsequent reproductive impairment, whereas cotreatment of the PCB-dosed fish with 5-hydroxytryptophane, which bypasses this biosynthetic step, reversed the PCB effects. Neuroendocrine disruption associated with alterations of neurotransmitter function has also been reported in croaker after exposure to lead.

The distinction between chemical exposures of the developing as opposed to the mature nervous system is of particular importance in the present context for both toxicological and neurobiological reasons. Both the nature and the adversity of outcome may depend on the time window during which chemical exposure occurs. Some hormones, such as sex steroids or thyroid hormones, are known to have a strong and strictly time-coupled organizational impact on brain development. From a neurobiological point of view, disruption of organizational factors during development in general and, more specifically, during brain development is important because long-lasting or irreversible neurobehavioral changes later in life may be the consequence of such interactions. For example, thyroid hormones are known to affect brain development:

a) by increasing the rate of neuronal proliferation in the cerebellum,

b) by timing neuronal proliferation and differentiation, and

c) by organizing the pattern of neuronal migration to specific brain areas.

In humans, endemic cretinism caused by iodine deficiency, congenital hypothyroidism, or maternal hypothyroidism is associated with well-known neurological and behavioral deficiencies, such as mental retardation, deaf-mutism, speech disorders, or motor deficits. However, the degree of thyroid dysfunction is clearly critical.

In the adult organism, endocrine disruption of the reproductive system is considered as a possible cause of neurobehavioral alterations either if gonadal hormones are shown to be affected in association with changes in reproductive behavior and nonreproductive neurobehavior, or if sexually dimorphic nonreproductive behavioral changes following chemical exposure are reported without endocrine data. A direct toxic effect on hormone-receptor-expressing neurons and glial cells must also be considered. Alterations of hormone concentrations may be caused by cytotoxic effects on hormoneproducing organs, resulting in impaired synthesis or release of hormones. For example, PCB exposure resulted in fine structural lesions in the thyroid and inhibition of proteolysis of thyroglobulin, thereby decreasing the release of T_4. In addition, thyroid hormone levels are influenced by increase in hormone metabolism due to PCB exposure and by blocking the binding sites for T_4 at its serum transport proteins, which causes enhanced clearance from serum and decreased availability to tissues.

The question of which mechanism underlies the effect of putative endocrine disruptors on a given neurobehavioral function ultimately depends on what is known about the regulation of that function at the cellular and subcellular level. However, the events that constitute the basis for higher neural functions are far from being understood for many of the end points investigated. The following are two examples of experimental studies in which attempts were made to delineate possible mechanisms for chemicalinduced alterations of neuroendocrine and neurobehavioral effects. However, these studies are only the first steps in the elucidation of the mechanisms.

SEXUAL DIFFERENTIATION OF THE NERVOUS SYSTEM

It is generally assumed that sexual differentiation of the brain in rodents depends on the activity of aromatase (CYP19), an enzyme that converts androgens to estrogens. Aromatase has been detected in all mammal brains so far examined, but its role in sexual differentiation in other than rodent species remains to be proven. Aromatase is expressed in several brain areas, including the HPOA, stria terminalis, amygdala, and striatum. Its regulation appears to differ in different brain areas regarding androgen dependence and the developmental phase of maximum activity. In the HPOA, a region with several sexually dimorphic nuclei, a sharp peak of activity was found at the end of gestation that declines to basal activity within the first 5 days after birth.

Maternal exposure to a mixture of PCBs, reconstituted according to the congener pattern found in breast milk and containing *ortho*-chlorinated and coplanar congeners, caused decreases in aromatase activity at birth of male rat pups together with an elevated sweet preference and reduced testes weights and testosterone levels in adult male offspring. Sweet preference behavior is more pronounced in female rats, suggesting that reductions in hypothalamic E_2 results in a more femalelike differentiation of the brain that in turn causes a feminization of behavior in adulthood.

EDC-RELATED MODES OF ACTION IN IMMUNOTOXICITY

The major function of the immune system is to defend against infectious agents and certain neoplastic cells. Various cell types and their soluble mediators execute the function of the immune system in finely tuned concert. The maintenance of homeostasis requires bidirectional communication between the neuroendocrine and immune systems. Most of the influence of the brain on the immune system is exerted by hormones released by the neuroendocrine system. Indeed, receptors for hormones have been detected on cells of the immune system, whereas receptors for cytokines have been detected in the endocrine glands and brain. It is also noteworthy that almost all lymphoid tissues are innervated, although the role of this neuroregulatory pathway is largely unknown.

The HPA axis represents the major pathway in the communication between the central nervous system and the immune system. Synthesis of glucocorticosteroid hormone (cortisol in man) by the adrenal gland, induced by ACTH from the pituitary gland, results in suppression of immune responses. Other mechanisms are those mediated by the direct action of neuropeptides, such as opioid peptides, on immune cells that are either stimulatory or inhibitory. For their communication, cells of the immune system carry receptors for a number of hormones, neuropeptides, and neurotransmitters, such as CRH, ACTH, PRL, β-endorphin, GH, and sex steroids. In addition, cells of the immune system produce inflammatory cytokines, specifically, tumor necrosis factor-α, IL-1, and IL-6, that may act as endocrine hormones of the immune system, produced at distant sites and acting upon the central components of the HPA axis and the sympathetic system.

Cortisol, the final effector of the HPA axis, has multiple and profound immunosuppressive effects. Histologically, the thymus is the first organ affected by this hormone. Cortisol affects production, traffic, and function of leukocytes; this often leads to lymphopenia and monocytopenia. In addition, monocyte chemotaxis, bactericidal activity, and T-lymphocyte proliferation can be inhibited by cortisol. Glucocorticoids also inhibit the production of many cytokines. In addition, glucocorticoids inhibit the expression of adhesion and adhesion receptor molecules on the surface of immune and other cells and potentiate the acute-phase reaction induced by cytokines, primarily IL-6.

PRL has been shown to regulate various aspects of the immune system. Hypoprolactinemia is associated with impaired lymphocyte proliferation and decreased production of macrophage-activating factors by T lymphocytes. The endogenous opioid peptides α-endorphin, β-endorphin, and γ-enkephalin are also produced in the pituitary gland. Endorphin receptors similar to those in the brain are present on spleen cells and probably several others types of leukocytes. β-Endorphin has been shown to enhance T-cell proliferation and IL-2 production. One biological activity of the thymus that is under neuroendocrine control is the secretion of thymic hormones. The secretion of thymulin, a nonapeptide produced by thymic epithelial cells, is modulated by GH and PRL.

The interaction between the pituitary and thymus is demonstrated by the immunodeficiency of the thymus-dependent immunity that occurs in mice following injection with antisomatotrope hormone serum. Modifying influences on immune responses have also been reported for sex steroids. The balance between male and female sex hormones, E_2 and testosterone, influences the extent of immune responsiveness. In general, the male sex hormone testosterone is immunostimulatory. E_2 and synthetic nonsteroidal estrogenic compounds such as DES are potent suppressors of specific immunity: the effects observed in rodents include thymic atrophy, suppression of thymus-dependent cellular immune responses, acceleration of autoimmune diseases, suppression of natural killer cell activity, myelotoxicity, and stimulation of the mononuclear phagocyte system. Considerable changes are seen in lymphoid organs during pregnancy, and increased serum E_2 levels during pregnancy correlate with lymphopenia and suppression of cellular immunity. By evaluation of steroidal and nonsteroidal compounds with varying degrees of estrogenicity, Luster et al. provided evidence that immunotoxicity correlated for the most part with estrogenicity.

In humans, both the neuroendocrine system and the immune system are immature at birth and fully develop at later stages in life. The immune system is highly sensitive to regulation by glucocorticoids in the human newborn, a period of life in which the capacity to generate a cortisol response is decreased, suggesting that this represents an adaptational response of the immune system that preserves the important regulatory effects of glucocorticoids on the immune system during this delicate developmental period. This may imply that the neuroendocrine system may also be very sensitive to EDCs during ontogeny. Regarding the immune system, its susceptibility to toxic compounds is most evident during the perinatal period of life, as shown in laboratory animal studies with various compounds, including TCDD and hexachlorobenzene. These considerations show that there are potentially multiple endocrine pathways that may influence the function of the developing and mature immune system and that these may be targets for EDCs.

REFERENCES

Buck, et. al., *Clinical and Diagnostic Veterinary Toxicology*. 2nd ed. 1976. pp. 25-37.

Casarett, L.J. and J. Doull. (eds.) *Toxicology: The Basic Science of Poisons*. 2nd Ed. Ch. 3-5, 9-12, 14-15.

Clarke, E. G. C. and M. L. Clarke. 1975. *Veterinary Toxicology*, 1st Edition. Williams and Wilkins. pp. 109-118.

Loomis, T.A. (ed). 1976, *Essentials of Toxicology*. 2nd Ed., pp. 1-23. Lea and Febiger, Philadelphia.

Mathew, H. and Lawson, A.A. 1980. *Treatment of Common Acute Poisoning*, 4th ed., Churchill Pub. New York.

Richards IS. 2008. *Principles and Practice of Toxicology in Public Health*. Jones and Bartlett Publisher, Sudbury Massachusetts.

Williams, P.L.; James, R.C.; and Roberts, S.M., eds. 2000. *Principles of Toxicology: Environmental and Industrial Applications*, 2nd edition. New York: John Wiley & Sons.

Bibliography

Alpin, T. E.H. *Poisonous Garden Plants and other Plants Harmful to Man in Australia*. Perth: Western Australia Dept. of Agriculture, 1976. Bot QK100 .A8 A655.

Aronson, A.L. 1972. *Chemical Poisonings in Small Animal Practice*. Veterinary Clinics of North America, 2:379-395.

Bailey, Frederick Manson. *Plants Reputed Poisonous and Injurious to Stock*. Brisbane: J.C. Beal, 1887. Bot QK100 .A8 B35.

Bailey,E.M., 1979. "Management and Treatment of Toxicoses in Cattle". *VM/SAC.*, pp 1650-1657.

Barkan, B.A. and F.W. Oehme. 1975. "A Classification of Common Midwestern Animal Toxicosis". *Vet. Tox.* 17:37-49.

Buck, et. al., *Clinical and Diagnostic Veterinary Toxicology*. 2nd ed. 1976. pp. 25-37.

Buck, W.B. and Bratich, P.M. 1986. "Activated charcoal: Preventing unnecessary death by poisoning". *Vet. Med.* 81:73-77.

Casarett, L.J. and J. Doull. (eds). *Toxicology: The Basic Science of Poisons*. 2nd Ed. Ch. 3-5, 9-12, 14-15.

Clarke, E. G. C. and M. L. Clarke. 1975. *Veterinary Toxicology*, 1st Edition. Williams and Wilkins. pp. 109-118.

Clarkson, T. W. 1977. *Factors Involved in Heavy Metal Poisoning*. Fed. Proc. 36: 1634-1639.

Colin, M.E.; Bonmatin, J.M.; Moineau, I., et al. 2004. "A method to quantify and analyze the foraging activity of honey bees: Relevance to the sublethal effects induced by systemic insecticides". *Archives of Environmental Contamination and Toxicology*. Volume: 47 Issue: 3 Pages: 387-395

Crosby, Donald G. 1998. *Environmental Toxicology and Chemistry*. New York: Oxford University Press.

de Padua, L.S. Plant Resources of South-East Asia. No. 12, *Medicinal and Poisonous Plants* 1. Leiden, The Netherlands: Backhuys, 1999. Bot SB108 .A785 P52 v.12:1.

Doull, J., C.D. Klaassen and M.O. Amdur, (eds.). 1980. *Casarett and Doull's Toxicology:The basic Science of Poisons*. 2nd. ed., pp. 3-27. Macmillan Publishing Company, New York.

Fane, L.R., Combs, H.F. and Decker, W.J. 1971. "Physical Parameters in Gastric Lavage". *Clinical Toxicology*, 4:389-395.

Forsyth, A. A. *British Poisonous Plants*. London: H.M.S.O., 1968. Bot QK100 .G7 F67 1968.

Foster, Steven. *A Field Guide to Venomous Animals and Poisonous Plants*, North America North of Mexico. Boston, MA: Houghton Mifflin, 1994. MAIN QL100 .F63 1994.

Hammond, P. B. and Beliles, R. P. 1980. *Metals in Doull, J.; Klassen, C.D. and Amdur, M.O.*(editors), *Casarett and Doull's Toxicology: The Basic Science of Poisons*. Second edition, New York, MacMillan p 409.

Hans P. Riemann and Dean O. Cliver. 2006. *Foodborne Infections and Intoxications*. Elsevier.

Hardin, James W. *Human Poisoning from Native and Cultivated Plants*. Durham, NC: Duke University Press, 1969. Bot QK100 .N6 H37.

Hocking A.D. et al. 2006. *Advances in Food Mycology* (Advances in Experimental Medicine and Biology) Springer .

Kingsbury, John Merriam. *Deadly Harvest: A Guide to Common Poisonous Plants*. New York: Holt, Rinehart and Winston,1965. Bot QK100 .A1 K55.

Lampe, Kenneth F. *AMA Handbook of Poisonous and Injurious Plants*. Chicago, IL: American Medical Association, 1985. Bot REF RA1250 .L27 1985.

Lee, D. H. K. 1973. "Biologic Effect of Metallic Contaminants-The Next Step". *Environ. Research* 6:121-131

Loomis, T.A. (ed). 1976, *Essentials of Toxicology*. 2nd Ed., pp. 1-23. Lea and Febiger, Philadelphia.

Mathew, H. and Lawson, A.A. 1980. *Treatment of Common Acute Poisoning*, 4th ed., Churchill Pub. New York.

Murphey, Edith Van Allen. *Stock Poisoning Plants, a Stockman's Pocket Book*. Corvallis, OR: Unnamed, 1947. Bot SB617.4 .M87.

Neatherly, M. W. and Miller W. J. 1975. "Metabolism and Toxicity of Cadmium, Mercuty, and Lead in Animals: A rewiew". *J. Diary Science* 58:1967-1982.

Needleman, H.L. 1998. "Clair Patterson and Robert Kehoe: Two Views of Lead Toxicity." *Environmental Research* 78(2):79-85.

Nelson, Lewis H.; Flomenbaum, Neal; Goldfrank, Lewis R.; Hoffman, Robert Louis; Howland, Mary Deems; Neal A. Lewin. 2006. *Goldfrank's toxicologic emergencies*. New York: McGraw-Hill, Medical Pub. Division.

Ohlendorf, H.M.; Hoffman, D.J.; Daiki, M.K.; and Aldrich, T.W. 1986. "Embryonic Mortality and Abnormalities of Aquatic Birds-Apprent Impacts of Selenium from Irrigation Drainwater." *Science of the Total Environment* 52(44).

Oldroyd BP. 2007. "What's Killing American Honey Bees"? *PLoS Biology* 5(6): e168 doi:10.1371/ journal.pbio.0050168) Retrieved on 2007-05-17.

Osweiler, G. D., T. L. Carson, W. B. Buck and G. A. Van Gelder (eds.) 1985. *Clinical and Diagnostic Veterinary Toxicology*, 3rd Edition, Kendall/Hunt Publishing Co., Iowa.

Palmer, WE, Bromley, PT, and Brandenburg, RL. 2007. *Wildlife & pesticides- Peanuts*. North Carolina Cooperative Extension Service.

Pina M, Fratamico et al. 2005. *Foodborne Pathogens: Microbiology And Molecular Biology*. Caister Academic Press.

Pond, W. G. 1975. *Mineral Interrelationships in Nutrition: Practical Implications*. Cornell Vet. 65:441-456.

Richards IS. 2008. *Principles and Practice of Toxicology in Public Health*. Jones and Bartlett Publisher, Sudbury Massachusetts.

Sharma, R. P. and Street, J. C. 1980. "Public Health Aspects of Toxic Heavy Metals in Animal Feeds". *JAVMA* 177:149-153.

Simon, N.M. and Krumlovsky, F.A. 1971. "The Role of Dialysis in the Treatment of Poisoning". *Rational Drug Therapy* 5(3). 7 pages.

Szabuniewicz, M.,Bailey, E.M. and Wiersig, D.O. 1971. "Treatment of some Common Poisoning in Animals". *VM/SAC.*, 66:1197-1205.

Thoman, M.E. 1970. "The Use of Emetics in Poison Ingestion". *Clinical Toxicology*, 3:185-188.

Ulmer, D. D. 1973. "Metals-from Provation to Pollution". *Fed. Proc.* 32:1758-1762.

Wilkinson,G.R. 1970. "Treatment of Drug Intoxication: A review of some Scientific Principles". *Clinical Toxicology*, 3:249-265.

Williams, P.L.; James, R.C.; and Roberts, S.M., eds. 2000. *Principles of Toxicology: Environmental and Industrial Applications*, 2nd edition. New York: John Wiley & Sons.

Index